ANESTHESIOLOGY AND THE CARDIOVASCULAR PATIENT

DEVELOPMENTS IN
CRITICAL CARE MEDICINE AND ANESTHESIOLOGY

Volume 31

The titles published in this series are listed at the end of this volume.

ANESTHESIOLOGY AND THE CARDIOVASCULAR PATIENT

Papers presented at the 41st Annual Postgraduate Course in Anesthesiology, February 1996

edited by

T. H. STANLEY AND P. L. BAILEY

Department of Anesthesiology,
The University of Utah Medical School,
Salt Lake City, Utah, U.S.A.

KLUWER ACADEMIC PUBLISHERS

DORDRECHT / BOSTON / LONDON

A C.I.P. Catalogue record for this book is available from the Library of Congress

ISBN 0-7923-3895-2

Published by Kluwer Academic Publishers,
P.O. Box 17, 3300 AA Dordrecht, The Netherlands.

Kluwer Academic Publishers incorporates
the publishing programmes of
D. Reidel, Martinus Nijhoff, Dr W. Junk and MTP Press.

Sold and distributed in the U.S.A. and Canada
by Kluwer Academic Publishers,
101 Philip Drive, Norwell, MA 02061, U.S.A.

In all other countries, sold and distributed
by Kluwer Academic Publishers Group,
P.O. Box 322, 3300 AH Dordrecht, The Netherlands.

Printed on acid-free paper

Printed in the Netherlands

Table of Contents

Preface

Peter L. Bailey, MD

ANESTHESIOLOGY AND THE CARDIOVASCULAR PATIENT contains the Refresher Course manuscripts of the presentations of the 41st Annual Postgraduate Course in Anesthesiology which took place at The Cliff Conference Center in Snowbird, Utah, February 23-27, 1996. The chapters reflect new data and concepts within the general framework of the pathophysiology and management of surgical candidates with cardiovascular disease. Each of the chapters is written by an authority in the field and has been edited only to the extent that was necessary to produce a coherent book. No effort has been made to provide a uniform presentation or style.

The purposes of the textbook are to 1) act as a reference for the anesthesiologists attending the meeting, and 2) serve as a vehicle to bring many of the latest concepts in anesthesiology to others within the short time of a formal presentation. Each chapter is a brief but sharply focused glimpse of the interests in anesthesia expressed at the conference. This book and its chapters should not be considered complete treatises on the subjects addressed but rather attempts to summarize the most salient points.

This textbook is the fourteenth in a continuing series documenting the proceedings of the Postgraduate Course in Salt Lake City. We hope that this and the past and future volumes reflect the rapid and continuing evolution of anesthesiology in the late twentieth century.

List of Contributors

Norbert de Bruijn, MD, FACC
Department of Anesthesiology, Duke University Medical Center, Durham, North Carolina, U.S.A.

John C. Drummond, MD
University of California, San Diego, Anesthesiology Service, VA Medical Center, San Diego, California, U.S.A.

Adre J. du Plessis, MD
Department of Neurology, Children's Hospital, Boston, Massachusetts, U.S.A.

Pierre Foëx, MD
Nuffield Department of Anaesthetics, University of Oxford, Radcliffe Infirmary, Oxford, U.K.

Paul R. Hickey, MD
Department of Anesthesia, Children's Hospital, and Department of Anaesthesia, Harvard Medical School, Boston, Massachusetts, U.S.A.

Richard A. Jonas, MD,
Department of Cardiovascular Surgery, Children's Hospital, Boston, Massachusetts, U.S.A.

Jerrold H. Levy, MD
Department of Anesthesiology, Emory University School of Medicine, and Emory University Hospital, Atlanta, Georgia, U.S.A.

Dennis T. Mangano, MD, Department of Anesthesiology, University of California, San Francisco, Anesthesiology Service, Veterans Administration Medical Center, San Francisco, California, U.S.A.

Jane W. Newburger, MD, MPH
Division of Cardiology, Department of Cardiovascular Surgery, Children's Hospital, Boston, Massachusetts, U.S.A.

Robert Neil Sladen, MD
Department of Anesthesiology, Division of Critical Care Medicine, Duke University Medical Center, Durham, North Carolina, U.S.A.

Bruce D. Spiess, MD
Department of Anesthesiology, Division of Cardiothoracic Anesthesia, University of Washington, Seattle, Washington, U.S.A.

Kenneth J. Tuman, MD
Department of Anesthesiology, Rush Medical College, Chicago, Illinois, U.S.A.

David C. Warltier, MD, PhD, Department of Anesthesiology, Medical College of Wisconsin, Milwaukee, Wisconsin, U.S.A.

Gil Wernovsky, MD
Department of Cardiovascular Surgery, Children's Hospital, Boston, Massachusetts, U.S.A.

PERIOPERATIVE CARDIAC MORBIDITY

Dennis T. Mangano, PhD, MD

Ischemic heart disease (IHD) can be complex in its clinical presentation. The patient with IHD usually has one of the many symptom complexes associated with varying degrees of ventricular dysfunction. As anesthesiologists, our assessment of a patient with IHD presenting for surgery is usually conducted over a very brief period of time and, therefore, requires a rather intense assessment of the patient's cardiac status. Several other factors add to the difficulties involved in this assessment: 1) The age of the population presenting for surgery is increasing; 2) surgical procedures are becoming more complex; and 3) cost containment procedures will limit the number and type of preoperative tests used to assess risk in patients with IHD, and there will be increasing pressure on us to expedite such an assessment (e.g., come-and-go, come-and-stay surgery). Thus, more than ever, we must know what specific tests are available for assessment of these patients and what information we can obtain from these tests to determine perioperative risk, preoperative therapeutics, intraoperative monitoring, choice of anesthetic, and postoperative care.

How significant is the problem of IHD in the United States? IHD appears to be a significant problem and will probably remain so well into the 1990s. This is substantiated by several statistics accumulated in the early 1980s from the United States. It is estimated that 10 million patients have IHD in the United States today, 4 million of whom have had previous myocardial infarctions. In any one year, approximately 1.3 million patients develop a new myocardial infarction and 700,000 deaths are attributed to IHD per year. Surgical procedures performed each year on these patients include approximately 400,000 cardiac catheterizations, with 175,000 coronary artery bypass grafts, and a rising number of coronary angioplasties. It is estimated that of the 20 million patients in the United States that undergo surgery each year, approximately 1 to 2 million have IHD or are at high risk for it. Thus, the problem is significant to anesthesiologists. It appears that the prognosis for patients with IHD is related to the development and severity of dysrhythmias, myocardial infarction and ventricular dysfunction. Before proceeding with a discussion of the tests used for IHD, it

T. H. Stanley and P. L. Bailey (eds.), Anesthesiology and the Cardiovascular Patient, 1–13.

is important to review the significance of dysrhythmias, infarction, and dysfunction in patients with IHD.

THE SIGNIFICANCE OF DYSRHYTHMIAS IN IHD

1. *Incidence*

In cases of acute myocardial infarction virtually all patients develop premature ventricular contractions within the first 5 days. Within one to three weeks following infarction, 73 to 94% of patients develop one or more dysrhythmias. In cases of chronic IHD, the incidence of patients in whom dysrhythmia is the predominant manifestation is unknown. It is known, however, that the most common dysrhythmias with chronic IHD are premature ventricular contractions (PVCs). Also, if chronic PVCs are frequent, multiform, or R-on-T, they are predictive of multivessel disease or significant ventricular dysfunction.

2. *Detection*

Detection of dysrhythmias depends on the duration of observation and the degree of stress.

Test	*Incidence of Ventricular Dysrhythmias*
EKG-rest (<1 min)	14%
EKG-rest (1 hr observation)	50%
EKG-routine activity (24-hr observation)	88%
EKG-stress testing (1 hr)	52-61%

Although 24-hour monitoring detects ventricular tachycardia approximately twice as often as stress testing, in 10% of the patients serious dysrhythmias (VT, VF) are detected only with stress testing.

3. *Prognosis*

The most serious dysrhythmias are ventricular fibrillation and tachycardia, and complex PVCs (R-on-T, multiform, repetitive). These carry the greatest risk of sudden death and are predictive of multivessel disease. Also significant are the conduction disturbances: complete heart block, Mobitz II, and bundle branch block (mortality 10 to 70%). Acute atrial dysrhythmias are usually indicative of concurrent disease, and are associated with significant risk if accompanied by acute ischemia or left ventricular failure.

4. Perioperative Risk

In patients with and without IHD, perioperative dysrhythmias commonly occur (17.9 to 61.7%), and are usually associated with stimulation, hypercarbia, hypertension, potassium loss, digitalis therapy and specific anesthetics. Most of these dysrhythmias are supraventricular or PVCs, and few (<1%) are associated with serious sequelae.

In patients with heart disease (IHD, hypertensive, valvular and congenital) or pre-existing dysrhythmias, the incidence of perioperative dysrhythmias (benign and serious) is increased by as much as 3-fold. The type of heart disease (IHD vs. valvular) and the severity of the disease (NYHA II vs. IV) appear to be the most critical factors. More informative data are lacking.

It thus seems reasonable to conclude that those patients with IHD who are at highest risk of developing serious perioperative dysrhythmias have: 1) prior infarction complicated by serious dysrhythmias, 2) evidence of ventricular dysfunction, or 3) recurrent or persistent dysrhythmias detected with the rest or exercise EKG.

THE SIGNIFICANCE OF INFARCTION IN IHD

1. Incidence

Approximately 4 million people in the United States have had one or more myocardial infarctions. Each year, 1.3 million patients develop a new myocardial infarction.

2. Detection

The hallmarks of the clinical diagnosis are history, EKG, and serum enzymes. The classical findings are well known and will not be discussed. But of note are the following:

a. History: Most patients have angina with infarction. However, 20-33% of infarcts are painless, and 35-90% have no prodromal symptoms. Silent extension of MIs has been reported in up to 57% of patients.

b. EKG: With infarction, acute changes in the EKG are characteristic. However, in 20-50% of patients the EKG is non-diagnostic (subendocardial MI, LBBB, WPW, LVH). Furthermore, only 25-50% of old myocardial infarctions can be detected by EKG.

c. Enzymes: In patients with a positive history for acute transmural MI and Q waves on EKG, SGOT, LDH and CPK-MB are elevated virtually all the time (94%, 100%, 100%, respectively). However, in patients with a history suggestive of an MI and with persistent ST-T wave changes (>24 hours), elevation of these same enzymes is not as frequent (63%,71%, 84%, respectively).

d. Other Diagnostic Tests: Echocardiography, nuclear radiology and cardiac catheterization are useful for detection of wall-motion abnormalities and evaluation of ventricular function. These are discussed in the last section.

3. *Prognosis*

For the past 20 years, the annual mortality following myocardial infarction has been 5-8%. The acute in-hospital mortality is 10-40%. Following infarction, short- and long-term prognoses are most significantly effected by:

a. The degree of ventricular dysfunction following infarction.
Highest risk: CHF symptoms, EF <.40, dyssynergy

b. The site of infarction/extent of disease.
Highest risk: anterior wall infarct, diffuse 3-vessel, left-main disease.

c. The type of post-infarction dysrhythmias and conduction disturbances.
Highest risk: fascicular block, complete heart block, serious ventricular dysrhythmias

4. *Perioperative Risk*

PREVIOUS STUDIES

	1962 (*Knapp*)	*1964* (*Tompkins*)	*1972* (*Tarhan*)	*1978* (*Steen*)	*1978* (*Goldman*)	*TOTAL* (*Average*)
Patients Studied	8,984	12,712	32,877	73,321	1,001	128,895
Previous MI	427	658	422	587	131	2,225
Reinfarction 1%	6.1%	6.5%	6.5%	6.1%	13.7%	6.8%
Reinfarction Mortality	58%	70%	54%	69%	67%	65%
% Reinfarction						
0-3 months	100%		37%	27%		
		55%			36%	
3-6 months	100%		16%	11%		

Previous studies have demonstrated that in patients with prior infarction: 1) the overall risk of reinfarction is 6-7% (vs. <1% without previous MI); 2) with recent infarction (within 6 months), the risk of reinfarction is high (36-100%); 3) mortality with reinfarction is high (54-70%); and 4) the statistics have not changed over the previous two decades. However, a recent study has found significantly reduced six-month reinfarction rates (5%) and mortality (2%) when aggressive monitoring and therapy are used. These results have significant implication, and certainly warrant independent verification.

Given a patient with a recent infarction, what risk factors place that patient at highest risk?

Preoperative Risk Factors.

History:	recent MI (<6 months), crescendo angina
Physical:	hypertension, CHF
EKG:	Q waves, BBB, CHB, LVH (strain), ventricular dysrhythmia
CXR:	cardiomegaly, CHF
Cath:	2-, 3-vessel disease, left-main disease, EF <.50, valve disease

In addition to these preoperative factors, the intraoperative factors associated with highest risk are: 1) surgery involving the great vessels, thorax, or upper abdomen; 2) emergency surgery; and 3) the degree and duration of intraoperative hypotension.

THE SIGNIFICANCE OF VENTRICULAR DYSFUNCTION IN IHD

1. *Incidence*

Approximately 700,000 patients die each year from IHD and its complications. With acute myocardial infarction, death usually results from ventricular dysrhythmias or failure. It appears that the mortality from dysrhythmias has been reduced by EKG monitoring and aggressive therapy. However, mortality from failure remains alarmingly high.

2. *Detection*

Quantitated ventriculography, nuclear cardiology and echocardiography provide sensitive measures of ventricular function: ejection fraction, wall motion, and myocardial compliance. The sensitivity of these is summarized by the following.

Measure	*Abnormality first appears with*
Ejection fraction	1-, 2-vessel disease (without MI)
Wall motion (dyssynergy)	3-vessel disease (without MI)
Compliance	MI
Cardiac output	MI + 3-vessel disease
End diastolic pressure	MI + 3-vessel disease

3. *Prognosis*

In patients with acute or chronic IHD, the degree of left ventricular dysfunction is of major prognostic importance. Ejection fraction and dyssynergy appear to be the best prognostic indicators of short- and long-term survival. One-year mortality is significantly higher (30%) in patients with ejection fractions <.40. In patients with three-vessel disease and EF <.50, the 2-year mortality is 36% (vs. 12% with EF >.50). With single-vessel disease, patients with markedly abnormal wall motion have a 5-year mortality of 60% (vs. 10% with normal wall motion). With three-vessel disease, the mortality is 90% (vs. 35% with normal wall motion).

4. Perioperative Risk

In patients with manifest symptoms and signs of left ventricular failure, the perioperative morbidity and mortality are markedly increased. Preoperative assessment is relatively straightforward. However, for the asymptomatic patient with IHD, assessment of the risk of ventricular failure is more difficult. In patients with IHD undergoing noncardiac surgery, there are no significant data. In patients undergoing myocardial revascularization, the studies indicate that of all the preoperative screening data (routine, EKG, and catheterization), ejection fraction and degree of dyssynergy are the best predictors of left and right ventricular dysfunction during the intraoperative and postoperative periods. Furthermore, studies of short- and long-term survival following cardiac surgery have demonstrated that the preoperative LV ejection fraction is the most useful prognostic guide compared with such measures as cardiac output and end-diastolic pressure.

PREOPERATIVE ASSESSMENT: ADDITIONAL INFORMATION

The preoperative screening data most relevant to the assessment of dysrhythmias, infarction and dysfunction are discussed above. In addition, the following appear to be informative and prognostic.

History

1. Anginal pattern - stable vs. unstable vs. variant
   - stress response, exercise tolerance
2. Dysrhythmia/failure symptoms with stress and effort.
3. Medication compliance (nitrates, beta blockers, Ca^{++} channel blockers)

The history is the focal point of the assessment. However, there does not appear to be a consistent relationship between the historical features of angina (location, duration, precipitation) and the extent of vessel involvement.

Physical Examination

On cardiac exam, the significance of the following four findings is noteworthy.

1. Displaced PMI: Cardiomegaly—usually indicates an EF <.50 and places the patient at increased risk.
2. Precordial systolic bulge: Wall motion abnormality—usually indicates a prior MI or acute ischemia.
3. S3: Increased LVEDP—usually indicates extensive MI.
4. S4: Decreased LV compliance—usually indicates a prior MI or ischemia.

Chest X-Ray

In patients with IHD, cardiomegaly (cardiothoracic ratio >.50) is predictive of poor ventricular function (EF <.50) in approximately 70% of patients. Other changes (increased LV volume, increased total heart volume) are equally predictive.

EKG (Resting)

Positive Findings: The EKG is a reliable predictor of IHD only when: 1) significant Q waves are present, or 2) ST changes occur with spontaneous angina (stable, unstable or variant). Other findings on the EKG (ST-T wave changes, LBBB, LVH) are non-specific.

Negative Findings: A normal EKG does not preclude IHD. In 25-50% of patients with IHD the resting EKG is normal. However, it is rarely normal in the patient with significant left ventricular dyssynergy.

EKG (Vector)

Vectorcardiography is useful in depicting infarction patterns where the scalar EKG is equivocal. There is also evidence that selected abnormal vector patterns are indicative of severe abnormality of left ventricular function.

EKG Ambulatory-Holter)

Compared with other methods of EKG monitoring, ambulatory monitoring significantly increases the yield of dysrhythmias. However, stress-response dysrhythmias may be missed. The yield of ST-segment changes is also increased, and a good correlation exists between ST depression occurring during normal activity and angiographic findings. However, the artifact problem is significant, and affects the reliability of ST interpretation.

EKG (Stress-testing)

For dysrhythmia detection, the "exercise EKG" (EEKG) increases the yield of PVCs 3-fold (over the rest EKG) and 8-fold for repetitive forms of ventricular dysrhythmias. Approximately 52% of patients with IHD exhibit PVCs on EEKG. The dysrhythmias usually occur not only at peak exercise, but also during the initial 3 minutes of recovery. In fact, ventricular fibrillation is most likely to occur during recovery.

For ischemia detection, the EEKG is informative if 1) the ST change is significant (>2 mm); 2) symptoms or hypotension occur with the ST change; or 3) the changes occur during the early testing period. Without these changes, it appears that exercise stress testing does not significantly improve diagnostic capability.

Echocardiography

One dimensional (M-mode) and two-dimensional (2D) echocardiography are safe and noninvasive techniques used in IHD primarily for assessing left ventricular wall motion and function (LV volumes, ejection fraction). They have also been used for detection of left-main stenosis, LV aneurysms, septal rupture, papillary muscle abnormality, and mural thrombus formation.

Wall Motion

1. M-mode echocardiography is not satisfactory. Although 1-2 mm sensitivity can be achieved, the beam is narrow (one dimensional) and only the basal LV is viewed.
2. 2D echocardiography is useful and reasonably accurate in 80-90% of patients with IHD. 2D wall-motion abnormalities correlate well with the location and extent of acute MI scarring (postmortem studies in dogs). Comparison with angiography demonstrates good correlation (84-97%), specificity (84%), and sensitivity (95%). Limitations include: 1) the technique varies from

laboratory to laboratory; 2) technical difficulties (COPD, anatomic abnormalities) limit use; 3) multiple cross-sectional views are necessary; and 4) inferior-posterior dyssynergy is more difficult to detect (vs. anterior).

Left Ventricular Function

1. M-mode echocardiography is inaccurate when dyssynergy is present. LV function is assessed by measuring the internal diameter of the LV along the beam at end-diastole ($LVID_d$) and end-systole ($LVID_s$). $LVID_d$ is accurate with or without dyssynergy. $LVID_s$, in the presence of dyssynergy, is inaccurate. Thus, estimates of ESV, SV, CO and EF may be inaccurate.
2. 2D echocardiography provides useful information if multiple cross-sections (>2) are used. 2D ejection fraction correlates well with angiographic ejection fraction (.78-.94). However, 2D left ventricular volumes consistently underestimate angiographic volumes by 30%, especially when less than four cross-sections are used. Thus, stroke volumes and cardiac outputs are underestimated. Estimates of ejection fraction are more accurate because of cancellation of errors. However, three or more cross-sections should be used for accurate estimation of ejection fraction.

Nuclear Cardiology

Radioisotope imaging for detection of myocardial infarction and quantitation of ventricular function is safe and relatively non-invasive.

Myocardial Infarction

Use of radioisotope imaging for detection of myocardial infarction is useful when conventional methods (symptoms, EKG, enzymes) are equivocal or untimely (LBBB, WPW, <6 hours or >48 hours post-MI). Two different techniques are used: "hot spot" and "cold spot" imaging.

	"Hot Spot" Imaging	*"Cold Spot" Imaging*
Radionuclide	Technetium ^{99}m-pyrophosphate	Thallium-201
Uptake by	Infarcted tissue	Normal tissue (normal perfusion and metabolism)
Positive with	Acute MI (>5 gm infarct)	Acute MI (>5 gm infarct) Old MI Ischemia
Timing:		
Earliest positive test	12-16 hours (post MI)	immediately
Most sensitive	48-72 hr	<24 hr
Other uses	RV MI Subendocardial MI Infarct size (+/-)	Chamber size LVH, RVH, ASH Stress testing

Left Ventricular Function. Two techniques are used: first pass radionuclide angiography and gated cardiac blood pool.

	First-Pass	*Gated-Pool*
Radionuclide	Any technetium (99m) labeled pharmaceutical	Technetium (99m) labeled albumin or rbc
Type of technique	Transient (30 sec) Multiple injections/hr	Steady state (6 hr) Single injection/hr
EF correlation with angiography	>.90	>.90
Uses	LVEF Exercise testing Dyskinesis RVEF Intracardiac shunt	LVEF Exercise testing Dyskinesis
Geometric Assumptions	None	Several

Cardiac Catheterization

Coronary angiography and ventriculography are the "gold standards" for definition of coronary anatomy and quantitation of ventricular function. In these regards, no other techniques are as accurate or informative.

Procedure

1. The catheter is advanced retrograde: peripheral artery to left ventricle.
2. Pressure D measurements (systemic, ventricular, atrial) are made.
3. Ventriculography (single-plane or bi-plane) is performed using a highly osmotic contrast dye (10-18 ml/sec over 3-4 sec).
4. Left ventricular volumes are measured (area-length method).
5. Segmental wall motion is quantitated (using hemiaxial shortening, segmental ejection fraction or percent asynergic segments).
6. Pressure measurements are repeated.
7. Selective coronary angiography is performed.

Information

Ventricular Function Data	*Angiographic Data*
1) Ejection fraction (most important)	1) Number and degree of vessel involvement
2) Dyssynergy	2) Presence of left main (equivalent) disease—especially with a high grade right coronary lesion or a left-dominant circulation.
3) Stroke work	
4) End-systolic volume	
5) End-diastolic volume	
6) Change in end-diastolic pressure (dye)	
7) Cardiac output	
8) End-diastolic pressure	

REFERENCES

Background

1. Kannel WB, McGee D, Gorden T: A general cardiovascular risk profile: The Framingham Study. Am J Cardiol 38:46, 1976
2. Gorleri R: Coronary Artery Disease. WB Saunders, Philadelphia, 1976
3. Cohn PF: Diagnosis and Therapy of Coronary Artery Disease. Little, Brown and Co, Boston, 1979

Dysrhythmia

1. Ruberman LD, Weinblatt E, Goldberg JE et al: Ventricular premature beats and mortality after myocardial infarction. N Engl J Med 279:759, 1977
2. Jelinek MV and Lown B: Exercise stress testing for exposure of cardiac arrhythmia. Prog Cardiovasc Dis 26:497, 1974
3. Angelini P, Feldman MI, Lufschanowski R et al: Cardiac arrhythmias during and after heart surgery. Prog Cardiovasc Dis 16:469, 1974

Myocardial Infarction

1. Tarhan S. Moffitt EA, Taylor WF et al: Myocardial infarction after general anesthesia. JAMA 220: 1451, 1972
2. Goldman L, Caldera DL, Nussbaum SB et al: Multifactorial index of cardiac risk in noncardiac surgical procedures. N Engl J Med 297:845, 1977
3. Rao TLK, El-Etra A: Myocardial reinfarction following anesthesia in patients with recent infarctions. Anesth Analg 60:271, 1981

Ventricular Dysfunction

1. Moraski RE, Russell RO, Smith M et al: Left ventricular function in patients with and without myocardial infarction and one, two or three vessel coronary artery disease. Am J Cardiol 35:1, 1975
2. Cohn PF, Gorlin R. Cohn LH et al: Left ventricular ejection fraction as a prognostic guide in surgical treatment of coronary and valvular heart disease. Am J Cardiol 34:136, 1979
3. Mangano DT, Van Dyke DC, Ellis RJ: The effect of increasing preload on ventricular output and ejection in man: Limitations of the Frank-Starling mechanism. Circulation 62:535, 1980

Assessment

1. Proudfit WL, Shirey EK, Sones FM: Selective cine coronary arteriography: Correlation with clinical findings in 1,000 patients. Circulation 33:901, 1966
2. Borer JS, Brensike JF, Redwood DR et al: Limitations of the electrocardiographic response to exercise in predicting coronary artery disease. NEJM 293:367, 1975
3. Reeder GS, Seward JB, Tajik AJ: The role of two-dimensional echocardiography in coronary artery disease. Mayo Clin Proc 57:247, 1982
4. Folland ED, Hamilton GW, Larson SM et al: The radionuclide ejection fraction: A comparison of three radionuclide techniques with contrast angiography. J Nucl Med 18:1159, 1977
5. Mangano DT: Preoperative assessment of cardiac catheterization data: Which parameters are most important? Anesthesiology 53:S106, 1980

THE CORONARY CIRCULATION

David C. Warltier, MD, PhD

An appreciation of the coronary circulation not only leads to more appropriate management of patients undergoing surgical procedures directly related to coronary artery disease, but is also required because of undiagnosed disease in patients otherwise presumed healthy. An understanding and an appreciation of the coronary circulation will lead to aggressive management of perioperative myocardial ischemia and ultimately reduce morbidity and mortality from such ischemic events.

ANATOMICAL RELATIONSHIPS

Left and right coronary arteries arise from ostia located in the aortic root and quickly subdivide into large epicardial branches. The left coronary artery has a left main segment before bifurcation into left anterior descending and left circumflex branches. The course of the left anterior descending artery is from base to apex along the anterior interventricular groove. This artery gives rise to a series of diagonal branches and septal branches which supply the anterolateral left ventricle, a portion of the right ventricle, the anterior two-thirds of the interventricular septum and occasionally the atrioventricular node. The left circumflex coronary artery courses in the left atrioventricular groove supplying several marginal branches and provides perfusion of the posterior and lateral walls of the left ventricle. In about 40% of individuals, the left circumflex gives rise to the sinus node artery.

The right coronary artery courses in a circumferential plane in the right atrioventricular groove. In half of individuals, this artery is considered "dominant" and continues onto the posterior aspect of the right ventricle, terminating on the diaphragmatic surface of the heart as the posterior descending artery. In this situation, this artery supplies the posterior one-third of the interventricular septum, as well as the muscle mass of the right ventricle and the inferior wall of the left ventricle. The right coronary artery supplies flow to the sinus node and atrioventricular node in 60% and 80% of individuals,

T. H. Stanley and P. L. Bailey (eds.), Anesthesiology and the Cardiovascular Patient, 15–26.

respectively. Ten to 15% of individuals have a dominant left coronary system in which the left circumflex coronary artery gives rise to the posterior descending artery. In 35 to 40% of humans, a "balanced" system is present in which neither the right nor the left coronary artery is dominant.

The large epicardial coronary arteries were once thought to simply represent conduit vessels since most of the regulation of flow in the coronary vasculature occurs at the level of the much smaller arteriole. It is now appreciated that the large epicardial arteries are subject to multiple hormonal and neural influences. The vascular endothelium of such vessels may give rise to constricting or relaxant substances (e.g., endothelium-derived relaxing factor or EDRF) which may modulate tone in such vessels. Thus, active vasomotion of the epicardial vessels readily occurs and, in the most obvious case, can lead to vasospasm of an apparently normal coronary artery.

The large epicardial left anterior descending, left circumflex and right coronary arteries give rise to intramural coronary vessels which penetrate into myocardium perpendicularly. These vessels traverse the left ventricular wall and give rise to nutritional circulation (extensive capillary networks) throughout the subepicardium, midmyocardium and subendocardium. The transmural vessels extending from subepicardium to subendocardium supply a series of collateral channels leading to a large interconnecting network of vessels (Fulton's Plexus) within the subendocardium (1). These branches are exposed to intramural tissue pressure and forces generated during contraction of the left ventricle, especially in the innermost layers. Because of the interaction of such forces with these vessels, a knowledge of the regional distribution of coronary blood flow between outer and inner layers of the left ventricle is as important as knowledge of the anatomic distribution of the large coronary arteries.

PHYSIOLOGY OF THE CORONARY CIRCULATION

Coronary blood flow is directly related to perfusion pressure and inversely related to resistance. There are a group of resistances that the coronary circulation is exposed to. This leads to an unusual phasic distribution of flow that is highest in diastole and lowest in systole. Conversely, coronary vascular resistance is maximal in systole and minimal in diastole.

The vascular resistance in the coronary circulation can be divided into three separate components on a functional rather than on an anatomic basis. The first component is represented by a basal viscous resistance of coronary vessels which would occur during maximum vasodilation without any external compressive forces on the coronary vessels. This represents only a small portion of the total coronary vascular resistance. The second component is the result of autoregulation. This is the major portion of coronary vascular resistance and is due to the constriction of arterioles which is subject to many influences, including tissue oxygen tension, products of metabolism such as adenosine, substances which may be released from vascular endothelium, circulating hormones, and sympathetic and parasympathetic nerve activity. Changes in autoregulated resistance occur over several cardiac cycles. Finally, compressive resistance is unique to the coronary circulation and is extravascular in nature. This resistance is instantaneous and occurs during each cardiac cycle. It is much greater in the subendocardium than the subepicardium. It is this compressive resistance that is primarily responsible for the unique phasic pattern of coronary blood flow.

In contrast to other tissues which have higher blood flow in systole than in diastole, the reverse situation occurs in left ventricular myocardium (Figure 1). A high intramyocardial tissue pressure (which can actually exceed intracavitary pressure) is generated within left ventricular myocardium during isovolumic contraction. As a consequence, intramural coronary vessels are abruptly compressed. Thus, left coronary flow remains low during early systole and may be momentarily reversed as blood is forced into the large epicardial coronary vessels during the compression of intramural vessels. Left coronary artery blood flow rises during isovolumic relaxation and reaches peak levels in diastole. Right coronary artery flow follows a more typical phasic pattern in

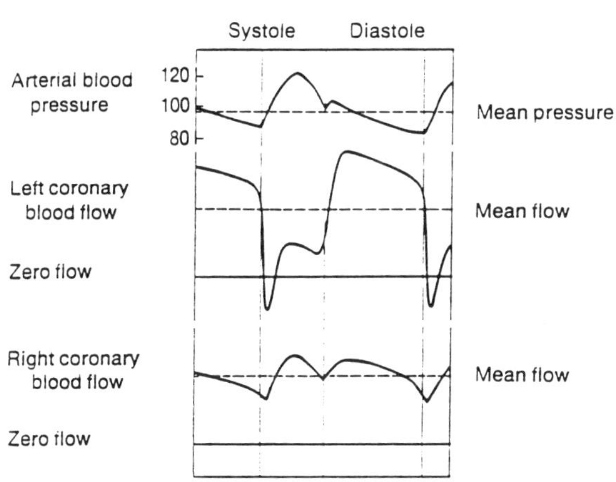

Figure 1. Phasic changes in left and right coronary blood flow during systole and diastole.

sequence with aortic pressure. This is because the right ventricle has a smaller muscle mass is present and less intracavitary pressures are generated.

The question of where and how total coronary blood flow is distributed within the left ventricular myocardium has been extensively studied. Ischemia and/or infarction is usually more extensive in the subendocardium than in corresponding subepicardial regions. The left ventricular subendocardium is sensitive to the development of ischemia and infarction because of the compressive forces that alter blood flow to this region. In systole, tissue pressure within the subepicardium remains relatively low, but within the subendocardium, intramyocardial tissue pressure rises to very high levels, as much as 30 to 50 mmHg greater than left ventricular intracavitary pressure. This pressure compressing the subendocardial vessels clearly exceeds the driving pressure for subendocardial perfusion. Therefore, the small amount of coronary flow that occurs in systole is preferentially distributed to the subepicardium. The subendocardium also exhibits increased energy expenditure, higher oxygen consumption and extraction, and as a consequence, a lower tissue oxygen tension.

The myocardium uses multiple substrates for production of ATP. The preferred substrates are free fatty acids and, to a lesser extent, lactate. Metabolism is strictly an oxidative process and utilization of glucose is negligible. Under ischemic conditions, however, a small degree of anaerobic metabolism of glucose (and subsequent lactate production) may occur. Although this is inadequate to sustain contractile function, it may offer some benefit to preserve vital cellular processes for short periods of time. There is a tight coupling of coronary blood flow to myocardial metabolism, and this has been termed metabolic autoregulation. Of the many mediators which have been proposed to be involved in this process, the most significant is adenosine. During periods of increased metabolic activity, more ATP is utilized and greater amounts of adenosine are produced. Adenosine diffuses through the interstitial space and interacts directly with vascular smooth muscle, producing arteriolar vasodilation. This could provide a moment-to-moment mechanism for vasodilation in the coronary circulation during increased myocardial oxygen demand.

As in other organs, myocardial blood flow is also autoregulated over a wide range of driving pressures providing a relatively constant coronary flow even in thel face of large changes in perfusion pressure (2) (Figure 2). As driving pressure increases, the coronary vasculature constricts, and flow remains constant. However, there is a point of maximum vasoconstriction, and coronary blood flow increases linearly with pressure beyond a mean driving pressure of 120 mm Hg. Conversely, as pressure is reduced, flow remains constant secondary to vasodilation. Maximum vasodilation is reached at a driving pressure of approximately 50 mm Hg. As pressure continues to decrease below this level, flow also decreases in a linear fashion. A regional difference in autoregulation also exists. The subepicardial vasculature has a greater ability to autoregulate than corresponding subendocardial vessels. Autoregulation is lost at higher perfusion pressures in the subendocardium than in the subepicardium(3). This may be partially due to the fact that the vessels in the subendocardium are relatively dilated under resting conditions.

Any factor which attenuates the ability of coronary vascular smooth muscle to alter arteriolar diameter, such as a vasodilator drug, will interfere with pressure autoregulation. When autoregulation is abolished by potent vasodilators, coronary blood flow will increase or decrease in a linear relationship with aortic pressure. Under these conditions, coronary pressure flow relations resemble those of an elastic or rigid tube (Figure 2). In theory, at least partial loss of autoregulation may occur with anesthetics that produce coronary vasodilation. A reduction in driving pressure for coronary flow might be expected to be accompanied by greater decreases in perfusion under these circumstances.

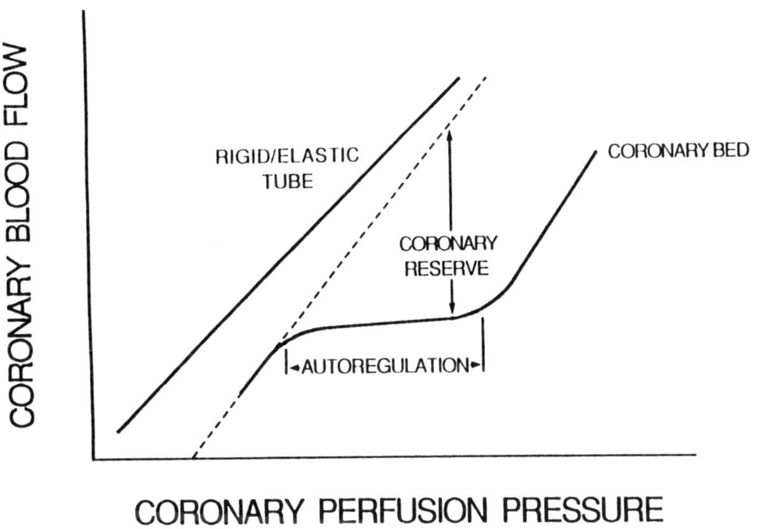

Figure 2. Pressure autoregulation in the normal coronary circulation. Note that at maximum vasodilation pressure autoregulation is abolished (dashed line) and pressure-flow relationships resemble that of a rigid/elastic tube. Also demonstrated is the concept of coronary vascular reserve. Coronary reserve represents the ability of coronary blood flow to be increased in response to stress (at a given driving pressure) and is the difference between maximum vasodilation and resting coronary flow.

If the linear relation between low perfusion pressure and coronary flow (or between higher pressure and flow during maximum vasodilation) is extrapolated, zero flow is found to occur at a finite diastolic arterial pressure. Therefore, the coronary arteries will not be perfused below a certain minimum perfusion pressure. This phenomenon can be demonstrated experimentally in the presence of high vagal tone and a prominent sinus arrhythmia resulting in prolonged RR intervals. Zero coronary flow has been found to be reached at diastolic aortic pressures as high as 40 mm Hg in experimental animals. This has been termed the "critical closing pressure" and is that pressure at which flow ceases in diastole. It is the minimum inflow pressure required for any diastolic coronary perfusion. This pressure most likely exceeds both coronary venous and left ventricular end diastolic pressures. The mechanism for "critical closure" depicts vessels as collapsible tubes which are kept distended by the driving pressure (4). When this pressure is exceeded by the intramyocardial tissue pressure, vessels collapse. It is likely that there is also a regional distribution of zero flow-pressure relations in the left ventricular wall. Flow to the subendocardium probably ceases at higher driving pressures than flow to subepicardial regions.

PATHOPHYSIOLOGY

Coronary vascular reserve allows coronary blood flow to increase (e.g., in response to a stress) without a change in driving pressure (Figure 2). Peak coronary vascular reserve occurs at maximum vasodilation. This flow is at least as high and may exceed that occurring during peak reactive hyperemia following brief coronary occlusion.

When coronary vascular reserve becomes diminished, susceptibility to myocardial ischemia develops during abrupt increases in oxygen demand. The most common cause for this is an obstruction or stenosis of a large epicardial coronary artery produced by atherosclerosis. With increasing severity of a coronary artery stenosis, the initial hemodynamic abnormality is a reduction in coronary vascular reserve. Only later with more severe degrees of coronary stenosis is resting coronary blood flow reduced. At 50% stenosis (reduction in vascular cross-sectional area), there is little effect on coronary reserve (or peak reactive hyperemia). Reactive hyperemia remains unaltered until approximately 60% stenosis is reached. At further degrees of severity of vascular obstruction (80-90% stenosis), the reactive hyperemic response is abolished ("critical stenosis"). In spite of this marked decrease in coronary vascular reserve, little change in resting coronary blood flow occurs secondary to vasodilation distal to the stenosis. At stenoses greater than 90% diastolic coronary flow becomes reduced, and coronary flow in systole is actually increased. Concomitant with these changes in diastolic and systolic total coronary blood flow, there is a redistribution of perfusion away from the subendocardium. Blood flow to subepicardial layers is relatively maintained until even higher levels of stenosis are reached.

Changes in systemic hemodynamics, such as a reduction in diastolic aortic pressure, an increase in heart rate, or elevation of left ventricular end diastolic pressure are compensated for by vasodilation in the normal coronary circulation. In the presence of a stenosis, however, such hemodynamic changes are met with marked alterations in the regional distribution of perfusion because vasodilation of the distal vascular bed is already present. For example, a factor of major importance involved in the regional distribution of coronary blood flow in the presence of a coronary artery stenosis, is left ventricular end-diastolic pressure (Figure 3). The driving pressure for subendocardial blood flow may be represented by P_A-P_T where P_A = diastolic arterial pressure and P_T = left ventricular end diastolic pressure. In a normal coronary artery, this may be 75-5 = 70 mm Hg. In the presence of a severe coronary stenosis, there is a large pressure drop across the vascular obstruction resulting in a much lower distal perfusion pressure of (75-45)-5 = 25 mmHg. If left ventricular end diastolic pressure increases (e.g., to 20 mmHg), the driving pressure for flow to the subendocardium is further reduced to (75-45)-20 = 10 mmHg and may fall below "critical closing" pressures. Therefore, left ventricular end diastolic pressure is as important a determinant of subendocardial perfusion as diastolic aortic pressure or heart rate in the presence of coronary artery disease.

When a coronary artery becomes totally occluded, blood flow may nevertheless be present in the perfusion territory of the occluded vessel. This flow arises from intra-arterial anastomoses, known as coronary collateral vessels. Collateral flow may be adequate to preserve structure and function of myocardium and prevent ischemia and/or infarction under resting conditions despite total coronary occlusion. This protection would depend on the magnitude of the collateral flow. Indeed, the limited capacity of these vessels to supply blood during periods of stress jeopardizes collateral-dependent myocardium.

Considerable research, primarily conducted in animals, has demonstrated that coronary collateral flow can be affected by drugs. Nitroglycerin and nifedipine which dilate large epicardial coronary arteries also dilate coronary collaterals and are capable of increasing perfusion of ischemic myocardium. Other drugs, such as adenosine and dipyridamole ("small vessel dilators"),

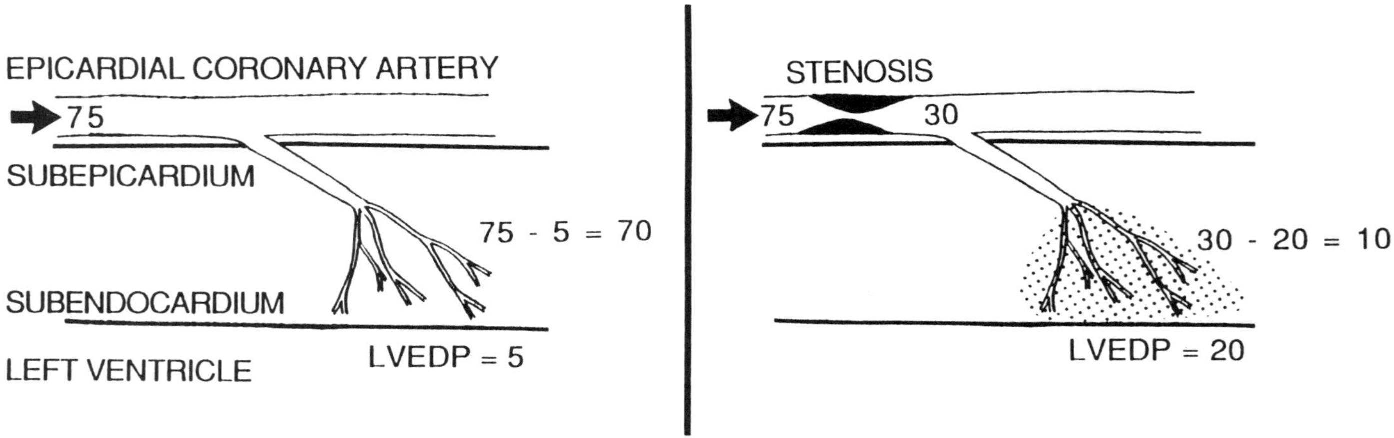

Figure 3. Schematic representation of pressure changes in a large epicardial coronary artery in the presence and absence of a stenosis. Left ventricular end diastolic pressure (LVEDP) becomes a significant factor in perfusion of subendocardium in the presence of a severe stenosis. Shaded area indicates a region in which the driving pressure for flow may be exceeded by intramyocardial tissue pressure (resulting in critical closure). See text for details.

decrease arteriolar resistance in normal areas. If the arterioles in the perfusion territory of a totally occluded coronary artery are near maximally dilated, no further decrease in the resistance of arterioles in ischemic areas will be produced by these drugs. In fact, the effect of the small vessel dilators to lower resistance in normal zones can reduce collateral flow by decreasing the driving pressure for collateral flow at the origin of the coronary collaterals. This phenomenon is termed "coronary steal" and is independent of change in systemic hemodynamics such as heart rate and diastolic aortic pressure. The redistribution of collateral perfusion away from certain regions partially contributes to the basis for "reversible perfusion defects" readily observable during persantine-thallium scans.

ANESTHETIC AGENTS

A major point of controversy in recent years is whether certain anesthetics cause "coronary steal" which may produce or exacerbate myocardial ischemia in patients with coronary artery disease. This would depend not only on the particular anesthetic agent but also on the presence of a "steal prone" anatomy. The latter is present in approximately 25% of patients presenting for coronary artery bypass graft surgery and consists of a totally occluded vessel with significant collateral perfusion and concomitant stenosis of the vessel of origin of the collaterals. The only anesthetic to be seriously implicated as a cause of this potential adverse effect is isoflurane, which is capable of producing coronary arteriolar vasodilation (5,6). Although production of ischemia has been demonstrated with isoflurane, it is unresolved whether the onset of ischemia was secondary to hemodynamic alterations such as decreases in aortic pressure and increases in heart rate or secondary to a direct redistribution of blood flow.

Some investigations have actually shown potentially beneficial effects of volatile anesthetics. Both halothane and isoflurane markedly improve recovery from regional wall motion abnormalities in postischemic, reperfused ("stunned") myocardium (7). Furthermore, these effects are unrelated to any anesthetic-induced change in myocardial oxygen supply or demand. Finally, studies using chronically instrumented dogs have shown little effect of isoflurane or desflurane on the regional distribution of coronary flow when anesthetized and conscious states are compared if hypotension is avoided (8).

CLINICAL MANAGEMENT

At present, there is no general consensus as to whether any specific anesthetic produces direct detrimental effects on myocardial perfusion. The most important clinical guideline for the anesthesiologist involved in the treatment of jeopardized myocardium is the production of the most beneficial myocardial oxygen supply/demand balance possible. Indeed, anesthetics may be useful in this regard, by their ability to reduce oxygen demand and decrease myocardial oxygen consumption and potentially redistribute perfusion to subendocardial regions.

Subendocardial perfusion is directly related to the difference between aortic and left ventricular pressures integrated over time during diastole. This is termed the diastolic pressure-time index (DPTI) and is directly related to oxygen supply. The demand for oxygen delivery is closely related to the area beneath the systolic portion of the aortic or ventricular pressure curves, i.e., the tension-time index (TTI). Thus, the ratio of DPTI to TTI has been used as an index of the relationship between subendocardial oxygen supply and demand.

In the presence of coronary artery disease, reference to the components of this ratio may serve as a useful reminder of the factors responsible for need and adequacy of perfusion. For example, DPTI may be decreased by an increase in left ventricular preload (excessive fluids, especially in the presence of a non-compliant ventricle; myocardial dysfunction) or by a decrease in the time spent in diastole (tachycardia) or by excessive reductions in aortic diastolic pressure (hypotension; aortic regurgitation). Similarly, TTI may be increased during tachycardia (more time spent each minute in systole) or by elevations of afterload (hypertension; aortic stenosis).

As a general rule, the patient with uncomplicated coronary artery disease can tolerate anesthetic agents, such as opioids, that decrease heart rate and maintain diastolic aortic pressure. Some patients with a hyperdynamic circulatory status (elevated ejection fraction and systemic arterial pressure) may benefit from an anesthetic technique which prevents excessive increases in myocardial oxygen demand. This would include simultaneous use of a volatile anesthetic as required to prevent sudden increases in heart rate, myocardial contractility and systolic arterial pressure in conjunction with an opioid. In contrast, a patient having a low stroke volume, ejection fraction and poor ventricular function may tolerate only low doses of an opioid with no added volatile inhaled agent.

Patients with coronary artery disease present a spectrum of hemodynamic profiles and responses to anesthesia and stress. Each patient must be managed individually to maintain optimum myocardial oxygen supply/demand balance. In most cases, particularly for major surgeries, this will require intra-arterial and pulmonary artery pressure monitoring with calculations of stroke volume, cardiac output, ventricular filling pressures and vascular resistances for optimum management. In particular, hemodynamic and electrocardiographic signs of myocardial ischemia should be carefully monitored. Myocardial ischemia should be aggressively treated with nitroglycerin, calcium entry blockers and/or beta-adrenergic antagonists. Table 1 lists some precipitating causes and potential management strategies of perioperative ischemia.

Table 1. Precipitating causes of perioperative ischemia.

Cause	*Management*
Increased heart rate	↑anesthetic depth beta blocker calcium entry blocker
Increased preload	nitroglycerin diuretic
Increased afterload	calcium entry blocker ↑anesthetic depth
Increased contractility	↑anesthetic depth beta blocker
Diastolic hypotension	↑preload (fluids) ↑afterload (vasopressor) ↓anesthetic depth
Coronary arterial spasm	calcium entry blocker nitroglycerin

The management of patients with coronary artery disease is a challenge for all anesthesiologists. Only through an understanding and an appreciation of those factors involved in oxygen supply and demand of compromised myocardium can expedient and appropriate intraoperative decisions be made.

REFERENCES

1. Fulton WFM: The Coronary Arteries. Springfield, Thomas, 1965
2. Marcus ML: The Coronary Circulation in Health and Disease. New York, McGraw Hill, 1983
3. Warltier DC, Gross GJ, Brooks HL: Pharmacologic- vs. ischemia-induced coronary artery vasodilation. Am J Physiol 240:H767-H774, 1981
4. Downey JM, Kirk ES: Inhibition of coronary blood flow by a vascular waterfall mechanism. Circ Res 36:753-760, 1975
5. Buffington CW, Romson JL, Levine A, et al: Isoflurane induces coronary steal in a canine model of chronic coronary occlusion. Anesthesiology 66:280-292, 1987

6. Moffitt E, Barker RA, Glenn JJ, et al: Myocardial metabolism and hemodynamic responses with isoflurane anesthesia for coronary arterial surgery. Anesth Analg 65:53-61, 1986
7. Warltier DC, Al-Wathiqui MH, Kampine JP, Schmeling WT: Recovery of contractile function of stunned myocardium in chronically instrumented dogs is enhanced by halothane or isoflurane. Anesthesiology 69:552-565, 1988
8. Hartman JC, Kampine JP, Schmeling WT, Warltier DC: Steal-prone coronary circulation in chronically instrumented dogs: isoflurane versus adenosine. Anesthesiology 74:744-56, 1991

DIASTOLIC FUNCTION: ANESTHESIA AND MYOCARDIAL ISCHEMIA

Pierre Foëx, MD

INTRODUCTION

Over the past decade, much interest has been focused on diastolic cardiac function because of the realization that alterations of diastolic function may be early markers of coronary heart disease, hypertensive heart disease, and many cardiomyopathies. As many as 40% of patients presenting with cardiac failure may have intact systolic function, implicating diastolic dysfunction as the major cause of failure (1). In addition to ischemia, hypertrophy and pericarditis, left ventricular filling may be impaired because of right ventricular failure associated with bulging of the septum into the cavity of the left ventricle.

There are many reasons why diastolic function has been studied much less extensively than systolic function. The first is that diastole was thought to be a purely passive phenomenon, and, therefore, of relative insignificance as a passive phenomenon is unlikely to be influenced by medication. It is now well recognized that relaxation of cardiac fibers requires approximately 15% of the total energy of the cardiac cycle. This energy is expended on a number of processes involving calcium. Relaxation involves the dissociation of calcium from the troponin-tropomyosin complex, and its re-uptake by the sarcoplasmic reticulum. This process is essential for the dissociation of the actin-myosin cross bridges and the restoration of the inhibitory action of the troponin-tropomyosin regulatory complex. In addition, calcium has to be extruded from the cardiac cells. These processes depend on the availability of ATP (2). If the balance of oxygen supply and demand is altered, reduced energy availability may impair ventricular relaxation before systolic function is disrupted. Several mechanisms may alter the calcium cycle: inadequate extrusion from the cell (calcium overload), leak from the sarcoplasmic reticulum, or excessive sensitivity of the troponin-tropomyosin complex to calcium. The resulting Ca^{2+} release-sequestration mismatch impairs relaxation, this in turn reduces the early diastolic filling (3). The second reason is that diastole is difficult to study because it is a

T. H. Stanley and P. L. Bailey (eds.), Anesthesiology and the Cardiovascular Patient, 27–38.

complex phenomenon. Its four main phases are isovolumic relaxation, rapid filling, diastasis, and atrial contraction.

PHASES OF DIASTOLE

I. Isovolumic Relaxation

Isovolumic relaxation is the interval between the closure of the aortic valve and the opening of the mitral valve. Relaxation of cardiac fibers causes a rapid reduction in pressure. Relaxation is controlled by a complex interaction of inactivation, changing loading conditions and nonuniformity in space and time (4,5). The major mechanisms of inactivation are the removal of myoplasmic calcium by the sarcoplasmic reticulum and the termination of the life-cycle of force generating sites. The low calcium concentration allows the actin-myosin dissociation as calcium moves away from the subunit C of the regulatory protein troponin to the sarcoplasmic reticulum.

In isolated heart muscle preparations, reductions of afterload abbreviate the relaxation phase, unless the sarcoplasmic reticulum is inactivated. In the working heart, changes in preload do not appear to alter the time constant of relaxation. By contrast, increases in afterload are associated with increases in the time constant of relaxation.

The architectural structure, the electrical activity, and the mechanical properties of the left ventricle are not uniform. Interventions which increase the nonuniformity (intracoronary isoprenaline infusion, regional ischemia) prolong the time constant of relaxation (6). In addition, many positive inotropic interventions reduce the time constant of relaxation possibly by stimulating the uptake of calcium by the sarcoplasmic reticulum.

Factors that influence the speed of isovolumic relaxation may affect the next phase of diastole, namely, the rapid filling that occurs immediately after mitral valve opening (4).

II. Rapid Filling Phase

This phase extends from the opening of the mitral valve until the left atrial and left ventricular pressures equilibrate. Myocardial relaxation, as an active process, continues during the rapid filling phase of the ventricle. The passive component is represented by the passive pressure-volume relation of the ventricle (7,8). Diastolic suction (elastic recoil), if present, is the expenditure of energy previously stored in the ventricular wall. Changes in shape and torsion can also store energy and contribute to diastolic suction (9). The atrioventricular pressure gradient is the motive force for ventricular filling. The best correlate of peak filling rate is the maximum atrioventricular pressure gradient (10).

Increases in preload increase the atrioventricular pressure gradient and augment the early ventricular filling. Chronically elevated afterload is associated with decreased early diastolic filling rate. Increases in inotropy are associated with increases in rapid filling. In addition, a close correlation exists between percentage of systolic shortening and early filling rate.

Rapid filling is decreased in patients with hypertrophic cardiomyopathy (11), hypertension and myocardial ischemia (8). Aging is also associated with an impairment of rapid filling (12). The rapid filling phase accounts for as much as 80% of the total filling. This phase ends with the equilibration of atrial and ventricular pressures.

III. Diastasis

In the absence of tachycardia, rapid filling ends after approximately one-third of the diastolic interval. Diastasis extends from the time of pressure equilibrium between atrium and ventricle until atrial contraction. Left ventricular filling is slow. The transmitral flow continues because of inertia (7). A small amount of blood returning from the pulmonary veins contributes usually less than 5% to ventricular filling (13). At fast heart rates, diastasis is shortened and atrial contraction occurs almost immediately after rapid filling.

IV. Atrial Contraction

Atrial contraction increases the atrioventricular pressure gradient. Currently it is estimated that no more than 25% of the left ventricular stroke volume (7,14) is accounted for by a properly timed atrial contraction. Both *in vitro* and *in vivo*, the Frank-Starling mechanism has been shown to operate in the atria (15). In patients with hypertrophic cardiomyopathy and in those with myocardial infarction, the contribution of atrial contraction to stroke volume is increased, and atrial systole may become a critical factor in the maintenance of an adequate stroke volume (16). In such circumstances, loss of atrial contraction may produce a dramatic reduction in cardiac output.

V. *Passive Properties of the Left Ventricle*

Passive properties refer to the pressure-volume relation when the ventricle is completely relaxed after the previous contraction and before the next systole. These properties are described as chamber stiffness and myocardial stiffness.

1. ***Chamber stiffness.*** Chamber stiffness describes the behaviour of the ventricle as a hollow structure. It is obtained from the passive pressure-volume relation or from a surrogate for volume such as segmental length, diameter or radius. The slope of the pressure-volume relation is an exponential. This indicates that the ventricle becomes stiffer at high dimensions. Geometry of the ventricle, wall thickness, characteristics of the myocardium, external constraints to filling, viscoelastic effects and changes in the coronary circulation influence the stiffness of the ventricle.

The chambers of the heart interact mechanically with each other especially during diastole. Acute shifts of the septum alter the stiffness of the cardiac chambers. The interaction between the ventricles is minimized in the absence of the pericardium. Conversely, when the pericardium is intact its effect on the pressure-volume relation of the ventricles depends upon the volume of the cavities. At low volumes, the effect of the pericardium is small. At high filling volumes, the stress imposed by the pericardium is high and contributes to the ventricular diastolic pressure (17).

The myocardium exhibits viscoelastic properties. This means that stresses in the wall depend upon both the magnitude of the deformation and the rate at which it occurs. Thus diastolic pressure depends on filling rate and ventricular volume. Viscous forces are greatest during the rapid filling in early diastole and during atrial systole.

An increase in coronary bed turgor increases ventricular stiffness. However, this effect is quite modest (17).

2. ***Myocardial stiffness.*** Myocardial stiffness represents the resistance of the myocardium to stretching when subjected to stress. It is determined by the relations between stress and strain. Because wall stress cannot be measured, there is little agreement on the best assumption for its estimation. Myocardial stiffness is thought to describe the material properties of the myocardium itself (18). It differs from chamber stiffness, which is a product of both myocardial stiffness and ventricular size.

Evaluation of Diastolic Function

All the phases of diastole can be analyzed and quantified. Indices of isovolumic relaxation include the time constant of isovolumic relaxation (τ) and the maximum rate of left ventricular pressure decline (-LV dP/dt_{max}). High-fidelity measurements of left ventricular pressure allow the first derivative of pressure with respect to time (-dP/dt) to be measured as well as the time constant (τ) of left ventricular pressure decline. As -dP/dt is highly dependent upon the developed left ventricular pressure, it is a less useful index of relaxation than the time constant τ. The latter is calculated from the time of maximum rate of pressure decline to the opening of the mitral valve, based on the valid assumption of a mono-exponential time course (19). Increases in heart rate, sympathetic stimulation and circulating catecholamines reduce the time constant of isovolumic relaxation. The latter is also sensitive to alterations in ventricular loading (4). Rapid filling is estimated as the peak filling rate or the peak change in dimensions (length, diameter) when dimensions rather than volume are measured. While in experimental animals continuous measurement of ventricular volume can be obtained using three-dimensional sonomicrometry or conductance catheters, non-invasive methods including echocardiography and radionuclide angiography are most often used in humans. More frequently, even in experimental animals, ventricular dimensions rather than volume are measured (diameter, segment length or wall thickness). The effects of atrial contraction can be determined using a number of complex indices in experimental studies and by Doppler flow measurements in echocardiographic studies. Finally, the relationship between pressure and dimensions at the end of diastole defines cardiac chamber stiffness (pressure-dimension) and myocardial stiffness (stress-strain). As these relationships are exponential, they can be quantified in terms of constants.

Two different approaches are used to describe these relationships. One relies on the instantaneous relationship between pressure and dimension during the early and middle part of diastole while the other relies on the relationship between individual pairs of pressure and dimensions at end-diastole, obtained by deliberately altering preload. While both methods yield stiffness constants it is clear that they do not represent the same properties of the ventricle. The instantaneous pressure dimension relationship is measured during the early to middle phase of diastole, while the other method examines only true end-diastolic measurements. Our preliminary data (unpublished observations) suggest that the instantaneous pressure dimension relationship during the early and middle part of diastole is highly sensitive to preload.

Effects of Anesthesia on Diastole

*1. **Time constant of relaxation.*** The pressure decline in the left ventricle is easy to measure. Many studies of the effects of inhaled anesthetics on isovolumic relaxation have been published. Most studies have shown that τ increases in a dose-related fashion as the concentration of the anesthetic agent is raised. This is true of comparisons in chronically instrumented animals in whom control data were obtained in the awake state (20) and in an acutely instrumented model in which control data were obtained under fentanyl anesthesia (21). The more recently introduced agents, sevoflurane (21) and desflurane (22), have effects similar to those of halothane, enflurane and isoflurane. Increasing infusion rates of propofol (23) or thiopentone also increase τ in a dose-related manner. As it is known that left ventricular relaxation depends upon load, inactivation and coronary filling, the effect of most anesthetic agents on τ is entirely predictable. Inhaled and intravenous anesthetics (at least propofol and sodium thiopental) decrease arterial pressure, an index of the load. Most anesthetic agents decrease calcium flux across the sarcolemma of cardiac cells and alter the release of calcium from the sarcoplasmic reticulum (24-27). It is logical to hypothesize that calcium flux preceding relaxation is also altered, resulting in impaired inactivation. Finally, with the exception of isoflurane, anesthetic agents cause dose-dependent reductions in coronary blood flow, hence they reduce coronary filling. Thus, the effects of many anesthetic agents on τ can be interpreted as a consequence of their effects on systolic function as mediated by their effect on calcium currents. The prolongation of τ may not be the expression of a specific effect of halogenated anesthetics, propofol, or sodium thiopental on relaxation.

In a study of the effect of halothane on phasic coronary flow, Doyle and colleagues (28) have shown that coronary flow during isovolumic relaxation is reduced more than total coronary blood flow. The exaggerated reduction of flow during isovolumic relaxation is probably a consequence of its slower time course.

2. ***Peak filling rate.*** Peak filling rate in most experimental models is replaced by peak lengthening or peak thinning rate. Pagel and colleagues have reported marked reductions in peak lengthening rate caused by halothane and isoflurane. These were reversed by calcium infusion (22). In experimental studies of the effects of graded concentrations of halothane, enflurane, isoflurane and sevoflurane, dose-dependent reductions in the peak lengthening rate were observed in both the apex and the base of the left ventricle (21). No differences between the four anesthetic agents were noted. However, marked differences

were noted between apex and base. The peak filling rate was much greater at the apex than the base. In addition, the effects of stepped increases in the concentration of the inhaled anesthetics were more significant at the apex than the base. These observations do not necessarily mean that halogenated anesthetics exert a specific effect on the peak lengthening rate of the left ventricle. This effect is likely to be a reflection of the effects of anesthetic agents on systolic function. As inhalational anesthetics depress myocardial contractility, they cause a dose-dependent reduction in systolic shortening. If segments shorten less, there is, as a consequence, less capacity for lengthening. If the duration of the cardiac cycle and its phases are little altered, peak lengthening rate must be reduced when systolic shortening is diminished. Thus, the effect of inhaled anesthetics on peak lengthening rate may, like their effect on τ, reflect changes in systolic function.

The regional differences in peak lengthening rate are the exact counterpart of the differences observed during systole (29) and not a specific effect of anesthetic agents on regional diastolic function. Also, the more significant depression of peak lengthening rate at the apex reflects the greater sensitivity of the apex to depression of its systolic function.

The importance of regional differences in systolic function and peak lengthening rate is that comparisons of studies are only meaningful if the same regions of the ventricle have been studied. Also, depending upon the area of the left ventricle studied, interventions may appear to exert a greater or lesser effect.

3. ***Ventricular stiffness.*** At the end of diastole, it is very unlikely that the relationships between pressure and dimensions are a direct function of events during the previous systole; thus, observations made at the end of diastole represent the true diastolic characteristics of the ventricle (chamber stiffness) or the cardiac muscle (myocardial stiffness).

Inhaled anesthetics cause an increase in cardiac stiffness when compared to the awake state in chronically instrumented dogs (20). By contrast, in an acutely instrumented canine model, with reference to fentanyl anesthesia, four inhaled anesthetics (halothane, enflurane, isoflurane and sevoflurane) did not appear to cause changes in cardiac stiffness. In these studies, two regions of the left ventricle were studied and the data showed stiffness to be greater at the base than at the apex (21). The greater stiffness of the base may reflect one of its roles, namely to support the aortic valve. This regional difference in cardiac stiffness makes it difficult to compare studies unless data refer to the same region. As to the difference between the studies of Pagel and colleagues (20) and our own studies (21), several factors may be implicated. First, one model used the awake state as control and the other used fentanyl anesthesia. Second, Pagel and colleagues studied the midwall and not the apex or the base. As neither apical nor basal region showed any change in our study, it is unlikely that changes would have been observed if the midwall had been studied. Third, Pagel and colleagues used the instantaneous pressure-length relationship (i.e., early and mid-diastole) while we obtained true end-diastolic points by acutely altering the preload by caval occlusion. It is very likely that the difference between models and the way in which stiffness was calculated explains the contrasting findings. It is worthwhile noting that in previous studies in the same model we have found that propofol did not cause changes in cardiac stiffness. However, at a high propofol infusion rate, the difference between apex and base was abolished (30).

Effects of Ischemia on Diastole

It has been long recognized that myocardial ischemia causes a reduction in systolic function associated with an increase in end-diastolic pressure and dimensions representing an increase in cardiac stiffness. The increase in end-diastolic dimension, termed "creep," is associated with a decrease in elastic distensibility. In a series of studies of the interactions between anesthesia and ischemia, we have shown that the increase in stiffness occurs when coronary flow decreases by 50% or more, and not only with coronary occlusion. Similarly, the unstressed length (at zero ventricular pressure) increases once coronary flow has been reduced by 50% or more, and left ventricular end-diastolic pressure (LVEDP) also increases (31). However, it is not easy to understand how an increase in stiffness in a limited area of the anterior wall of the left ventricle, representing less than 25% of its mass, could cause an increase in LVEDP, as the latter should occur only when a generalized increase in stiffness has occurred. Indeed, our study showed that ischemia in the apical region was associated with an increase in stiffness in both the apical (ischemic) and basal (remote, non-ischemic) region of the left ventricle. In the latter region this increase in stiffness was accompanied by an increase in unstressed length. This observation of an effect of ischemia at a distance is not specific to halothane anesthesia; we have observed it in studies carried out using isoflurane or fentanyl anesthesia with or without nitrous oxide.

What are the mechanisms of the remote effect of regional ischemia? Decrease in myocardial perfusion cannot be implicated as coronary blood flow is not reduced. Altered metabolism is also unlikely as there is no reason for an imbalance between oxygen demand and supply in a territory perfused by normal coronary arteries. Mechanical interactions between ischemic and non-ischemic regions have been demonstrated for systolic function. Usually, overall systolic shortening is increased (32), mostly because of an increase in isovolumic shortening associated with systolic lengthening in the ischemic area. After the end of systole, early lengthening is usually observed in the non-ischemic region, while post-systolic shortening occurs in the ischemic region. It is difficult to imagine how early lengthening could result in stiffening of the remote nonischemic myocardium. However, no study, thus far, has attempted to determine whether altered loading conditions might influence the effect of ischemia on remote, well perfused, myocardium. An alternative hypothesis is that mediators are released by the ischemic myocardium, especially the endocardium. Such mediators could be transported by the coronary circulation to the normally perfused region. Amongst the mediators released by ischemia, endothelins, platelet activating factor (PAF) and adenosine may play a role. The latter, though released by ischemic myocardium, is unlikely to increase myocardial stiffness as no such effect has been seen in response to its intracoronary administration (unpublished observations). PAF, in studies using an isolated heart preparation, has little effect on cardiac stiffness (33). However, endothelin-1 given as intracoronary infusion, increases cardiac stiffness at concentrations that have little effect on coronary blood flow. This effect is not simply an effect of the infusion of fluid in the coronary circulation, because it is prevented by the prior administration of the endothelin blocker BQ123 (unpublished observations). Therefore, it is possible that endothelins, known to be released during ischemia, may exert an effect on the remote myocardium.

Is the finding of an increase in stiffness of the ischemic and remote non-ischemic myocardium of any relevance to anesthesia? If the effect of ischemia on the myocardium, ischemic or remote, was observed exclusively during the period of ischemia, it would probably be of little relevance. However, this effect outlasts the duration of ischemia, suggesting that diastolic stunning occurs in the ischemic and in the remote non-ischemic myocardium (34). How long diastolic stunning lasts has not been established. If it were shown to be long lasting, the effects of brief periods of ischemia may contribute to the development of a major delayed complication of anesthesia and surgery, i.e., ischemia-induced pulmonary edema. This problem can be exacerbated by errors in fluid management, as the same volume load causes substantially greater increases in left ventricular end-diastolic pressure during episodes of regional ischemia (35).

Assuming that endothelin plays a role in the stiffening of remote myocardium, prevention of this effect may be possible by selective blockade of endothelin receptors or by using drugs that prevent its release.

REFERENCES

1. Soufer R, Wohlgelertner D, Vita NA, et al. Intact systolic left ventricular function in clinical congestive heart failure. Am J Cardiol 55:1032-36, 1985
2. Morgan JP, Mackinnon R, Briggs M, Gwathney JK. Calcium and cardiac relaxation. In: Diastolic Relaxation of the Heart. Basic Research and Applications for Clinical Cardiology, W Grossman and BH Lorell eds. Martinus Nijhoff, Boston, pp 17-26, 1988
3. Smith VE, Katz AM. Inotropic and lusitropic abnormalities in the genesis of heart failure. Eur Heart J 4 (Suppl A):7-17, 1983
4. Brutsaert DL, Rademackers FS, Suys SU. Triple control of relaxation; implications in cardiac disease. Circulation 64:190-196, 1984
5. Brutsaert DL, Rademakers FE, Sys SU, Gillebert TC, Housman PR. Analysis of relaxation in the evaluation of ventricular function of the heart. Prog Cardiovasc Dis 28:143-163, 1985
6. Lew WY, Rasmussen CM. Influence of nonuniformity on rate of left ventricular pressure fall in the dog. Am J Physiol 256:H222-232, 1989
7. Yellin EL, Nikolic S, Frater RWM. Left ventricular filling dynamics and diastolic function. Prog Cardiovasc Dis 32:247-271, 1990
8. Mirsky I, Pasipoularides A. Clinical assessment of diastolic function. Prog Cardiovasc Dis 32:291-318, 1990
9. Nikolic S, Yellin EL, Tamura K, Tamura T, Frater RWM. Effect of early diastolic loading on myocardial relaxation in the intact canine left ventricle. Circ Res 66:1217-1226, 1990
10. Ishida Y, Meisner JS, Tsujioka K, et al. Left ventricular filling dynamics: influence of left ventricular relaxation and left atrial pressure. Circulation 74:187-196, 1986
11. Louie EK, Edwards-LC. Hypertrophic cardiomyopathy. Prog Cardiovasc Dis 36:275-308, 1994
12. Arrighi JA, Dilsizian V, Perrone-Filardi P, et al. Improvement of the age-related impairment in left ventricular diastolic filling with verapamil in the normal human heart. Circulation 90:213-219, 1994
13. Keren G, Meisner JS, Sherez J, Yellin EL, Laniado S. Interrelationship of mid-diastolic mitral valve motion, pulmonary venous flow, and transmitral flow. Circulation 74:36-44, 1986
14. Little WC, Downes TR. Clinical evaluation of left ventricular diastolic performance. Prog Cardiovasc Dis 32:273-290, 1990
15. Matsuda Y, Toma Y, Ogawa H, et al. Importance of left atrial function in patients with myocardial infarction. Circulation 67:566-571, 1983
16. Rahimtoola SH, Ehsani A, Sinno MZ, et al. Left atrial transport function in myocardial infarction: importance of its booster function. Am J Med 59:686-694, 1975
17. Gilbert JC, Glantz SA. Determinants of left ventricular filling and of the diastolic pressure-volume relation. Circ Res 64:827-852, 1989
18. Lew WYW. Evaluation of left ventricular diastolic function. Circulation 79:1393-1397, 1989

19. Weiss JL, Fredericksen JW, Weisfeldt ML. Hemodynamic determinants of the time course of fall in canine left ventricular pressure. J Clin Invest 58:751-760, 1976
20. Pagel PS, Kampine JP, Schmeling WT, Warltier DC. Alteration of left ventricular diastolic function by desflurane, isoflurane, and halothane in the chronically instrumented dog with autonomic nervous system blockade. Anesthesiology 74:1103-1114, 1991
21. Munoz HR, Marsch SCU, Foëx P. Regional diastolic left ventricular function under inhalation anaesthesia in dogs. Br J Anaesth 74:479P, 1995
22. Pagel PS, Kampine JP, Schmeling WT, Warltier DL. Reversal of volatile anesthetic-induced depression of myocardial contractility by extracellular calcium also enhances left ventricular diastolic function. Anesthesiology 78:141-154,1993
23. Puttick RM, Diedericks J, Sear JW, et al. Effect of graded infusion rates of propofol on regional and global left ventricular function in the dog. Br J Anaesth 69:375-381, 1992
24. Terrar DA, Victory JGG. Effects of halothane on membrane currents associated with contraction in single myocytes isolated from guinea-pig ventricle. Br J Pharmacol 94:500-508, 1988
25. Terrar DA, Victory JGG. Isoflurane depresses membrane currents associated with contraction in myocytes isolated from guinea-pig ventricle. Anesthesiology 69:742-749, 1988
26. Puttick RM, Terrar DA. Effects of propofol and enflurane on action potentials, membrane currents and contraction of guinea-pig isolated ventricular myocytes. Br J Pharmacol 107:559-565, 1992
27. Takahashi H, Terrar DA. Effects of etomidate on whole-cell and single L-type calcium channel currents in guinea-pig isolated ventricular myocytes. Br J Anaesth 73:812-819, 1994
28. Doyle RL, Foëx P, Ryder WA, Jones LA. Effects of halothane on left ventricular relaxation and early diastolic coronary blood flow in the dog. Anesthesiology 70:660-666, 1989
29. Diedericks J, Leone BJ, Foëx P. Regional differences in left ventricular wall motion in the anesthetized dog. Anesthesiology 70:82-89, 1989
30. Sohma A, Foëx P, Ryder WA. Regional distensibility, chamber stiffness, and elastic stiffness constant in halothane and propofol anesthesia. J Cardiothor Vasc Anesth 7:188-194, 1993
31. Marsch SCU, Wanigasekera VA, Ryder WA, Wong LSS, Foëx P. Graded myocardial ischemia is associated with a decrease in diastolic distensibility of remote non-ischemic myocardium in anesthetized dog. J Am Coll Cardiol 22:899-906, 1993
32. Meyer T, Foëx P, Ryder WA. Regional interaction and its effect on patterns of myocardial segmental shortening and lengthening during different models of asynchronous contraction in the dog. Cardiovasc Res 26:476-486, 1992
33. Munoz HR, Evans RD, Marsch SCU, Foëx P. Platelet-activating factor does not affect diastolic function in isolated rat hearts. Cardiovasc Res (1995, in press)

34. Marsch SCU, Dalmas S, Philbin DM, Wanigasekera VA, Ryder WA, Wong LSS, Foëx P. Postischemic diastolic dysfunction. J Cardiothor Vasc Anesth 8:611-617, 1994
35. Dalmas S, Wanigasekera VA, Marsch SCU, Ryder WA, Wong LSS, Foëx P. The influence of preload on post-systolic shortening in ischaemic myocardium. Eur J Anaesthesiology 12:127-133, 1995

VENTRICULAR FUNCTION

David C. Warltier, MD, PhD

The measurement and significance of ventricular contractile function forms the basis for understanding cardiac performance under normal conditions and of abnormalities of the heart that can lead to pump failure. Only recently has the importance of ventricular function in diastole to overall cardiac performance been described. To date, investigations of the influence of anesthetic agents on diastolic function are few.

CELLULAR BASIS OF CARDIAC CONTRACTILE FUNCTION

Cardiac muscle is composed of myocytes in a syncytium of interconnected cells. Although the direction of this interconnecting network of muscle cells is dependent upon transmural depth within the ventricle, there is a general orientation of the muscle cells at any given depth. Collagen fibers surround these cells and form an interstitial architectural framework. The cardiac cells are thus extensively tied to one another and supported by this collagen mesh. Abnormalities of the collagen cytoarchitecture have only recently been recognized as underlying a variety of cardiomyopathies.

The ultrastructure of the myocyte is complex. Around each cell is a plasma membrane or sarcolemma. Intercalated discs form junctions between myocytes and permit electrical, chemical and physical communication between cells. Within each myocyte, there are myofibrils made up of two types of myofilaments (thin and thick) which run in a direction parallel to the long axis of the cell in a regularly repeating unit known as a sarcomere. Analogous to the interconnection of myocytes by the intercalated discs, each sarcomere is interconnected with adjacent sarcomeres by Z lines. The thin filaments are composed of actin and extend from the Z line to cross with thick filaments composed of myosin. Two proteins, troponin and tropomyosin, are bound to actin and during diastole inhibit the crosslinking of actin and myosin. Microscopically, the thin filaments not overlapped with thick filaments form a region known as the I band. The A band consists of the thick myosin filaments and those thin actin filaments that overlap. Changes in the length of the myocyte are directly related

T. H. Stanley and P. L. Bailey (eds.), Anesthesiology and the Cardiovascular Patient, 39–50.

to the degree of interdigitation of the actin and myosin filaments. The myofibrils in each cell are surrounded by an extensive network of intracellular tubules called the sarcoplasmic reticulum which serves as a storage depot for calcium. In addition, invaginations of the sarcolemma also course inward and form a transverse tubular system (T tubules). Thus, the T tubule is a direct extension of the sarcolemma. Finally, there are numerous mitochondria within the myocyte that function to supply the adenosine triphosphate (ATP) required for both contraction and relaxation of cardiac muscle.

Following initiation of the action potential in cardiac muscle, there is a rapid influx of sodium into the myocyte which produces the quick upstroke and overshoot (phase 0) of the action potential. The depolarization sweeps over the entire plasma membrane and down transversely through the T tubule system to the internal milieu of the myocyte. Depolarization of the sarcolemma and T tubule system results in an intracellular influx of calcium across the plasma membrane *via* slow channels during the plateau phase (phase 2) of the action potential. The transsarcolemmal entry of calcium then triggers a further release of calcium from the sarcoplasmic reticulum. This increase in intracellular free calcium concentration (from 10^{-7} to 10^{-5} M) secondary to depolarization initiates the contractile process and is the basis for excitation-contraction coupling. The cytosolic calcium combines with troponin C subunits located on the actin filament, resulting in a conformational change of the tropomyosin molecule and exposure of the binding sites for the myosin and actin filaments. Subsequent binding of actin and myosin (formation of crossbridges) results in a greater overlap of thin and thick filaments. The I band dimension is reduced as the length of the sarcomere is decreased and contraction occurs. The process requires energy obtained from ATP *via* an actomyosin ATPase.

During repolarization, energy-dependent pumping and extrusion of calcium from the cytoplasm into the sarcoplasmic reticulum occurs. In addition, the intracellular calcium concentration is also lowered by transsarcolemmal exchange of extracellular sodium for calcium. This process results in a loss of calcium from troponin binding sites. The troponin-tropomyosin complex in the presence of the reduced cytosolic calcium concentration inhibits the interaction of actin with myosin. As a consequence, relaxation of the myocyte occurs. It is of significance that the relaxation process requires ATP and is not a passive process. Relaxation can be markedly prolonged in the presence of limited supplies of ATP as occurs in ischemia or hypoxia.

THE CARDIAC CYCLE

The left ventricular cardiac cycle initially depicted by Carl J. Wiggers (1) (Figure 1) represents a combination of mechanical, electrical and valvular events in a complex relationship. At a sinus rate of 75 beats per minute, the complete cycle for filling and emptying takes approximately 800 msec. The contractile period of the left ventricle (systole) begins with the initial rise of ventricular pressure and closure of the mitral valve following ventricular depolarization (QRS complex). During systole when left ventricular pressure exceeds that in the aorta, there is an opening of the aortic valve and ejection of blood. Systole ends concomitant with closure of the aortic valve. Closure of the aortic valve also begins the period of diastole during which ventricular relaxation and

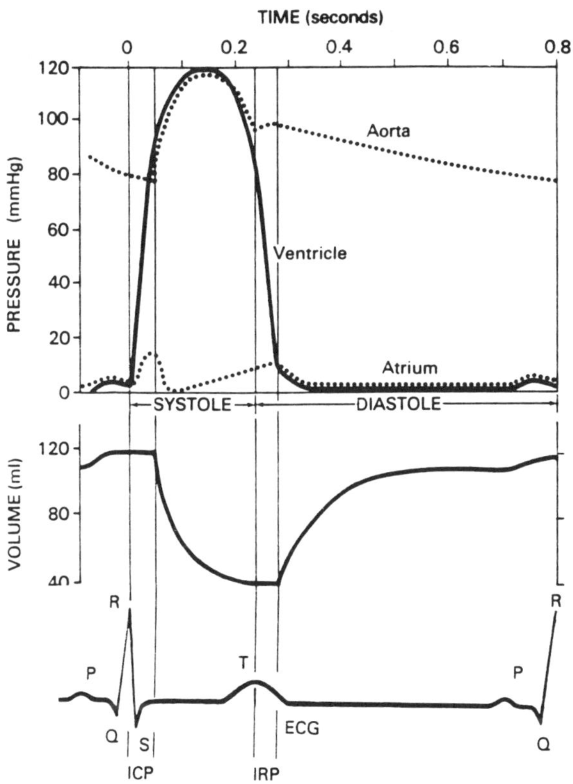

Figure 1. Changes in aortic, left ventricular and atrial pressures, left ventricular volume and electrocardiogram during the cardiac cycle. ICP and IRP = volume and electrocardiogram during the cardiac cycle. ICP and IRP = isovolumic contraction and isovolumic relaxation periods, respectively.

filling occur. During normal sinus rhythm, systole and diastole compose approximately one-third and two-thirds of the cardiac cycle, respectively. At higher rates, significant reductions occur primarily in the time spent in diastole.

Under normal conditions, the atrial pressure waveform is composed of three major deflections (Figure 1). After the P-wave of atrial depolarization recorded electrocardiographically, the atria contract causing an *a* wave which occurs late in diastole. With initiation of systole, ventricular contraction causes a pressure wave to be transmitted in a retrograde fashion through the atrioventricular valve resulting in the atrial *c* wave. In the final portion of systole and continuing into early diastole, as venous blood returns from the periphery, atrial filling proceeds. The atrioventricular valve remains closed, and there is a slow increase in atrial pressure which results in the atrial *v* wave. Under normal conditions, atrial contraction (*a* wave) occurring late in diastole is responsible for approximately 15 to 20% of left ventricular filling. The contribution of the atria to filling may be more significant in disease states having a significantly reduced ventricular compliance.

Ventricular systole is subdivided into a number of components. Isovolumic contraction occurs between closure of the mitral valve and opening of the aortic valve, and little change in ventricular volume occurs during this period. The upstroke of the ventricular pressure waveform is maximal at this time and is often used to estimate the contractility of the ventricle (left ventricular $+dP/dt_{max}$). Unfortunately, $+dP/dt_{max}$ is preload-, afterload-, and heart rate-dependent and as such is, at best, only a poor index of contractility. After isovolumic contraction and opening of the aortic valve, a period of rapid ejection occurs. About two-thirds of the ventricular volume is emptied into the aorta during the period of rapid ejection. This is followed by a slowing of ejection at the end of which aortic pressure exceeds that in the left ventricle and the aortic valve closes. Thus, the changes in ventricular volume that take place are large during the first third of ejection and decrease in an exponential fashion until the end of systole. The normal end diastolic left ventricular volume (EDV) is approximately 120 ml and end systolic volume (ESV) is 40 ml. Therefore, normal stroke volume (ESV) is about 80 ml. Ejection fraction [(EDV-ESV)·100/EDV] is normally approximately 67%.

Ventricular relaxation occurs initially in an isovolumic fashion characterized by a rapid fall in ventricular pressure with a relatively constant ventricular volume. When ventricular pressure falls below that in the atrium, the atrioventricular valve opens and a period of filling occurs. Early in diastole, there is a rapid filling phase during which most of the filling of the left ventricular chamber takes place. This is followed by a slower filling phase known as diastasis. Finally, near the end of diastole, ventricular filling is once again augmented by atrial contraction.

VENTRICULAR PRESSURE-VOLUME RELATIONS

Measurement of the instantaneous change in ventricular volume and pressure forms the basis for analysis of ventricular function by the pressure-volume diagram or loop. If the recorded ventricular pressure and volumes from the Wiggers diagram are plotted simultaneously, a loop results which can be used to display various phases of the cardiac cycle (Figure 2). The changes in pressure versus volume occur in a counter-clockwise fashion over the time course of a single cardiac cycle. Beginning with mitral valve opening, the first phase of the left ventricular pressure-volume diagram demonstrates large increases in volume with minimal changes in pressure. Diastolic filling is primarily through passive means with filling in late diastole augmented by contraction of the atrium. The second phase of the ventricular pressure-volume loop is characterized by an abrupt increase in pressure with minimal change in

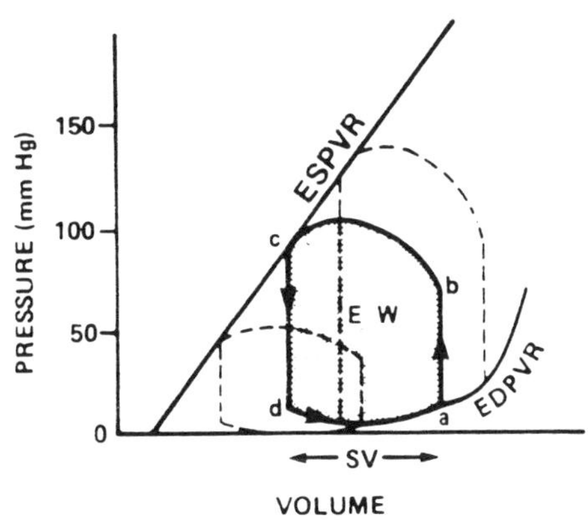

Figure 2. Plot of left ventricular pressure versus volume during the cardiac cycle. The width of a single cardiac cycle = stroke volume (SV). The shaded area of the loop corresponds to stroke work (EW). Arrows indicate the direction of movement through the loop. Phases da, ab, bc, and cd represent left ventricular filling, isovolumic contraction, systolic ejection, and isovolumic relaxation, respectively. Points d and a represent opening and closing of the mitral valve, respectively. Points b and c represent opening and closing of the aortic valve, respectively. Note that a family of loops can be constructed by alterations in afterload and preload (dashed loops) and the end systolic pressure-volume relationship (ESPVR) or end diastolic pressure-volume relationship (EDPVR) determined.

volume (isovolumic contraction). Isovolumic contraction begins with closure of the mitral valve. The third phase of the diagram corresponds to systolic ejection and begins with opening of the aortic valve. Ventricular volume during this phase rapidly declines secondary to ejection into the aorta. Following closure of the aortic valve, the final phase of the loop is characterized by a rapid decline in ventricular pressure with little change in volume (isovolumic relaxation). Isovolumic relaxation ends with the opening of the mitral valve.

Analysis of pressure-volume relationships by such diagrams offers advantages over simple plots of pressure and volume waveforms over time (2). For example, the area within the loop can be determined and is equal to the ventricular stroke work completed in a single cardiac cycle. A series of left ventricular pressure-volume loops can be obtained by transient alterations in preload or afterload and used to estimate the contractile state of the ventricle. Sagawa et al. (3,4) described the end systolic pressure-volume relationship (ESPVR) as linear (Figure 2), and the slope of the ESPVR was suggested to be directly related to inotropic state. Although the ESPVR is probably curvilinear, it has been used to quantify positive inotropic effects. For example, sympathetic stimulation of the heart will shift the ESPVR to a steeper slope. End diastolic pressure-volume relationships in the fully relaxed ventricle can also be determined from loops. Incomplete relaxation from excessive heart rates, myocardial ischemia or hypertrophic states will shift the diastolic pressure-volume relationship in an upward fashion. A family of loops can be constructed by alteration of left ventricular preload to yield the Frank-Starling relationship demonstrating stroke work to be directly related to end diastolic volume (providing a constant heart rate and afterload). The subsequent plot of preload recruitable stroke work (PRSW) versus end diastolic dimension (Figure 3) has recently been advocated as a more sensitive measure of contractility (especially for the study of negative inotropes such as volatile anesthetics) (2,5).

Ventricular pressure-volume diagrams have not only been used in the experimental laboratory but also have recently been constructed for humans using an impedance catheter (to measure instantaneous ventricular volume) positioned within the left ventricle in the cardiac catheterization laboratory. Kass et al (6) has obtained families of such loops through alterations in left ventricular preload and investigated the influence of percutaneous transluminal coronary angioplasty (PTCA) on left ventricular function. Brief coronary artery occlusion decreased the slope of the ESPVR, which quickly returned to preocclusion levels during reperfusion. Monitoring of such loops can be used clinically to assess adequacy of PTCA.

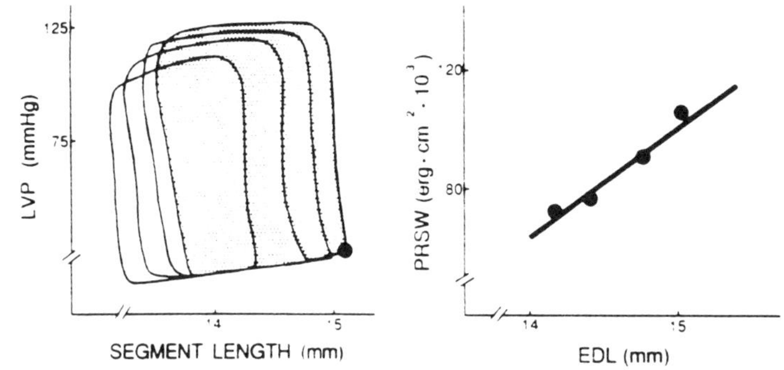

Figure 3. Calculation of the preload recruitable stroke work (PRSW)-end diastolic length (EDL) relationship form left ventricular pressure-dimension (segment length) loops. A family of loops was generated by reduction in left ventricular preload via inferior vena caval constriction. The stroke work (shaded area) of each of four loops versus the end diastolic length (large dot) for that loop is plotted to yield a straight line, the slope and intercept of which are related to myocardial contractility.

LEFT VENTRICULAR PRESSURE-SEGMENT LENGTH LOOPS

The pressure-volume relationship can be extrapolated to a single region within the left ventricle and analogous pressure-segment length relationships determined (2,5,7). Ultrasonic piezoelectric transducers placed within left ventricular subendocardium can be used experimentally to measure changes in the length of a segment of myocardium during the cardiac cycle. The time for ultrasound to be transmitted between a pair of transducers is directly proportional to the length between the transducers. Normally, segment length increases during diastole and shortens during systole analogous to changes in ventricular volume. Abrupt increases in afterload by administration of phenylephrine or decreases in preload by inferior vena caval constriction can be used to generate a series of diagrams for measurement of end systolic pressure-length and PRSW-end diastolic length relationships (5).

Because myocardial ischemia is a regional phenomenon, there may only be small changes reflected in the global ventricular pressure-volume loop whereas the pressure-ischemic segment length loop will be dramatically altered. During acute ischemia, the pressure-length loop is tilted to the right from lengthening of the segment during isovolumic contraction (systolic lengthening) and shortening during isovolumic relaxation (post systolic shortening). Systolic lengthening is secondary to passive stretch on the ischemic segment produced by the normally contracting surrounding myocardium to which it is tethered. Any shortening that occurs after systole in the ischemic segment cannot contribute to overall left ventricular function because it occurs after the end of the ejection period. The pressure-length loop from a moderately ischemic zone can be divided into three regions corresponding to an area of postsystolic shortening, systolic lengthening and the area between each that contributes to ventricular function. Paradoxical aneurysmal bulging of a region during systole is readily observable from the pressure-length diagram, especially during periods of severe ischemia when the loop may become extremely deformed.

ANALYSIS OF LEFT VENTRICULAR DIASTOLIC FUNCTION

Over the last ten years, there has been an increasing awareness of the importance of diastolic function in overall left ventricular performanc (8). For example, a significant number of patients with poor systolic function may be asymptomatic or easily medically managed. In contrast, a significant group of patients with normal ejection fractions have overt signs and symptoms of cardiac failure (9). It is this latter group of patients that may have impairment of ventricular relaxation or reduced ventricular compliance. Abnormalities of diastolic function may be manifested in the absence or preceding significant impairment of systolic function. Schematic pressure-volume diagrams describing hemodynamics in pure systolic versus pure diastolic failure are depicted in Figure 4.

Diastole is a complex sequence of interrelated dynamic processes that remains incompletely understood. The study of left ventricular diastolic function has been seriously hampered in man because of the limited access to ventricular pressure measurements. Recent developments, however, using pulsed Doppler flow velocity measurements across the mitral valve have led to considerable investigation in this area (10). With this technique peak filling velocity during early diastole and during atrial contraction can be measured noninvasively. Presently, a large number of indices (11) determined *via* invasive or noninvasive means have been used to quantify diastolic function in different studies. All indices are dependent upon the phase of diastole in which the measurements are made. These indices have been used to describe active (ventricular relaxation) or passive (viscoelastic properties: chamber and myocardial stiffness) components.

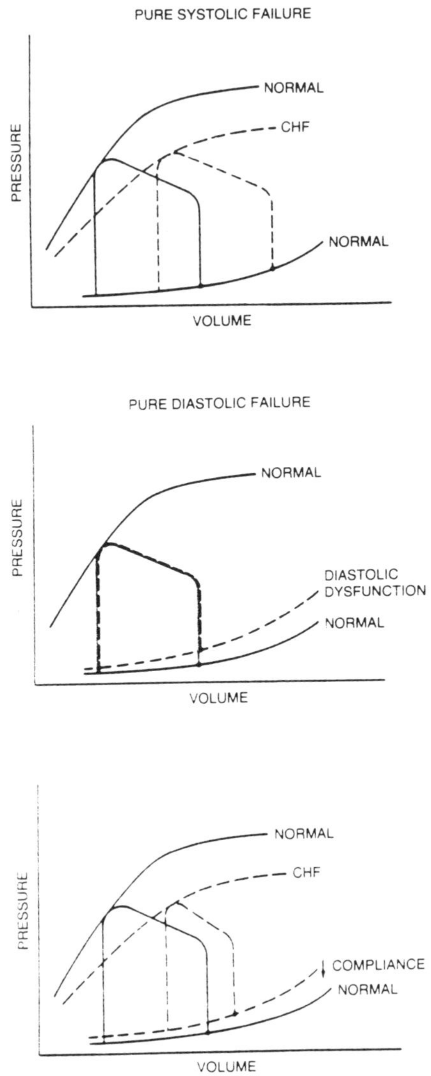

Figure 4. Schematic diagram of left ventricular pressure-volume relationships as derived from loops in pure systolic heart failure (top panel), pure diastolic heart failure (middle panel), and mixed systolic and diastolic failure (lower panel). Note depression of the ESPVR when congestive heart failure (CHF) is due to systolic failure versus maintenance of ESPVR during diastolic dysfunction (characterized by an upward shift of the pressure-volume relationship to diastole). Solid lines represent pressure-volume data from normal hearts and dashed lines represent data from heart in failure.

Diastole is composed of four different phases. Initially, isovolumic relaxation occurs when the aortic valve closes and ends when ventricular pressure falls below atrial pressure and the mitral valve opens. The early rapid filling period begins after opening of the mitral valve. Most of left ventricular filling occurs during this period of time despite the fact that it composes only one-third of diastole. Filling during this time is directly dependent on the left atrial-left ventricular (transmitral) pressure gradient. Pressure and volume curves may diverge in the initial portion of rapid filling such that pressure decreases during expansion of volume. This has been described as a "suction mechanism" which aids in the filling process. The rapid filling phase is followed by a period during which the increases in ventricular volume begin to slow (diastasis). Only a small amount of filling occurs during diastasis, and tachycardia severely limits filling during this period. During the final phase of diastole, atrial systole occurs and further augments ventricular filling. Rapid heart rate causes diastasis to be markedly shortened, but rapid filling and atrial systole remain relatively unchanged as the major components of filling. Ischemia can produce profound alterations in ventricular pressure-dimension relationships in diastole because ATP is required to restore cytosolic calcium levels to 10^{-7} M during relaxation.

Measures of isovolumic relaxation include the maximum rate of left ventricular pressure decline (left ventricular -dP/dt) or -dP/dt at 25 or 50 mmHg and the time constant of pressure decay (tau; τ). The latter is usually derived by plotting the natural logarithm of pressure decline against time. Ventricular filling phases of diastole are most often described by relationships between pressure and volume (or dimension) to provide information regarding chamber and myocardial stiffness characteristics. Many of these indices of diastolic function can only be completed in experimental settings because very accurate measures of volume and pressure that are required.

The ease of filling (compliance) of the left ventricle during diastole can be influenced by a number of factors including the completeness of isovolumic relaxation, coronary vascular turgor, constraint of ventricular enlargement by the pericardium, impingement by the right ventricle *via* the intraventricular septum, or by relative elasticity of the myocardium itself. From a purely mechanical standpoint, ventricular myocardium resists rapid changes in length similar to a nonlinear spring, a property known as viscoelasticity. The higher the filling rate of the left ventricle or the greater the left ventricular volume, the greater the viscoelastic effects on diastolic function. These elastic effects are apparent in the left ventricle during early rapid filling and atrial systole when the rate of filling and subsequent stretch of the myocardium is most rapid. Left ventricular chamber stiffness is defined as the change in pressure for a given change in volume (dP/dV) and is usually measured by indices derived from relationships between minimum left ventricular pressure and the onset of atrial systole. The inverse of chamber stiffness is termed compliance (dV/dP). Myocardial stiffness provides an index of late diastolic function and denotes resistance to stretching (stress) when cardiac muscle is subjected to a strain at end diastole. Alterations in chamber stiffness may cause a change in shape of or shift in the entire diastolic pressure-volume curve.

Myocardial ischemia, hypertrophic cardiomyopathy and left ventricular hypertrophy associated with hypertension have all been described to adversely influence diastolic function of the left ventricle (12). For example, myocardial ischemia may cause transient abnormalities in diastolic function, especially in relaxation and ventricular compliance. Ischemia produces an upward shift of the pressure-volume relationship. At any given volume, higher left ventricular diastolic pressures will occur, and thus, filling can be markedly impaired.

Volatile anesthetics significantly influence left ventricular diastolic function. Halothane, isoflurane and the new anesthetic, desflurane, have been shown to prolong isovolumic relaxation to an equal degree in chronically instrumented dogs. Desflurane and isoflurane produce no effect on regional chamber stiffness or myocardial stress-strain relationships indicating that these agents do not alter ventricular compliance. In contrast, halothane causes an increase in chamber stiffness suggesting that this anesthetic may affect ventricular viscoelastic properties. Whether the effects of volatile anesthetics on diastolic function are exacerbated in disease processes manifesting abnormal baseline diastolic function is currently unknown.

SUMMARY

An understanding of ventricular function is essential for the practicing anesthesiologist. Before an appreciation of the influence of anesthetics on the circulation can be gained, an understanding of the basis for normal hemodynamics is required. The former "passive" period of the cardiac cycle, diastole, is now established as a complex, active process of many separate but interrelated phases. Left ventricular function and interrelationships of volume and pressure during the cardiac cycle are best understood through the pressure-volume diagram. The actions of anesthetics and ischemia can produce alterations in both systole and diastole which are reflected in changes in the shape and dimensions of such diagrams. Finally, analysis of pressure-dimension diagrams provides experimentalists with a rational foundation for investigations of anesthetic agents in the basic research laboratory.

REFERENCES

1. Wiggers CJ: The Henry Jackson Memorial Lecture. Dynamics of ventricular contraction under abnormal conditions. Circulation 5:321-348, 1952
2. Pagel PS, Kampine JP, Schmeling WT, Warltier DC: Effects of nitrous oxide on myocardial contractility as evaluated by the preload recruitable stroke work relationship in chronically instrumented dogs. Anesthesiology 73:1148-1157, 1990
3. Sagawa K, Suga H, Shoukas AA, Bakalar KM: End-systolic pressure/volume ratio: A new index of ventricular contractility. Am J Cardiol 40:748-753, 1977
4. Sagawa K: The ventricular pressure-volume diagram revisited. Circ Res 43:677-687, 1978
5. Pagel PS, Kampine JP, Schmeling WT, Warltier DC: Comparison of end-systolic pressure-length relations and preload recruitable stroke work as indices of myocardial contractility in the conscious and anesthetized, chronically instrumented dog. Anesthesiology 73:278-290, 1990
6. Kass DA, Midei M, Brinker J, Maughan L: Influence of coronary occlusion during PTCA on end-systolic and end-diastolic pressure-volume relations in humans. Ciruclation 81:447-460, 1990
7. Foëx P, Francis CM, Cutfield GR, Leone B: The pressure-length loop. Br J Anaesth 60:65S-71S, 1988
8. Grossman W: Diastolic dysfunction and congestive heart failure. Circulation 81:III-1-III-7, 1990
9. Grossman W, McLaurin LP: Diastolic properties of the left ventricle. Ann Intern Med 84:316-326, 1976
10. Quinones MA: How to assess diastolic function by Doppler echocardiography, Heart Disease Update. Edited by Braunwald E. Philadelphia, WB Saunders, 1991, pp. 351-358
11. Lew WYW: Evaluation of left ventricular diastolic function. Circulation 79:1393-1397, 1989
12. Harizi RC, Bianco JA, Alpert JS: Diastolic function of the heart in clinical cardiology. Arch Intern Med 148:99-109, 1988

MYOCARDIAL ISCHEMIA AND HYPOXEMIA

Pierre Foëx, MD

INTRODUCTION

Silent myocardial ischemia may occur in totally asymptomatic patients, in patients who have suffered myocardial infarction, and in patients with angina (1,2). In all groups of patients with silent myocardial ischemia, the risk of cardiovascular events is increased. Silent ischemia may result from an imbalance between increased oxygen demand and limited supply (demand ischemia) or from an acute reduction in oxygen supply (supply ischemia). Why it is silent is not understood. While it has been suggested that release of β-endorphin may be increased in patients with silent ischemia, this has not been always confirmed (3). However, recent evidence suggests that sympathetic autonomic dysfunction may play a role (4).

Perioperative silent myocardial ischemia is a frequent event in surgical patients with coronary artery disease. Its incidence is highest in those presenting for coronary artery bypass surgery (5) and those undergoing vascular surgery (6). The incidence of preoperative silent ischemia, documented with ambulatory ECG monitoring is between 15 and 90%. Predictors for silent ischemia include a history of previous myocardial infarction, ECG evidence of previous infarction and nonspecific changes (7), as well as hypertension and left ventricular hypertrophy (8). There is also an association between low ejection fraction (less than 40%) and silent ischemia (7).

Recent studies have shown that silent ischemia is more common in poorly controlled hypertensive patients (patients with currently elevated blood pressure) than in normotensive patients, treated hypertensives and untreated hypertensives (9). The higher incidence of silent ischemia in the poorly controlled hypertensive patient is not dependent upon the definition of hypertension as this observation remains true when different definitions are used (10).

It is well documented that silent ischemia is more common (more frequent episodes, longer duration) in the postoperative period than preopera-

T. H. Stanley and P. L. Bailey (eds.), Anesthesiology and the Cardiovascular Patient, 51–60.

tively (11,12). Thus, the postoperative ischemic burden is greater in terms of minutes of ischemia per hour monitored.

SILENT MYOCARDIAL ISCHEMIA AND ADVERSE OUTCOME

Several studies have shown an association between silent myocardial ischemia and postoperative adverse cardiovascular outcome. Raby and colleagues reported that 12 out of 13 major cardiac events occurred in patients with preoperative silent ischemia and only 1 in those without silent ischemia (13). As the group with silent ischemia represented only 20% of the patients studied, the association between silent ischemia and adverse events was striking. Even more impressive is the association between postoperative silent ischemia and adverse outcome. Indeed, in a further study, Raby and colleagues showed that the odds ratio for adverse cardiovascular events rose from 2.7 (preoperative ischemia) to 16 in those patients with postoperative silent ischemia (14). Even more disquieting is the observation by Mangano and colleagues of the longterm effects of postoperative ischemia. Longterm follow-up revealed that over the two years after surgery, mortality was substantially greater in patients with than in patients without postoperative silent ischemia. Longterm adverse outcome was even worse when the patient had suffered myocardial infarction after their operation (15). Whether postoperative silent ischemia is a marker of more severe coronary disease (hence the worse longterm prognosis) or represents a further insult to the myocardium worsening the prognosis is unsettled. Intuitively, both factors may contribute to the longterm adverse outcome and it is tempting to postulate that prevention and/or treatment of perioperative silent ischemia may improve outcome. This hypothesis is supported by the known temporal association between duration of ischemia and cardiac events (16), as well as the temporal association between silent ischemia and adverse outcome (14).

It is well established that cardiovascular complications of anesthesia and surgery occur predominantly during the second, third and fourth postoperative days (17,18). This is also the time at which silent myocardial ischemia is more frequently observed, and episodes of ischemia are of longer duration (5,11).

CAUSES OF POSTOPERATIVE MYOCARDIAL ISCHEMIA

What are the possible causes of the increased incidence of silent ischemia in the postoperative period? At least three major causes should be considered: cardiovascular instability, altered blood coagulation, and hypoxemia.

The association between hemodynamic aberrations such as tachycardia, hypertension, hypotension, left ventricular dilatation and myocardial ischemia is well known (19). It is also well documented that during the postoperative period heart rate is substantially faster than preoperatively (5), and that episodes of silent ischemia are frequently, but not always associated with tachycardia. In the anesthetic setting, Slogoff and Keats (19) showed a clear association between cardiovascular instability and intraoperative ischemia and between silent ischemia and postoperative myocardial infarction. Outside the surgical setting, the extent of the adverse role of an increase in heart rate can be inferred from studies of outcome after myocardial infarction. Heart rates above 120 beats per minute increase mortality after infarction by a factor of 7.5 (20).

After surgery, changes in both coagulation and fibrinolysis are known to occur after surgery. The increase in coagulation factors peaks after 7 to 14 days, while the nadir of fibrinolysis occurs at 1 to 5 days after surgery. Not surprisingly, this is associated with an increased risk of deep venous thrombosis and arterial occlusion. These changes in coagulation may be responsible for postoperative myocardial ischemia and/or infarction. Indeed, it is increasingly recognized that transient occlusion followed by lysis of small clots may be responsible for myocardial ischemia.

Role of Hypoxemia

Another important factor is hypoxemia. The advent of pulse oximetry and computerized data collection has made it possible to obtain a continuous record of arterial oxygen saturation after operation and in patients with sleep disorders. Studies have documented severe episodic desaturation in the early postoperative period associated with significantly decreased mean arterial oxygen saturation. Hypoxemia is most likely to appear during sleep, when external environmental stimulation is minimized, and central or obstructive apnea may occur in susceptible individuals. Not surprisingly, nocturnal hypoxemia occurs frequently in patients recovering from major surgery. Indeed, in the absence of administration of supplementary oxygen, postoperative hypoxemia is very common and the lowest level of hypoxemia is noted during the second night, while episodic hypoxemia is more common during the third night (21). The causes of hypoxemia include sleep apnea, obstructive apnea and respiratory depression caused by opioids. When supplementary oxygen is given according to perceived clinical needs, very low saturations may occur during the night after surgery of the abdominal aorta. However, the most dramatic episodes of desaturation are likely to occur during the third or fourth postoperative nights, as, at that time, supplementary oxygen is unlikely to be given routinely. We reported in 1991 a temporal association between hypoxemia and silent myocardial ischemia in three patients who had undergone surgery of their abdominal aorta (22). In each patient administration of supplementary oxygen corrected their saturation and suppressed the signs of ischemia. In these patients postoperative tachycardia was a persistent phenomenon. This study was extended to 34 patients who had undergone major vascular surgery and revealed the high incidence and considerable severity of postoperative hypoxemia especially during the third and fourth postoperative nights (23). Most patients were receiving supplementary oxygen for the first two nights, but oxygen use was much more variable on the following three nights. Not surprisingly the portion of the night during which saturation was below 90% was highest during the third and fourth rather than first and second night. However, episodes of hypoxemia were still observed until the fifth postoperative night. It is clear that without supplementary oxygen, major abdominal vascular surgical patients are at risk of significant hypoxemia until the fifth night after their operation. Note that the pattern of hypoxemia consisted of periods of relatively stable baseline hypoxemia (between 80 and 90%) lasting for 30 to 90 minutes, alternating with repetitive cyclic desaturations of short (30 to 60 sec) duration.

The pathogenesis of postoperative hypoxemia is unlikely to be uniform. In the early postoperative phase it is likely to be caused by the reduction in FRC consequent to anesthesia and surgery, and the development of atelectasis in dependent lung regions (24). The respiratory depressant effect of anesthesia and opioids contributes to early postoperative hypoxemia. Later, hypoxemia is more likely to relate to persistent reductions in FRC, impaired diaphragmatic function, abdominal distention and additional chest wall splinting due to pain. In our patients, the pattern of periods of relatively stable baseline hypoxemia and repetitive cyclic desaturations of short duration was identical to that reported in patients with sleep apnea. While we did not record the EEG, others have investigated the association between REM sleep and hypoxemia. The highest incidence of hypoxemia may coincide with the rebound of REM sleep or in association with REM sleep; sleep disordered breathing and episodic hypoxemia has been observed during the second and third postoperative nights (25).

The risk of hypoxemia is also a function of the type of surgery. Upper abdominal surgery is associated with a prolonged reduction of respiratory function. Lung volumes are reduced in a restrictive pattern and the decreased functional residual capacity can contribute to hypoxemia and atelectasis. The site of the surgical incision is an important factor as well as the extent of the transection of the abdominal muscles and the severity of the postoperative pain (26).

Not surprisingly, disordered patterns of breathing have also been reported after thoracotomy, resulting in hypoxemia that was either stable and improving hypoxemia, stable and constant, or unstable and deteriorating (27). The development of laparoscopic surgery may reduce the incidence of postoperative hypoxemia. Laparoscopic cholecystectomy, for example, is associated with smaller reductions in vital capacity and forced expiratory volume than conventional cholecystectomy (28).

That nocturnal respiratory disorders and hypoxemia are associated with adverse outcome is strongly suggested by the circadian variation in unexpected postoperative deaths. In a report by Rosenberg and colleagues (29) 13 of 18 unexpected deaths occurred during the night.

Postoperative hypoxemia has been shown to be associated not only with myocardial ischemia and cardiac arrhythmias but also with mental confusion, postoperative delirium and poor wound healing. That postoperative delirium is caused, at least in part by hypoxemia, can be inferred from the efficacy of supplementary oxygen as reported recently by Aakerlund and Rosenberg (30). Hypoxemia may also exert an adverse effect on wound healing and resistance to bacterial infection (31).

The association between nocturnal hypoxemia and cardiovascular accidents is not unique to the perioperative period. There is abundant evidence for an association between disordered breathing and cardiac events. Disordered breathing is common during sleep in patients suffering from coronary artery disease, even in those who do not have associated symptomatic pulmonary disease. The disorder consists of obstructive apnea or Cheyne-Stokes breathing. The episodes of disordered breathing can be as frequent as 20 times per hour and are associated with marked reductions of hemoglobin oxygen saturation (32). In patients with chronic obstructive airways disease, the low basal mean saturation is exacerbated by episodes of more severe hypoxemia. During such episodes, atrial or ventricular ectopy, tachycardia, prolongation of the Q-T interval, and ST segment depression have been reported and are corrected by oxygen therapy (33). In addition to hypoxemia, central or obstructive sleep apnea is associated with modest hypercarbia, systemic hyper- or hypotension and cyclic acceleration and slowing of heart rate. These effects in themselves may precipitate myocardial ischemia in patients with coronary artery disease, and, in the longer term, together with hypoxemia, may accelerate the progression of atherosclerosis. Indeed, sleep apnea has been found to be more severe in male survivors of acute myocardial infarction than in male subjects without evidence of coronary artery disease. Both average and minimum oxyhemoglobin saturation values were lower in patients with acute myocardial infarction. These patients also spent longer periods of time with a saturation below 90% (34). Similarly, a case control study has revealed that snoring is a strong risk factor for acute myocardial infarction (35). At the time of acute myocardial infarction, sleep apnea is common and is particularly prominent in patients with low cardiac index. The episodes of sleep apnea are associated with desaturation in 40% of patients. In these patients cardiac rhythm disturbances are frequently observed confirming the association between hypoxemia and adverse cardiac events (36). In the case of obstructive apnea, cardiac effects include an association between hypoxemia and periodic fluctuations in both heart rate and blood pressure

Ischemia occurs more frequently when episodes of hypoxemia are prolonged and when the desaturation is severe (12). In addition, myocardial ischemia may be facilitated by the changes in blood pressure and heart rate that attend episodes of sleep apnea. Under these circumstances both hemodynamic factors and hypoxemia contribute to the development of myocardial ischemia. While many studies have focused on groups of patients at risk for coronary heart disease, a relationship between hypoxemia and ischemia has also been documented in patients without evidence of coronary artery disease (37).

MANAGEMENT OF PERIOPERATIVE HYPOXEMIA/ISCHEMIA

Because postoperative hypoxemia and associated myocardial ischemia increase the risk of complications of anesthesia and surgery, the question of its prevention is important. It can be argued that better methods of pain relief should minimize the risk of hypoxemia. The epidural route of administration of opioids is popular, effective, and its effects on oxygenation have been studied. Even in patients with normal preoperative saturation, hypoxemia may occur postoperatively at a time patients are receiving opioids intramuscularly or epidurally (38). While epidural opioids usually provide better pain relief, as assessed by pain scores, than parenteral modalities of opioid administration, epidural opioids can be associated with more hypoxemia, particularly when given as continuous infusions (39).

Because the extent of postoperative nocturnal hypoxemia is variable, it would be useful to be able to predict which patients are most at risk for severe desaturation. In this respect the mean overnight saturation is a useful predictor, while the awake saturation is not (21,40).

As cardiovascular complications (myocardial infarction, life-threatening arrhythmias, acute left ventricular failure and cerebrovascular accidents) often occur after episodes of desaturation associated with prolonged episodes of ischemia (16), the role of monitoring saturation and myocardial ischemia during the postoperative period must be considered.

The increasing availability of pulse oximeters and of ECG monitors with ST-segment analysis may offer new avenues for the detection of both arterial hypoxemia and myocardial ischemia. If the risk of complications relates to severity and duration of both hypoxemia and silent ischemia, detection of hypoxemia and ischemia within a short period of their development may be sufficient, as "instantaneous" detection is logistically impossible outside intensive care or telemetry units. If periods of hypoxemia and ischemia of less than 15 minutes are much less likely to cause major cardiovascular events than more prolonged episodes, then monitors with the appropriate alarms could be used on ordinary wards provided protocols were available for the management of hypoxemia and ischemia. Clearly, for hypoxemia, oxygen supplementation can easily be implemented. For ischemia, drug regimes are available with a central role still played by glyceryl trinitrates, and beta-adrenergic blockers (41,42).

The question of prevention of hypoxemia and ischemia is more complex as there is no ideal method of pain relief known to prevent their occurrence. Though it is effective (43) it would be impractical and disruptive to use supplementary oxygen for several nights in all patients. Similarly it would be difficult to justify the use of drugs to minimize the risk of ischemia in all surgical patients. Some groups of patients are more likely to benefit from prevention and monitoring: those with known coronary artery disease; those at high risk for coronary artery disease, especially when they are to undergo and have undergone vascular surgery; and patients with poorly controlled hypertension.

REFERENCES

1. Deanfield JE, Maseri A, Selwyn AP, et al. Myocardial ischaemia during daily life in patients with stable angina: its relation to symptoms and heart rate changes. Lancet ii: 753-758, 1983
2. Fox K, Mulcahy D. Silent ischaemia—to treat or not to treat? Arch Mal Coeur Vaiss 86:41-44, 1993
3. Marchant B, Umachandran V, Wilkinson P, Medbak S, Kopelman PG, Timmis AD. Reexamination of the role of endogenous opiates in silent myocardial ischemia. J Am Coll Cardiol 23:645-651, 1994
4. Shakespeare CF, Katritsis D, Crowther A, Cooper IC, Coltart JD, Webb-Peploe MW. Differences in autonomic nerve function in patients with silent and symptomatic myocardial ischaemia. Br Heart J 71:22-29, 1994
5. Knight AA, Hollenberg M, London MJ, Tubau J, Verrier E, Browner W, Mandano DT. Perioperative myocardial ischemia: importance of the preoperative ischemic pattern. Anesthesiology 68:681-688, 1988

6. Pasternack PF, Grossi EA, Baumann FG, Riles TS, Lamparello PJ, Giangola G, Yu AY, Mintzer R, Imparato AM. The value of silent ischemia monitoring in the prediction of perioperative myocardial infarction in patients undergoing peripheral vascular surgery. J Vasc Surg 10:617-625, 1989
7. Muir AD, Reeder MK, Foëx P, Ormerod OJM, Sear JW, Johnston C. Preoperative silent myocardial ischaemia: Incidence and predictors in a general surgical population. Br J Anaesth 67:373-377, 1991
8. Hollenberg M, Mangano D, Browner W, London M, Tubau J, Tateo I. Predictors of postoperative myocardial ischaemia in patients undergoing noncardiac surgery. JAMA 268:205-209, 1992
9. Hemming AE, Howell S, Sear JW, Foëx P. Admission blood pressure is predictive of silent myocardial ischaemia in treated hypertension. Br J Anaesth 71:760P, 1993
10. Allman KG, Muir A, Howell SJ, Hemming AE, Sear JW, Foëx P. Resistant hypertension and preoperative silent myocardial ischaemia in surgical patients. Br J Anaesth 73:574-578, 1994
11. Mangano DT, Hollenberg M, Fegert G, Meyer ML, London MJ, Tubau JF, Krupski WC. Perioperative myocardial ischemia in patients undergoing noncardiac surgery. I: Incidence and severity during the 4 day perioperative period. The Study of Perioperative Ischemia (SPI) Research Group. J Am Coll Cardiol 17:843-850, 1991
12. Gill NP, Wright B, Reilly CS. Relationship between hypoxaemic and cardiac ischaemic events in the perioperative period. Br J Anaesth 68:471-473, 1992
13. Raby KE, Goldman L, Creager MA, Cook EF, Weisberg MC, Whittemore AD, Selwyn AP. Correlation between preoperative ischemia and major cardiac events after peripheral vascular surgery. N Engl J Med 321:1296-1300, 1989
14. Raby KE, Barry J, Creager MA, Crook F, Weisberg MC, Goldman L. Detection and significance of intraoperative and postoperative myocardial ischemia in peripheral vascular surgery. JAMA 268:222-227, 1992
15. Mangano DT, Browner WS, Hollenberg M, Tateo IM. Long-term cardiac prognosis following noncardiac surgery. JAMA 268:233-239, 1992
16. Landesberg G, Luria MH, Cotev S, Eidelman LA, Anner H, Mosseri M, Schechter D, Assaf J, Erel J, Berlatzky Y. Importance of long-duration postoperative ST-segment depression in cardiac morbidity after vascular surgery. Lancet 341:715-719, 1993
17. Haagensen R, Steen PA. Perioperative myocardial infarction. Br J Anaesth 61:24-37, 1988
18. Metzler H, Mahla E, Rotman B, Rehak P, Potisk S, List WF. Postoperative myocardial ischaemia in patients with recent myocardial infarction. Br J Anaesth 67:317-319, 1991
19. Slogoff S, Keats AS. Does perioperative myocardial ischemia lead to postoperative myocardial infarction? Anesthesiology 62:107-114, 1985
20. Parsons RW, Jamrozik KD, Hobbs MS, Thompson PL. Early identification of patients at low risk of death after myocardial infarction and potentially suitable for early hospital discharge. Br Med J 308:1006-1010, 1994

21. Rosenberg J, Ullstad T, Rasmussen J, Hjorne FP, Poulsen NJ, Goldman MD. Time course of postoperative hypoxaemia. Eur J Surg 160:137-143, 1994
22. Reeder MK, Muir AD, Foëx P, Goldman MD, Loh L, Smart D. Postoperative myocardial ischaemia: temporal association with nocturnal hypoxaemia. Br J Anaesth 67:626-631, 1991
23. Reeder MK, Goldman MD, Loh L, Muir AD, Foëx P, Casey KR, McKenzie PJ. Postoperative hypoxaemia after major abdominal vascular surgery. Br J Anaesth 68:23-26, 1992
24. Hedenstierna G. Gas exchange during anaesthesia. Br J Anaesth 64:507-514, 1990
25. Rosenberg J, Wildschiodtz G, Pedersen MH, von Jessen F, Kehlet H. Late postoperative nocturnal episodic hypoxaemia and associated sleep pattern. Br J Anaesth 72:145-150, 1994
26. Craig DB. Postoperative recovery of respiratory function. Anesth Analg 60:46-52, 1981
27. Entwistle MD, Roe PG, Sapsford DJ, Berrisford RG, Jones JG. Patterns of oxygenation after thoracotomy. Br J Anaesth 67:704-711, 1991
28. Putensen-Himmer G, Putensen C, Lammer H, Lingnau W, Aigner F, Benzer H. Comparison of postoperative respiratory function after laparoscopy or open laparotomy for cholecystectomy. Anesthesiology 77:675-80, 1992
29. Rosenberg J, Pedersen MH, Ramsing T, Kehlet H. Circadian variation in unexpected postoperative death. Br J Surg 79:1300-1302, 1992
30. Aakerlund LP, Rosenberg J. Postoperative delirium: treatment with supplementary oxygen. Br J Anaesth 72:286-290, 1994
31. Rosenberg J Hypoxaemia in the general surgical ward—a potential risk factor? Eur J Surg 160:657-661. 1994
32. De Olazabal JR, Miller MJ, Cook WR, Mithoefer JC. Disordered breathing and hypoxia during sleep in coronary artery disease. Chest 82:548-552, 1982
33. Tirlapur VG, Mir MA. Nocturnal hypoxemia and associated electrocardiographic changes in patients with chronic obstructive airways disease. N Engl J Med 306:125-130, 1982
34. Hung J, Whitford EG, Parsons RW, Hillman DR. Association sleep apnoea with myocardial infarction in men. Lancet 336:262-264, 1990
35. D'Alessandro R, Magelli C, Gamberini G, Bacchelli S, Cristina E, Magnani B, Lugaresi E. Snoring every night as a risk factor for myocardial infarction: a case-control study. Br Med J 300:1557-1558, 1990
36. Saito T, Yoshikawa T, Sakamoto Y, Tanaka K, Inoue T, Ogawa R. Sleep apnoea in patients with acute myocardial infarction. Crit Care Med 19:938-941, 1991
37. Rosenberg J, Rasmussen V, van Jensen F, Ullstad T, Kehlet H. Late postoperative episodic and constant hypoxaemia and associated ECG abnormalities. Br J Anaesth 65:684-691, 1990
38. Wheatley RG, Somerville ID, Sapsford DJ, Jones JG. Postoperative hypoxaemia: comparison of extradural, i.m. and patient-controlled opioid analgesia. Br J Anaesth 64:267-275, 1990

39. Madej TH, Wheatley RG, Jackson JB, Hunter D. Hypoxaemia and pain relief after lower abdominal surgery: comparison of extradural and patient-controlled analgesia. Br J Anaesth 69:554-557, 1992
40. Reeder MK, Goldman MD, Loh L, Muir AD, Casey KR, Lehane JR. Late postoperative nocturnal dips in oxygen saturation in patients undergoing major abdominal vascular surgery. Predictive value of pre-operative overnight pulse oximetry. Anaesthesia 47:110-115, 1992
41. Pepine CJ, Cohn PF, Deedwania PC, Gibson RS, Handberg E, Hill JA, Miller E, Marks RG, Thadani U. Effects of treatment on outcome in mildly symptomatic patients with ischemia during daily life. The Atenolol Silent Ischemia Study (ASIST) Circulation 90:762-768, 1994
42. Wallace A, Layug E, Browner W, Hollenberg M, Jain U, Tateo I, Mangano D and SPI Research Group. Randomized, double blinded, placebo controlled trial of perioperative myocardial ischemia in high risk patients scheduled for noncardiac surgery. Anesthesiology 81:A99, 1994
43. Rosenberg J, Pedersen MH, Gebuhr P, Kehlet H. Effect of oxygen therapy on late postoperative episodic and constant hypoxaemia. Br J Anaesth 68:18-22, 1992

RIGHT VENTRICULAR FUNCTION: IMPORTANCE AND ASSESSMENT

Norbert P. de Bruijn, MD, FACC

RIGHT VENTRICULAR ANATOMY

The right ventricle consists of a muscle mass approximately 15% the size of the left ventricle. It forms a crescent shaped chamber attached to the left ventricle/interventricular septum. The right ventricular chamber anatomically and functionally consists of an inflow portion, the "body," and an outflow tract. Although the left and right ventricles appear as almost separate entities, they are bound together by common, spiraling muscle bundles (1).

The pattern of right ventricular contraction, under normal circumstances, is a peristalsis-like motion, working its way from the inflow portion and the apex toward the outflow tract. Outflow tract contraction is delayed 25-50 ms.

Most of the right ventricular free wall is perfused by the right coronary artery, while a small part of the anterior wall and the anterior portion of the interventricular septum are supplied by the left anterior descending coronary artery. The posterior (or inferior) part of the septum is also perfused by the right coronary artery. The conus artery perfuses the right ventricular outflow tract. The venous drainage system of the right ventricle allows delivery of cardioplegia to the right ventricle, although it has been suggested that it is not very suitable for this purpose. A large conus vein accompanies the conus artery and communicates with the coronary sinus via the small cardiac vein, which is in fact often absent. The main branch draining blood from the right ventricle is the right posterior interventricular vein, which empties directly into the coronary sinus (2).

RIGHT VENTRICULAR PHYSIOLOGY

The left ventricle, due to its heavy muscle mass and ellipsoidal concentric shape, is eminently suited for pumping blood into a high resistance circuit. In

T. H. Stanley and P. L. Bailey (eds.), Anesthesiology and the Cardiovascular Patient, 61–64.

contrast, the right ventricle, which is thinwalled and functions as a bellows, i more suited for volume displacement into the low resistance pulmonary vascu lar circuit. Mean pulmonary artery pressure and pulmonary vascular resistanc are about one sixth of systemic values.

Right ventricular pump function has been difficult to study, in part du to its complex geometry. Also, the right ventricle lacks an isovolumic systoli phase and the end of systole is difficult to define. These complexities contribut to the paucity of data on right ventricular pump function.

The basis of the most useful methods to assess ventricular pump functio has been a quantification of ventricular capacity to generate mechanical energ as a function of initial muscle fiber length. In the intact heart this translates int the assessment of generated stroke volume or pressure as a function of end diastolic volume (or pressure). Morris et al. (3) examined the temporal an quantitative relationships between dynamic right ventricular free wall chor dimension and right ventricular pressure in the working canine heart. Th instantaneous right ventricular pressure-dimension relationship has a shap similar to that of the left ventricle but is more triangular in comparison to th rectangular left ventricular pressure-dimension loop, suggesting that righ ventricular ejection, unlike that of the left ventricle, continues somewha beyond the point of peak ventricular pressure.

Under a variety of circumstances right ventricular contractile perfor mance has been shown to be hemodynamically unimportant in maintainin adequate circulation. In health, contraction of the interventricular septur appears to be sufficient for the development of right ventricular work Cauterization of the right ventricular free wall has been shown to result in n detectable impairment of right ventricular pressure generation or global righ ventricular performance (4). The success of surgical bypass of the right ventricl as in Fontan-type operations also shows that a pumping right ventricle is nc necessary in the face of normal right ventricular afterload. In the presence c abnormal right ventricular afterload, however, right ventricular dysfunctio can lead to hemodynamic instability. An impaired right ventricle may fail i the presence of elevated resistance in the pulmonary circulation and left ver tricular preload will subsequently become inadequate.

Due to their arrangement in series, left ventricular hemodynamics signi icantly influences right ventricular function. Preload and afterload of both ver tricles influence each other. Left ventricular volume and pressure overloa decrease right ventricular compliance. This effect is probably enhanced by th presence of an intact pericardium and has been attributed to geometric rea rangement of the right ventricle and rightward shift of the interventricular septum.

ASSESSMENT OF RIGHT VENTRICULAR FUNCTION

The assessment of left ventricular pump function is well established in the operating room and ICU setting as well as in other less acute settings. Recently, there has been a desire to better assess right ventricular function independently. Part of the reason for this has been that recent studies have emphasized the importance of the right ventricle in ischemic heart disease, congenital heart disease and pulmonary hypertension. Until recently the only satisfactory way to obtain right ventricular volumes and ejection fraction had been by angiography, nuclear and echocardiographic methods, especially biplane contrast ventriculography. None of these methods, with the exception of echocardiography, is practical in the operating room.

In recent years the thermodilution method used for the measurement of cardiac output has been modified to enable the user to estimate right ventricular volumes by the use of a fast response thermistor. The method is based on the conservation of (thermal) energy during a few consecutive systoles: injection of a bolus of cold fluid into the right atrium induces a transient fall in blood temperature. Measurement of the blood temperature by a fast response thermistor allows the recognition of a series of plateaus, along with the rewarming phase of the thermodilution curve, due to the pulsatile ejection of blood from the right ventricle. At any time, the thermal energy content of the right ventricle is a function of the temperature and its volume. The colder blood in the ventricle is diluted by the inflow of warm venous blood. Thus during this rewarming phase, the thermal energy in the ventricle immediately prior to systole, at the end-diastolic volume, is equal to the thermal energy present during the previous systole, at end-systolic volume, plus the thermal energy of the blood flowing into the ventricle at diastole. From this principle end-systolic volume, end-diastolic volume and thus ejection fraction can be derived mathematically.

A number of factors determine the reliability of the RVEF measurement. The optimal position of the rapid response thermistor has been determined to be approximately 2 cm distal to the pulmonic valve (5). Another factor is adequate mixing of the cold fluid bolus with the chamber blood; it has been shown that right atrial injection is the superior method to accomplish this. The effect of the presence of tricuspid regurgitation on the measurement is not quite clear; until recently there seemed to be agreement that regurgitant tricuspid flow invalidated the RVEF measurement. Very recent studies seem to conclude that the inaccuracy introduced by regurgitant flow is acceptable. RVEF measurements also markedly dependent on the respiratory cycle, especially in patient being mechanically ventilated. Lastly, the measurement is unreliable in the fac of clinically significant tachycardia in adult respiratory distress syndrome an atrial fibrillation (6).

RIGHT VENTRICULAR DYSFUNCTION

It appears that right ventricular dysfunction is almost always caused b some degree of pulmonary arterial hypertension. In adult respiratory distres syndrome (ARDS), it has been shown that mortality is increased when complicated by pulmonary arterial hypertension (7). Whether the pulmonary hypertension is due to circulating humoral factors, microembolization of the pulmonary microvascular bed or the effects of alveolar hypoxia, its adverse effec on right ventricular pump function has been well documented.

REFERENCES

1. Dries DJ, Mathru M. The right ventricle: selected issues. In: Righ Ventricle: the Neglected Neighbor of the Left. Dries DJ and Mathru M (eds.). RG Landes, Austin 1994, pp 1-14
2. McAlpine WA. Heart and Coronary Arteries. Springer-Verlag, Berlin 197(pp 190-191
3. Morris JJ III, Pellom GL, Hamm DP et al. Dynamic right ventricula dimension. J Thorac Cardiovasc Surg 91:879-887, 1986
4. Sade RM, Castaneda AR. The dispensable right ventricle. Surgery 77: 62 1975
5. Spinale FG, Smith AC, Carabello BA et al. Right ventricular functio computed by thermodilution and ventriculography. J Thorac Cardiova Surg 99:141-152, 1990
6. Vincent JL, Jankowski S, Friedman G. Thermodilution assessment of rigl ventricular function. In: Right Ventricle: the neglected Neighbor of th Left. Dries DJ and Mathru M (eds.). RG Landes, Austin 1994, pp 75-86
7. Sibbald WJ, Paterson NA, Holliday RL et al. Pulmonary hypertension i sepsis: measurement by the pulmonary arterial diastolic-pulmonary wedg pressure gradient and the influence of passive and active factors. Che 73:583, 1978

PERIOPERATIVE MYOCARDIAL ISCHEMIA AND STROKE—NEW DEVELOPMENTS

Dennis T. Mangano, PhD, MD

INTRODUCTION

Cardiovascular disease continues to be the most significant healthcare risk. In the United States, more than 25% of the population has cardiovascular disease, with one out of every two deaths attributable to cardiovascular disease, and with more than one-third of the healthcare resources appropriated to the diagnosis and treatment of cardiovascular disease. The impact of cardiovascular disease on the surgical patients is substantial, as well. Regarding cardiac surgery, more than 350,000 coronary artery bypass graft procedures are performed annually in the United States, consuming over $10 billion a year in resources, and more than $1 billion for in-house and long-term costs of treating cardiovascular complications following surgery. Regarding noncardiac surgery, of the 25 million patients undergoing such surgery, approximately one-third have coronary artery disease, risk factors, or are over the age of 65 years. Four percent of this entire population, or approximately one million patients, suffer cardiovascular morbidity during the perioperative period, resulting in an overall in-hospital and long-term cost exceeding $22 billion annually in the United States.

Regarding perioperative stroke, approximately 3 to 5% of patients undergoing CABG surgery suffer stroked, with an additional 30% or more suffering in-hospital CNS dysfunction, and 10% suffering moderately-severe long-term CNS dysfunction. In patients undergoing noncardiac surgery, approximately 75,000 suffer CNS adverse outcome. The resulting cost of CNS stroke and dysfunction following cardiac and noncardiac surgery is approximately $6 billion annually, which compares with the $18 billion annually expended on stroke in the ambulatory population.

The problems, therefore, of perioperative myocardial infarction in stroke are challenging, serious, and result in substantial healthcare expenditures, and warrant serious attention.

T. H. Stanley and P. L. Bailey (eds.), Anesthesiology and the Cardiovascular Patient, 65–69.

PERIOPERATIVE MYOCARDIAL INFARCTION

Adverse cardiovascular outcome associated with surgery was recognized as an important healthcare problem in the 1950s to 1960s. Over the ensuing two decades, numerous studies addressed identification of the predictors of such adverse outcome. These studies focused particularly on a limited set of preoperative potential predictors, and identified recent myocardial infarction and ventricular dysfunction as important predictors. As a result, standards of care were developed. The next major advance was the effort associated with the identification of multivariate predictors of outcome, led by Goldman et al. These studies identified a series of predictors, and used composite scores to assess risk.

During the period from 1980 to 1990, attention was redirected from the preoperative to intraoperative identification of predictors. In these regards, the occurrences of changes in hemodynamics and ischemia, as detected by multiple-lead electrocardiography and transesophageal echocardiography, were proven to have benefit in subsets of populations. Finally, beginning in the late 1980s and continuing to the present, it has become recognized that the early postoperative period is perhaps the most important, with early ischemia on emergence from anesthesia being the strongest predictor of both in-hospital and long-term outcome. These studies emphasize, as well, the importance of perioperative morbidity, demonstrating a 15-fold increase in risk in those who suffered myocardial infarction following operation, but survived, over those who did not. Those patients who did suffer infarction had a substantially greater risk of suffering further infarction over the 2-year follow-up, as well as increased risk of unstable angina requiring revascularization, and cardiac death.

Thus, the approach to the problem of perioperative cardiovascular morbidity has been redirected from identification of preoperative predictors, to intraoperative diagnostic testing, and finally to the important postoperative period. With these factors now identified, the challenge is in therapeutic trials to identify approaches to mitigating adverse cardiovascular outcome both in-hospital and long term.

Four classes of therapeutic approaches appear to be the rational directions for future research and development. These are 1) control of hemodynamics; 2) investigation of the present and new anti-ischemic therapies (nitrates, β-blockers, calcium channel blockers, adenosine regulating agents); 3) anti-thrombotics; and 4) stress modulation (α_2 agonists). Each of these areas is under active investigation. It appears that following subset identification, patients will be maintained on a combination of these therapies depending on the preoperative chronic disease state and the anticipated stress types that will be induced perioperatively. The approaches are exciting, for the early trials have demonstrated that both ischemia and infarction are preventable in high-risk patients undergoing surgery, and that therapeutic agents such as adenosine-related agents, α_2 agonists, and other stress modulators can be safely administered to these patients following surgery.

PERIOPERATIVE STROKE AND CNS DYSFUNCTION

As previously noted, it can be estimated that stroke results in a healthcare expenditure of approximately $6 billion annually over the acute phase and 4-year poststroke rehabilitation phase. Thus, given 350,000 CABG patients (of the 500,000 cardiac surgery patients) and a stroke rate of 3 to 5%, the cost of stroke following CABG surgery ranges between $600 million and $1 billion per year in the United States. For the 75,000 patients undergoing valve replacement repair, the stroke rate is 5 to 7%, resulting in an annual cost of $225 to $315 million. Regarding CNS dysfunction following cardiac surgery, it is difficult to estimate costs; however, because of the high incidences of CNS dysfunction, the costs may prove to be substantial as well.

For noncardiac surgery, it is unfortunate that few data are available. From the data available, however, it does appear that the incidence of stroke and dysfunction are much less than for cardiac surgery. Given the large population of patients undergoing noncardiac surgery (25 million in the United States and an equal number in Western Europe, Canada, and Japan), the financial and social impact may be even more impressive than for cardiac surgery. For example, if we assume that of the 25 million patients, the 16 million without major risk factors for cardiovascular disease have a 0% stroke rate incidence, and for the remaining 8 million the incidence is 1%, then approximately 80,000 patients will suffer perioperative stroke following noncardiac surgery, resulting in a cost of nearly $5 billion annually. Regarding CNS dysfunction following noncardiac surgery, few data are available and no estimates can even be approximated at this time.

For cardiac surgery, a number of approaches to the solution of perioperative stroke and CNS dysfunction have been made. These include: *Preoperatively*—Carotid revascularization and *Intraoperatively*—Use of arterial filters and membrane oxygenators, control of acid-base balance and glucose; regulation of blood pressure, use of barbiturates (thiopental) and calcium channel blockers (nifedipine); and, more recently, use of adenosine-regulating agents (acadesine). Clearly, the rationale for some of these techniques, such as use of arterial filters and membrane oxygenators appears to be well-based; however, the number of outcome studies addressing these techniques and therapies is quite limited. For example, the beneficial effect of barbiturates was established in only one study involving valve replacement under special conditions, and refuted in patients undergoing CABG surgery. Similarly, the calcium channel blocker results have not been established in large-scale study. In fact, only one recent study has established that perioperative stroke is preventable. In 634 CABG patients, the use of an adenosine-regulating agent (acadesine) reduced the stroke rate from 4.5% to 0.5%. However, the results of this study, though encouraging, require confirmation. Regarding CNS dysfunction, no large-scale study has been performed.

Thus, therapeutic trials are quite limited; however, based on the acadesine results, it appears that stroke may be preventable, calling for outcome studies using similar agents, as well as other potentially useful agents.

In addition to the potential role of adenosine in cytotoxicity, other promising anti-stroke therapies include glutamate pathway-modulating compounds (NMDA-antagonists, AMPA-antagonists, calcium channel blockers, phospholipid breakdown antagonists), central sympathetic-modulating compounds (α_2 agonists) and other agents (propofol). A substantial amount of research in animals is presently underway, and it is expected that clinical trials involving such agents will be performed over the next 3 to 5 years.

Three million patients in this country have suffered stroke, and an additional 500,000 annually suffer stroke with 150,000 deaths, incurring costs of over $18 billion annually. Thus the problem is substantial, and will continue to be so. Of particular importance is the subset undergoing surgery, affecting nearly 100,000 patients and costing more than $5 billion annually. Clearly, the development of anti-stroke therapy is worthwhile.

Because of the incidence of stroke, scientific proof of the efficacy of such agents mandates large-scale multicenter clinical trials. However, substantial limitations exist regarding clinical trial design in the non-surgical-ambulatory population, given either a prophylactic approach or acute intervention approach to stroke therapy. The patient undergoing surgery represents not only an important patient population because of the costs of stroke in that population, but also because the surgical patient can serve as a model for assessment of stroke therapy. Surgical patients are already in-hospital allowing pre-event and immediate post-event assessment and reasonably predictable stroke rates. Thus, both prophylaxis trials and acute intervention trials can be performed in hospitalized populations. These trials, however, are complicated by the multiple confounders, and, therefore, mandate meticulous attention for successful completion.

In conclusion, because of the aging of our population, and the medical, financial and social impact of stroke and dysfunction, the development of anti-stroke therapy, particularly in the surgical patient, will be a critical area of medical research over the next several decades.

REFERENCES

1. Mangano DT. Perioperative cardiac morbidity. Anesthesiology 72: 153-184, 1990
2. National Center for Health Statistics: Health, United States 1099 DHHS Publication No. (PHS) 89-1232. Public Health Service, Washington, US Government Printing Office, March 1989, pp. 10-17, 66-67, 100-101
3. Frye RL, Higgins, MW, Beller GA, et al. Curry Task Force III: Major demographic and epidemiologic trends affecting adult cardiology. J Am Coll Cardio 12:840-846, 1988
4. Mangano DT, Browner W, Hollenberg M, et al. Association of perioperative myocardial ischemia with cardiac morbidity and mortality in men undergoing noncardiac surgery. N Engl J Med 323:1781-1788, 1990
5. Mangano DT. Multicenter outcome research. J Cardiovasc Anesth 8(Suppl 1):1-3, 1994
6. *McSPI* Research Group Organizational Plan, 1992
7. Mangano DT, Hollenberg M, Fegert G, et al. Perioperative myocardial ischemia in patients undergoing noncardiac surgery. I. Incidence and severity during the four-day perioperative period. J Am Coll Cardiol 17:843-850, 1991
8. Mangano DT, Wong MG, London MJ, et al. Perioperative myocardial ischemia in patients undergoing noncardiac surgery. II. Incidence and severity during the first week following surgery. J Am Coll Cardiol 17:851-857, 1991
9. The *McSPI* Research Group: Effects of acadesine on morbidity and mortality following coronary artery bypass graft surgery. Circulation (in review, 1994)
10. Leung JM, Stanley T 3rd, Mathew J, Curling P, Barash P, Salmenpera M, Reves G, Hollenberg M, Mangano DT, SPI Research Group: An initial multicenter, randomized controlled trial on the safety and efficacy of acadesine in patients undergoing coronary artery bypass graft surgery. Anesth Analg 78:420-434, 1994

STRESS RESPONSES IN NEONATAL AND FETAL CARDIAC SURGERY

Paul R. Hickey, MD

Survey of the neuroanatomical, neurophysiological, and neurochemical development of the nociceptive pathways in the central nervous system of the human fetus and newborn has shown that the structural and functional machinery necessary for the perception of pain and the production of stress responses are present at birth (1). Substantial cardiovascular, humoral, metabolic, and behavioral responses to painful and stressful stimulation have been documented in newborns and infants (1-4). These data contradict traditional beliefs that infants do not possess the physiological machinery to feel pain, that they are somehow "protected" from pain and operative stress by unexplained endogenous mechanisms, or that neonates do not perceive nociceptive stimuli as painful. On a humane basis alone, these data argue that all small children, infants and neonates need control of stress responses and adequate anesthesia and analgesia in the perioperative period. Thus modulation of stress responses is an important goal of pediatric anesthesia and may be of particular importance in the youngest of patients, infants and neonates. In cardiac surgical procedures involving cardiopulmonary bypass where stress responses are known to be increased by as much as an order of magnitude, stress responses in the neonate and fetus can assume a proportionately large and even lethal role.

EFFECTS OF PAIN AND STRESS IN INFANTS

The cardiopulmonary, hormonal, metabolic and behavioral responses of infants and small children to painful stimuli during and after operations have be shown to be deleterious in at least some cases. Increases in heart rate and blood pressure, increases in intracranial pressure, along with high osmotic loads caused by high blood glucose levels which result from stress in the operating room and intensive care unit have been suggested as a cause of intracranial hemorrhage in newborn infants. Deleterious decreases in arterial oxygen satura-

T. H. Stanley and P. L. Bailey (eds.), Anesthesiology and the Cardiovascular Patient, 71–75.

tion and increases serum cortisol levels result even from the stress of minor procedures such as circumcision in the unanesthetized infant (5,6).

Hormonal and metabolic responses after thoracotomy in premature infants have been documented to continue for several days postoperatively (2-4). Responses in beta endorphins, catecholamines, growth hormone, cortisol, glucagon, and insulin all have been documented. These hormonal responses result in changes in oxygen consumption and in alterations in blood glucose, lactate, pyruvate, tissue glycogen levels, and protein metabolism. Particularly during and after major operative procedures, the magnitude of stress responses in neonates and older infants may reach levels considered pathologic, resulting in protein breakdown and negative nitrogen balance, impaired immune responses, hypercoagulable states, and poor tissue perfusion.

Recent evidence from clinical studies suggests that anesthetic techniques directed at reducing stress responses intraoperatively and postoperatively such as high dose narcotic techniques and epidural techniques for procedures in the lower half of the body, can modify stress responses and result in improved hospital morbidity in both adults and children (2-6). These deleterious stress responses, when unmodified by adequate anesthesia, may be associated with postoperative complications or even death in the human neonate (4-6). From the viewpoint of the anesthesiologist trying to preserve normal homeostasis during the perioperative period, anesthesia and stress control for the fetus, neonates, and infants is mandatory, particularly during and after major cardiac procedures when substantial physiological derangements are expected to occur.

ROLE OF STRESS RESPONSES IN MINOR SURGERY

In less extreme cases of relatively minor surgery in the infant and neonate, the importance of modulating stress responses is less certain and few data are available. Certainly studies of circumcision in neonates have shown that substantial stress responses to such "minor" procedures occur, but their significance, other than documented short term behavioral changes, remains unknown (1,7,8). Because the mechanisms by which stress responses affect post-operative morbidity and recovery are poorly understood, it is difficult to detect subtle effects of inadequate protection from stress on the intra- and postoperative clinical course. Whether perioperative control of pain and stress are equally valuable and important factors in morbidity resulting from minor surgical procedures in infants and neonates will require considerable investigation in very large numbers of patients. Nevertheless, both clinical and experimental data clearly show that substantial and clinically significant stress responses result from surgical procedures in infant and even in the fetus and that such stress responses can alter postoperative outcome after uncomplicated anesthesia and surgery.

INFANT STRESS RESPONSES AND POSTOPERATIVE OUTCOME

The concept of anesthetic technique having an impact on postoperative morbidity and mortality in an uncomplicated anesthetic and surgical procedure through modulation of stress response is relatively novel and by no means universally accepted. However it is becoming clear that extremes of stress and pain, in addition to modulating classic humoral and metabolic responses through activation of the sympathetic nervous system, also have effects on the immune system, cytokine production by various cell populations, protein synthesis and wound healing, coagulation, and tissue energy stores. These effects all have been demonstrated in isolated systems and in some clinical studies. All or some of these mechanisms might well mediate effects on mortality and morbidity.

Studies of neonates undergoing cardiac surgery at our institution show that in cases of extreme stress in neonates, morbidity and even hospital mortality may be affected by how well pain and stress are controlled in the perioperative period (4). In these studies, patients randomized to receive deep levels of opiate anesthesia and postoperative analgesia had statistically lower incidence of both morbidity and mortality than those receiving light levels of inhalation with halothane which is known to be ineffective in attenuating stress responses. Prior to the era of high dose narcotic anesthesia, there was some question whether sick neonates and infants could tolerate levels of anesthesia adequate to suppress stress responses (9). However, a number of recent studies have documented the safe use of high dose narcotic anesthesia in neonates, infants and small children (3,4,10,11).

POSTOPERATIVE STRESS

In the postoperative period, stress responses can continue and anesthetic/analgesic techniques designed to minimize postoperative stress response can be important in preventing complications. In infants undergoing major cardiac surgery, critical hemodynamic crises may be triggered by inadequate pain control. High risk infants who have had complex intracardiac repairs and high pulmonary vascular resistance frequently have pulmonary hypertensive crises in the early postoperative period which result in severe systemic hypotension and sometimes sudden death. These are seen most frequently in agitated children and often respond to sedative and analgesic agents which block the stress of tracheal suctioning (11,12). Thus, control of pain and stress in the postoperative period can potentially prevent deleterious hemodynamic crises in addition to their role in attenuating metabolic and hormonal stress responses.

STRESS RESPONSES AND OUTCOME IN FETAL SURGERY

With the coming era of fetal surgery, considerations of pain and stress responses in the human fetus have important potential clinical applications. Despite the lack of universal acceptance of the concept that modulation of stress responses can impact postoperative mortality, even in critically ill neonates undergoing high risk surgical procedures, recent experimental studies published in the fetal surgery literature unequivocally link anesthetic technique and postoperative mortality. These studies support the notion that unmodulated stress responses, even in the fetus, can result in postoperative mortality (13-15). Using total spinal anesthesia and indomethacin to inhibit fetal stress responses and block placental vasoconstriction, surgical procedures and cardiac bypass can be performed at 80% of full gestational age in fetal lambs, with subsequent continuation of the pregnancy to full term and normal delivery. Other anesthetic techniques used in these studies that did not inhibit fetal stress resulted in progressive placental vasoconstriction after cardiac bypass resulting in decreased cardiac output and placental gas exchange. The outcome of this process was progressive increases in arterial pCO_2, decreases in arterial pH, and finally fetal death. Inhibition of stress responses by appropriate anesthetic management in this experimental fetal surgery was critical to postoperative fetal survival (15).

SUMMARY

Stress responses to surgical procedures are important considerations in pediatric anesthesia because even the youngest of premature neonates and the fetus in utero, have been shown to mount substantial classical stress responses to surgical procedures. Appropriate anesthetic techniques in infants and neonates have been shown to modulate these stress responses to both minor and major surgical procedures and have important implications for the anesthetic care of pediatric patients undergoing cardiac surgery. In the case of major cardiac surgical procedures in neonates, postoperative outcome has been demonstrated to be linked to stress responses and can be modified by anesthetic techniques attenuating stress responses. In experimental fetal cardiac surgery procedures, anesthetic techniques inhibiting fetal stress responses are critical in averting postoperative mortality.

REFERENCES

1. Anand KJS and Hickey PR: Pain and its effects in the human fetus and neonate. New Engl J Med 317:1321-1329, 1987
2. Anand KJS, Sippell WG, Aynsley-Green A: Randomized trial of fentanyl anaesthesia in preterm babies undergoing surgery: effects on the stress response. Lancet 1:243-248, 1987
3. Anand KJS, Hansen DD, Hickey PR: Hormonal-metabolic stress responses in neonates undergoing cardiac surgery. Anesthesiology 73:661-670, 1990
4. Anand KJS, Hickey PR: Halothane-morphine vs. high-dose sufentanil anesthesia and postoperative analgesia: stress responses and clinical outcome in neonatal cardiac surgery. New Engl J Med 326:1-9, 1992.
5. Tuman KJ, et al: Effects of epidural anesthesia and analgesia on coagulation and outcome after major vascular surgery. Anesth Analg 73:696-704, 1991.
6. Yeager MP, et al: Epidural anesthesia and analgesia in high-risk surgical patients. Anesthesiology 66:729-736, 1987
7. Maxwell LG, et al: Penile nerve block for circumcision. Obst-Gynecol 70:415-419, 1987.
8. Stang HJ, et al: Local anesthesia for circumcision:stress and cortisol responses. J Am Med Ass 259:1507-1511, 1988.
9. Berry FA and Gregory GA: Do premature infants require anesthesia for surgery? Anesthesiology 67:291-293, 1987
10. Yaster M, Koehler RC, Traystman RJ: Effects of fentanyl on peripheral and cerebral hemodynamics in neonatal lambs. Anesthesiology 66:524-530, 1987
11. Hansen DD & Hickey PR: Anesthesia for hypoplastic left heart syndrome: use of high dose fentanyl in 30 neonates. Anesth Analg 65:127-132, 1986
12. Del Nido PJ, Williams WG, Villamater J, et al: Changes in pericardial surface pressure during pulmonary hypertensive crises after cardiac surgery. Circulation 76:(Suppl III)93 96, 1987
13. Fenton KN, Heinemann MK, Hickey PR, Hanley FL: The stress response during fetal surgery is blocked by total spinal anesthesia. Surg Forum 1992;43:631-4.
14. Fenton KN, Heinemann MK, Hickey PR, et al: Inhibition of the fetal stress response improves cardiac output and gas exchange after fetal cardiac bypass. J Thorac Cardiovasc Surg 1994;107:1416-22.
15. Fenton KN, Zinn HE, Heinemann MK, et al: Long-term survivors of fetal cardiac bypass in lambs. J Thorac Cardiovasc Surg 1994;107:1423-7.

COST CONTAINMENT AND EFFICIENCY IN PERIOPERATIVE CARE

Kenneth J. Tuman, MD

THE MAGNITUDE OF THE PROBLEM

One trillion dollars will be spent in the U.S. on health care during 1996, the result of five consecutive double digit annual increases. Health care costs have risen faster than the Gross Domestic Product (GDP) in all but 3 years since 1960 and at the current growth rate are projected to be 18% of the GNP by the year 2000. Factors affecting the increase in health care expenditures include an increase in population number with a shift in population age and severity of illness, medical inflation in excess of the economy-wide inflation, and advanced (expensive) technological innovation as well as ineffectiveness of current cost-containment measures. In addition, the greatest contributor to the rising costs of health care may be the administration of health care delivery, estimated to be upwards of 30-40% of recent increases in health care costs.

Currently, most decisions on how to conserve medical resources focus on monetary costs and high prices. Unfortunately, looking solely at price can be dangerous and naive, since this may not reflect the value of a service. Despite these limitations, physicians must consider monetary charges in addition to the risks and benefits of the health care rendered. Surveys of managed care plans indicate that outcomes data are important but usually limited or unavailable and that price, patient satisfaction and provider access are currently the measures most critical to their competitive edge. Although consideration of costs is neither unethical nor immoral, this should not be done without losing sight of quality. It is unavoidable that physicians must include economic considerations in their clinical decision making, and when presented with more than one option for patient assessment or therapeutic intervention, their duty is not to choose the more expensive alternative unless there is compelling evidence that it will be of greater benefit.

Anesthesiologists are not and will not be immune to conserving health care dollars. More and more they are confronted with difficult decisions about

T. H. Stanley and P. L. Bailey (eds.), Anesthesiology and the Cardiovascular Patient, 77–98.

which patients are appropriate for outpatient surgical procedures, what pre-anesthetic evaluations are actually required, what anesthetic drugs or techniques are most cost effective, and what advances in (usually high cost) monitoring technology are really necessary to equip their operating rooms. These strategies have become a necessity as cost containment becomes an increasingly pressing goal, especially in the low-cost provider, contracted care scenario. Despite the objections of most to "economic credentialing," physicians with expensive practice patterns are increasingly at risk of losing their privileges in a low-cost provider unit if they are unable to change to more cost-effective practice patterns.

VALUE-BASED ANESTHESIA MANAGEMENT

The relationship between the costs of anesthetic management strategies and perioperative outcomes and efficiency forms the basis to define value-based anesthesia care (1). Implicit in this definition of the appraisal of costs and outcomes is the application of information to determine which anesthetic management paradigms are associated with the best achievable outcome at a reasonable cost, acknowledging that economic resources are limited. Although the relationship between outcome and costs is not a simple one, it is generally accepted that the cost-benefit relationship has a diminishing slope, with additional investment of resources generally resulting in only marginal increments of improvement. The slope of this relationship depends on the efficiency with which anesthesia services are provided. Efficiency can be defined either as operational efficiency or allocative efficiency, both of which are concerned with improving the use of available resources. Operational efficiency addresses the question of how to meet some given objective at the least cost. Allocative efficiency considers the ethical question of maximizing the overall benefit to society, given that resources are limited and that not all desirable objectives can be met. The latter issue is often a central feature of the argument between providing "adequate and acceptable" care and the "best possible" care. Indeed, efficiency ultimately involves an assessment of the costs and benefits of different uses of resources and subsequently defines those potential alternative utilizations of resources known as opportunity costs.

The assessment of the value basis of anesthesia management refers not only to the drugs, devices and medical procedures employed by anesthesiologists involved in the practice of medicine both within and outside of the operating room, but also includes the important role of administrative and organizational support for health care delivery. In the current market where insurers increasingly identify and contract for services with a "provider unit" that gets a single, prospectively determined and often slightly discounted payment covering all costs (and more commonly) professional fees, anesthesiologists are compelled to define the value of their services.

METHODS OF CLINICAL ECONOMIC ANALYSIS

Pre-anesthetic evaluation, intra-operative management and postoperative care are three major areas where the basics of clinical economic analysis can be applied. Although there are currently little data to help the clinician decide on the best way to spend the health care dollar, a few basic analytic techniques can help in the assessment of the clinical economic effects of various testing paradigms, drugs, new technologies, and other services. These include the use of cost-minimization, cost-benefit, cost-effectiveness, or cost-utility analysis and examination of outcome data which are needed to perform these analyses (2). Cost-minimization analysis does not consider indirect costs and is the least useful of these techniques because it assumes that the consequences of each intervention are identical. Such analysis would lead to the distorted conclusion that ketamine and morphine should be used in preference to propofol and fentanyl for outpatient surgery. Traditional cost-benefit analysis uses simple economic values, comparing dollar differences between competing costs with the economic values of benefits. The central feature of cost-benefit analysis is the translation of outcome quantities into dollar values. While this concept is appealing, there are major practical limitations in placing monetary values on theoretic benefits to patients. For example, a healthy patient undergoing a brief surgical procedure probably places less value on avoidance of nausea than a patient undergoing intensive chemotherapy. Cost-effectiveness analysis does the same but tries to relate these dollar amounts to other attributes of health benefits. Effectiveness is not valued in monetary terms, therefore, value judgments must be made by a decision maker, not the cost-effectiveness analyst. Even if interventions are associated with additional costs, they may be preferable if improvement in outcome decreases unit costs. Cost-utility analysis relates economic costs to utility units—for example, dollars spent per quality adjusted years of life (QALY) obtained.

When evaluating these types of economic analyses, direct benefits and costs are the easiest terms to quantitate. We can examine short- or long-term survival or reduction of hospital or overall direct costs as markers of benefit. In contrast, a given technology or health care intervention may have certain indirect benefits which are often difficult to measure. How do we quantitate the avoidance of future morbidity? For example, better coagulation monitoring or the use of drugs such as aprotinin may mean less blood product usage and a lower incidence of hepatitis in the future. Potential reduction of future morbidity and improvement of quality of life are indirect benefits of health care interventions which are rarely evaluated. Indirect costs are just as difficult to measure as indirect benefits. When a monitor or test is used to obtain physiologic data which prompt the performance of multiple additional tests and interventions, how do we figure in these costs? This difficulty is faced when assessing nearly every technology and testing protocol in the current high-tech practice of medicine.

COST-EFFECTIVE PREOPERATIVE PRACTICES

Laboratory testing is a common aspect of both inpatient and outpatient preoperative assessment, as well as postoperative care, especially in the critically ill surgical patient. It is estimated that more than $30-40 billion are spent in North America on preoperative testing and the subsequent follow-up evaluations initiated secondary to that testing. It has also been estimated that over 50% of these costs could be saved by the appropriate ordering of tests in a selective fashion based upon the history or physical exam (3). A number of studies have indicated that non-selective ordering of tests does not result in beneficial changes in perioperative care nor serve as an effective screen for detection of unsuspected disease (3,4). Indiscriminate preoperative testing basically serves as random screening, which has never been shown to be of benefit, in contrast to selective testing (e.g., mammograms for females over the age of 50). Consider the preoperative ECG in this context. Although most clinicians agree that many preoperative tests can be safely eliminated by ordering only those based on specific abnormalities in the history and physical exam, the preoperative ECG continues to be recommended by many "experts" before elective surgery, even in asymptomatic males older than 40 years and females older than 50 years, despite the lack of firm data regarding the utility of routine electrocardiography prior to anesthesia and surgery (5). In the absence of abnormalities based on the history or physical exam, a single resting ECG serves as an insensitive screen of significant coronary artery disease. The insensitivity of the resting ECG as a marker for significant coronary artery disease, coupled with a finite incidence of false positives which occasionally lead to further expensive testing without any change in perioperative risk or management, begs the question of the relative value of such preoperative testing of asymptomatic surgical patients. Firm documentation of significant benefit of routine preoperative ECG testing to patient health is absent. Further, the degree to which the preoperative ECG significantly influences decision making in the perioperative period, as well as the degree to which ECG abnormalities generate additional preoperative testing costs, are currently unknown. A randomized, controlled trial of the safety of a strategy of selective preoperative ECG testing is unlikely to be done in patients older than 50 years of age and sample size considerations indicate that the conduct of such a study in younger patients would be impractical.

The argument that such testing is required for "medical-legal reasons" appears to have questionable basis since there are now several reports which indicate that between 30 and 60% percent of all unexpected abnormalities found on preoperative testing are not noted or pursued (5). Testing which is not indicated by history or physical findings is likely to not only bear additional direct cost, but extra indirect costs in the form of greater liability risks, if abnormalities detected on preoperative screening are not appropriately pursued. In addition, assuming that the results of laboratory results are independent of one another, the more tests ordered the greater likelihood that abnormal results will appear. For example, assuming the specificity of a laboratory test is 97%, if six tests are ordered, there is almost a 20% chance that at least one of the tests will be abnormal. Such abnormalities often generate hidden preoperative costs in addition to the cost of the screening tests themselves. It appears that in general, in the future, less preoperative testing is in order to reduce direct costs, and to potentially improve the efficiency of operating room schedules by eliminating the need to pursue falsely positive or slightly abnormal results which do not affect perioperative management, as well as potentially reduce medical-legal liability. Recent data indicate that there is no greater incidence of abnormalities for many laboratory tests in asymptomatic elderly patients compared to younger ones and suggest that age alone is probably not a good criteria for ordering batteries of laboratory tests (6). Use of a portable computer or video health questionnaire and a preoperative evaluation clinic have been recommended as methods to reduce inefficiency and the cost of inappropriate preoperative assessments and test selection.

Other preoperative practices have been evaluated because of cost and efficiency concerns. Routine preoperative hospital admission of medically stable patients prior to major operations including cardiac, thoracic, joint replacement and major abdominal or urologic procedures has been questioned. The use of "a.m. admission" has probably reduced costs without any demonstrable reported effect on surgical or anesthetic outcome. Other routinely accepted practices are also now being evaluated for cost-effectiveness. For example, the cost-effectiveness of preoperative autologous blood donation has been examined both for total joint replacement as well as cardiac surgery (7,8). Birkmeyer et al. utilized a large number of variables in a decision analysis and determined that the cost of autologous blood donation varied from $40,000 to $1.5 million per QALY (dollars spent per quality adjusted years of life) saved, with the differences between autologous blood collections and transfusion requirements explaining the majority of the variation in cost effectiveness among the types of joint replacements studied (7). The collection of a large number of autologous units with a low transfusion requirement in primary unilateral knee replacement makes autologous blood donation the least cost effective for that procedure ($1.1-1.5 million per QALY). By contrast to other common medical practices, this compares to cost effectiveness (utility) estimates of $6,000/QALY for coronary revascularization to treat three vessel or left main coronary disease and $11,000/QALY to screen for cervical cancer every 4 years (7).

COST CONSIDERATIONS IN THE OPERATING ROOM

Costs of Anesthetic Drugs and Supplies

Anesthesia drug expenses are a small part of the total health care budget. Although the cost for anesthetic drugs is relatively small when considered on a single-case basis, the large number of doses administered contributes to enormous aggregate costs. Lampotang et al. calculated that if U.S. prices are representative, total annual world expenditure on the currently available inhaled anesthetics (excluding nitrous oxide) is roughly $450 million (9). Uniformly reducing fresh gas flows from 5 to 2.5 L/minute would save approximately $225 million yearly worldwide and about $100 million annually in the U.S. Relatively simple measures can have significant impact on cost reduction without markedly impairing styles of clinical practice. Cost saving measures such as this are likely to generate relatively little controversy, are easy to implement, and apply to large numbers of cases. In the future, however, anesthesiologists will likely be faced with choosing between modes of anesthesia care which produce similar acceptable outcomes but at different levels of cost-effectiveness. The decisions involved in making these choices are significantly more complicated, controversial, and emotion-evoking than resolving to conserve resources by reducing fresh gas flows while delivering the same inhaled anesthetics.

When considering the costs of anesthetic drugs, a number of variables must be evaluated when comparing "expensive" drugs to apparently cheaper alternatives (Table 1). The costs of anesthetic drugs include the cost of the drug itself, as well as adjuvant agents; equipment and supplies (e.g., infusion devices

Table 1. Representative costs of anesthesia drugs and monitors.

Direct Costs	Indirect Costs
acquisition of drug or monitor	'rescue' therapy for complications
adjuvant agents or required materials	delay in resumption of normal activities (lost productivity)
drug or material wastage	extended recovery room, ICU or hospital stay
consumable equipment and supplies for drug delivery or application of monitoring	excess operating room or facility turnover time (drug preparation/drug recovery and preparation/initiation of monitors)
monitors and other capital equipment	drug & equipment storage, preparation & set-up, including labor
labor related to insertion and use of PAC, SSEP, TEE, etc.)	maintenance and repair of monitoring and drug delivery monitors (e.g., equipment, including labor
	drug- or monitoring-related complications

PAC, pulmonary artery catheter; SSEP, somatosensory-evoked potentials; TEE, transesophageal echocardiography

or special vaporizers); and the amount of drug wastage that occurs during a typical use. In addition, there may be other indirect costs associated with a given anesthetic drug that are either difficult to quantitate or simply not considered. These include the indirect cost of drug preparation and setup time which may prolong operating room turnover time, as well as the costs of extended recovery room stay or additional drug therapy to treat postoperative side effects.

Careful evaluation of such information about drug costs and alternative therapeutic agents is essential for cost-efficient anesthesia practice. For example, newer induction agents like propofol (which moved into the top 20 hospital pharmacy dollar volume leaders in 1993)(10) may have greater acquisition costs but can potentially save overall hospital costs when used appropriately for outpatient surgery and when patient care protocols allow for less intense and shorter duration nursing care with earlier dismissal of these patients (11,12). Conversely, propofol infusions utilized for long, major operations in patients who require postoperative hospitalization will not provide for earlier ambulation and discharge (13) and may cost significantly more than most inhaled anesthetics. Similarly, considerable savings may be seen with the use of older but effective opioids and muscle relaxants, especially during longer operations. While newer, often shorter duration and more specific acting drugs are often very useful in short to intermediate duration procedures, the benefit of their use may be reduced or eliminated in longer operations, especially in healthy patients. While there is little doubt that the newer and more expensive drugs are often easier to use, there are essentially no data to suggest that most patients would not have an equally satisfactory experience when older, less expensive drugs are titrated to effect based upon an understanding of pharmacokinetics, pharmacodynamics and physiology. There are some data to support the bias of many clinicians that equally prompt awakening can be achieved with a variety of general anesthetics, if they are utilized optimally by experienced clinicians and not compared in a rigid, artificial study protocol (14).

Our specialty must help develop the pharmacoeconomic and pharmacoepidemiologic foundation to define the relative value of new drugs. This will necessitate evaluation not only of efficacy and side effects, but will also involve assessment of parameters such as the time until resumption of normal physical or mental activity as well as other measures of "outcome." Studies evaluating recovery-related productivity losses are important because these losses have the same economic impact on society as direct health care expenditures (15). Prevention of postoperative side effects such as nausea and vomiting with an expensive antiemetic or a given anesthetic drug may cost more than the medical costs of treatment of this problem, but if the economic losses of patients are considered, the preventive approach might be far more economically favorable. It is evident that such analyses are complex and difficult to perform, and that the value of a given intervention will vary among patients in relation to their underlying condition, and the anticipated surgical procedure, as well as the postoperative care requirements.

Even when published studies provide data to evaluate new therapies or interventions, we are often faced with the dilemma of determining relative clinical utility. Statistical power, sample size requirements, and related analytical issues are often confusing and can make it difficult to place study results in proper perspective. What may appear to be a large clinically important difference might not be significant if a study's sample size is small; less meaningful clinical differences may be highly statistically significant if the sample size is large enough. Caution is merited if the clinical differences are reported as a relative change or risk reduction. For example, if intervention 'A' is associated with a 25% actual reduction in the incidence of a complication (e.g., 0.5-0.25) and intervention 'B' is associated with a 1% actual reduction in the incidence of another complication (e.g., 0.02-0.01), both could still be described as producing the same relative improvement (50%) despite a different clinical utility. This has profound importance for the assessment of cost-effectiveness. We might only need to administer a given anesthetic or antiemetic to four patients to prevent one episode of nausea and vomiting (hypothetical intervention 'A') while we might have to use 100 or more costly spinal needles to prevent one case of postdural puncture headache (hypothetical intervention 'B'). Calculation of the number of patients requiring a treatment is an important concept when examining cost differences between clinical alternatives (16).

In the aggregate, cost savings associated with prudent drug selection can be substantial. If only $20 were saved with every anesthetic delivered in the U.S., about $500 million would be saved annually; This represents less than 0.05% of national health care expenditures but is approximately the estimated reduction in anesthesiologists' Medicare reimbursements between 1993 and 1996. Although the costs of anesthetic drugs are important to consider, it should be acknowledged that they usually represent a minor fraction of the costs of a surgical procedure. In addition to drug costs, there is significant potential for cost savings associated with reduction of waste in disposable equipment and materials. Behavior modification programs based upon education of staff about costs and general guidelines for equipment and drug utilization have reported widely variable long-term success (17,18). This success may be enhanced if clinicians are cognizant of the concept of opportunity costs: with limited resources, those utilized for one commodity cannot be used for others which might produce potentially greater benefits. In the prospective payor market, opportunity costs have become an important focus when deciding how to spend limited resources. Nonetheless, cost savings associated with prudent selection of anesthetic drugs and avoidance of material waste, although important, pales by comparison with decreasing operating room time by a few minutes (10 min translates to $100-$150), restricting use of expensive technology to those patients in whom outcome benefits are likely, and modifying some of our current postoperative care practices.

Costs of Monitoring

The costs of monitoring include anesthesiologists' professional fees, the cost of monitors, consumable items, operating room time, maintenance costs, and the costs of complications (Table 1). The cost of capital equipment used for monitoring, assuming a long operational period and a high degree of utilization, generally does not contribute to significant cost on a per case or per hour basis. On the other hand, the costs of consumables as well as the cost of operating time during the placement of invasive monitors can be significant, especially if no other patient-related activity is simultaneously occurring.

The magnitude of problems related to evaluating the use of high cost technology in health care is exemplified by the PAC; nearly one million PACs are sold annually in the U.S. and more than $2 billion are spent on hospital charges for the catheter and introducer sheath, sterile setup, transducers and disposable thermodilution cardiac output supplies, physician charges for insertion of the catheter, and lab charges for mixed venous blood gas tension analyses. Despite the presence of only a few prospective, randomized trials suggesting beneficial outcome effects with use of the PAC to achieve specific therapeutic goals (19, 20), application of this technology is widespread. The largest studies to date which have examined the impact of PAC on outcome after coronary artery bypass graft (CABG) surgery, although not randomized, have been unable to demonstrate any significant effect on morbidity or mortality compared to CVP monitoring (21,22). While the economic issues associated with the routine use of PACs are obviously important, analysis of its use is extremely complex (23).

Superficial analysis would suggest tremendous cost savings if significant numbers of patients with good ventricular function underwent CABG surgery without the routine use of a PAC. In at least two studies, more than 1200 patients (68%) did not receive routine PAC monitoring (21,22), which conservatively translates into more than 3/4-million dollars of direct cost savings in those studies alone. If one-half of the nearly 300,000-400,000 patients undergoing CABG annually in the U.S. did not routinely receive a PAC, this would represent approximately $150 million in direct cost reduction each year. However, the indirect costs of use and, if not used, the indirect costs of failure to provide optimal cardiopulmonary support must be assessed. For example, if invasive monitoring only contributes to delaying the demise of terminally ill patients, it will be associated with enormous increases in direct costs and provide no benefit. On the other hand, if patients who would have died or suffered life-threatening complications can be spared those outcomes because of the precisely titrated care made possible by invasive monitoring, then benefit can be significant. The direct costs of using PACs can be trivial compared with the potential indirect savings. Although the "conservative" approach of selectively using invasive monitors is encouraged in the current medical-economic climate, a small body of knowledge suggests that conservatism may represent a false economy both fiscally and in terms of outcome (19,20). The dilemma is further complicated by Iberti's finding that physicians' (including anesthesiologists') understanding of the use of the PAC is "extremely variable and frighteningly low" (24). Practice parameters which guide physicians to the proper use of such technology may not only improve quality of care but help decrease costs by reducing unnecessary variability and suboptimal application of technology in clinical practice.

Another example of a technology which has undergone widespread use because of the belief that it contributes to better patient outcome is the pulse oximeter. In contrast to the PAC, however, simple amortization of the acquisition and maintenance costs (estimated at $3500 and $500, respectively) of a pulse oximeter with a finger probe reused in a single operating room for 2000 patients over 2 years, yields a cost of approximately $2 per patient. Although the specific cost per case will vary depending upon the purchase price, maintenance costs and utilization rate, the estimated cost per patient of the pulse oximeter is orders of magnitude less than the cost of a PAC. Pulse oximeters are now present in most critical care areas and essentially every operating room in the U.S. Annual world sales of pulse oximeters exceeded $200 million in 1989. Analogous to the predicament of widespread use of the PAC, there are yet no prospective, controlled investigations which have conclusively demonstrated that pulse oximetry itself actually makes a difference in morbidity and mortality. A randomized, multicenter trial of pulse oximetry in Denmark, which involved 20,802 patients divided into two groups, was unable to demonstrate an effect of that monitoring on actual morbidity and mortality, except for a decreased incidence of intraoperative myocardial ischemia (25). For the most serious postoperative complications, anesthesia-related death and myocardial infarction, with incidences of 0.034% and 0.15%, respectively, the sample size requirement to achieve a statistical power of 90% in the latter study would have been more than 1,000,000 and 500,000, respectively. To effectively assess the utility of pulse oximetry, an outcome study would need a sample size many-fold larger than that used in the Danish study, would have to include a significantly greater proportion of patients at risk for adverse outcomes (e.g., ASA status III and IV, age >60 years, etc.), and will probably never be conducted.

In the absence of such outcome studies, the decision to incorporate pulse oximetry as an ASA standard for basic intraoperative (as well as postanesthesia care unit) monitoring has been motivated primarily by evidence that pulse oximetry is superior to clinical judgment in providing an early warning of hypoxic events. Also, retrospective review of anesthetic management associated with adverse events indicates that a large fraction of negative outcomes could be prevented by application of this technology. Cooper et al. demonstrated that significantly fewer patients experienced "recovery room impact events" such as hypotension or arrhythmias after pulse oximetry was introduced into the operating room (26). Another study from the same institution found 11 major anesthesia-related mishaps in an analysis of more than one million anesthetics administered to ASA I and II patients (27). In this study 8 anesthetic-related accidents, involving inadequate ventilation or oxygenation, and 5 deaths occurred during the 9.5 years before routine use of pulse oximetry and only one accident and no deaths occurred during the 3 years since implementation of pulse oximetry. More recently, Cullen et al. provided evidence indicating that pulse oximetry is associated with a reduction in anesthetic-related complications and unanticipated ICU admissions, primarily those related to the need to rule-out-MI (28). Cullen et al. postulated that this may have occurred because pulse oximetry probably allows early identification of hypoxemic, hypotensive or low perfusion states before subsequent ischemic changes become manifest or persist too long. This postulate is consistent with the Danish multicenter study demonstrating that angina or ECG ischemia occur in significantly fewer patients monitored with pulse oximetry than in a control group not monitored with pulse oximetry. Although the marginal cost of additional ICU time was not quantified in the Cullen et al. study, a tremendous cost savings is likely even if we only consider the reduction in the rate of questionable myocardial infarction associated with the use of pulse oximetry.

Another retrospective analysis of the benefits of pulse oximetry by the Closed Claims Project of the Professional Liability Committee of the ASA determined that of 348 "preventable" injuries or deaths, "pulse oximetry. . . would have been efficacious in preventing injury in 138 cases" (29). In contrast, monitors other than pulse oximetry or capnometry (e.g., the PAC or automated BP devices) were considered potentially preventative in only 7% of the preventable injuries or deaths. The findings of the Closed Claims Project as well as the studies conducted at the Harvard hospitals could have considerable economic impact. If use of pulse oximetry is associated with a reduction in preventable injuries or deaths, not only will the indirect cost savings to patients and their families be great (especially in the case of permanently disabling injury), but the direct cost savings will also be substantial. The median total cost of settlement or judgment has been 11 times greater for injuries judged preventable by additional monitoring ($250,000) compared with those judged not preventable ($22,500). This reduction in the cost of adverse outcomes has been recognized by medical liability insurance underwriters and the "liability insurance relativity factor," an industry index of relative risk, decreased from 5.0 to 2.5-3.0 for the specialty of anesthesiology between 1985 and 1990.

While there is still no published cost-benefit analysis of pulse oximetry, the type of data reviewed above are strongly suggestive that pulse oximetry improves the safety and outcome of anesthesia care and is probably cost-effective in this manner. Because of the low incidence of critical events and the presence of confounding factors such as other changes in technology, new drugs and an overall increased awareness of risk management issues with an emphasis on increased vigilance, we will probably never be able to prove that pulse oximetry is an independent factor improving safety and outcome after anesthesia. Nonetheless, the weight of evidence supports the contention that the widespread application of pulse oximetry during anesthesia is associated with fewer cases of serious anesthesia-related morbidity and mortality and subsequently with significant cost savings. In contrast, widespread reduction in liability costs will probably never be attributed to devices such as the PAC; to the contrary, complications associated with the insertion and use of this monitor could increase medical-legal liability costs.

POSTOPERATIVE ANESTHETIC & CRITICAL CARE MANAGEMENT: WHAT ARE THE COST ISSUES?

The problems associated with the rapidly rising costs of delivering anesthesia and intensive care and limited resources to pay for them are interwoven with a third problem: the almost universal lack of reported measures of quality. Despite our convictions that using certain anesthetic techniques, drugs or monitors have improved patient care, there are little objective data to support many of these beliefs. Objective measures of quality in the health care industry have become issues of great economic, as well as medical, significance. Efforts to understand, measure, and improve "quality" of health care not only make it possible to sort out what works in medicine but also are the key to controlling the utilization and, hence, the costs of medical services. Outcomes research will allow development of practice guidelines, which in turn will help produce a leaner, trimmer health care economy (Figure 1).

Assessment of high volume, high cost medical activities such as CABG surgery, for example, must include measures of several distinct aspects of quality: necessity, appropriateness, effectiveness, satisfaction and efficiency. We can measure the impact of anesthesia and critical care of CABG patients on at least three of these characteristics. Most techniques currently employed to anesthetize patients for CABG surgery are "effective" in producing the basic elements of general anesthesia: unconsciousness, muscular relaxation, and attenuation of reflex responses to noxious surgical stimuli. Although choice of anesthetic agent per se has not been demonstrated to critically influence cardiac or noncardiac outcome after CABG surgery, anesthesiologists can anticipate that in the future they will be asked to make decisions about choice of anesthetic based in part upon evaluation of patient satisfaction and the overall efficiency of

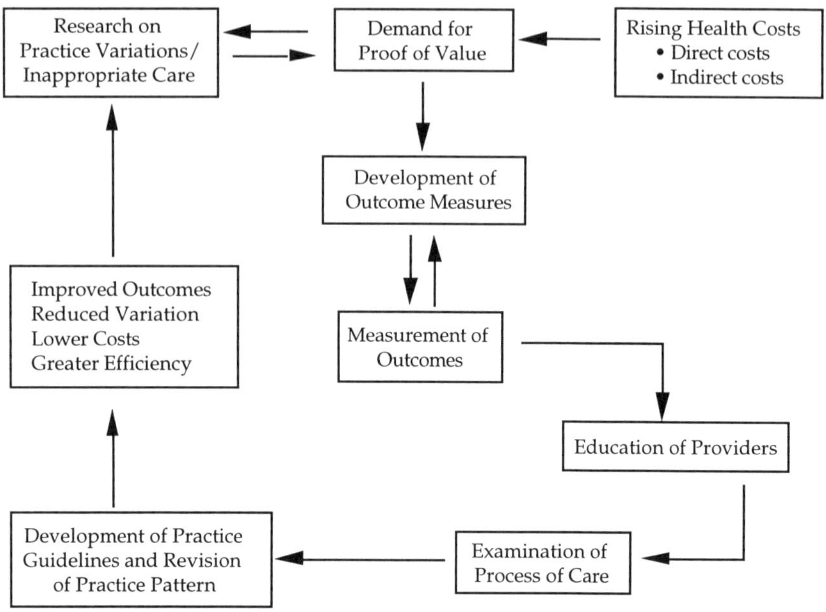

Figure 1. Use of outcome data to improve efficiency and reduce costs.

patient care during and after operations such as CABG. Outcomes research is necessary for successful development of practice guidelines to streamline peri-operative management and make the recovery process as efficient as possible.

Medical managers and efficiency experts are suggesting that we can shorten ICU stays if ventilator time is reduced and extubation is performed within a few hours after CABG surgery in awake, stable patients who have acceptable cardiopulmonary status and minimal chest tube drainage. While potentially reducing ICU costs significantly , this approach is not universally accepted. The issue is further clouded by recent data suggesting that "intensive postoperative analgesia" with an extended period of opioid infusion after CABG may result in much less postoperative myocardial ischemia than routine intermittent opioid administration (30). Until well-conducted studies validate well-defined differences in outcome (incidence of myocardial infarction, heart failure, life-threatening arrhythmias, length of ICU stay, 30-day mortality and total cost), clinicians actually have little data to help them decide on the actual benefits versus the risks of "fast track" protocols compared to conventional management or more prolonged intubation with extended periods of sedation and analgesia after CABG surgery. In the absence of such validation, timing of extubation after CABG surgery still remains an important question and more information is needed to characterize the cost-benefit aspects of early extubation. Without such data, we have little objective basis to evaluate the suggestions of medical efficiency consultants who might suggest that using lower opioid doses or opioids with shorter duration of action may help reduce ventilatory time, ICU stay, and costs for some patients. These types of suggestions are currently being offered by national consulting firms with the intent of reducing overall costs and improving efficiency of recovery after CABG surgery. If no difference in ultimate outcome can be demonstrated among a variety of anesthetic or postoperative sedation techniques, it may be unacceptable to choose an anesthetic technique which results in prolonged ventilatory depression and eliminates the cost savings associated with early patient discharge from an ICU to a "step-down" unit. If similar degrees of intraoperative hemodynamic stability can be achieved with lower as well as higher doses of opioid, administration of large doses of fentanyl may be inefficient from a cost-benefit perspective. In contrast, the use of so-called "balanced anesthesia" with titration of dose-to-effect and the use of short acting drugs, which may have greater acquisition costs, may reduce the likelihood (and overall costs) of prolonged recovery after anesthesia for cardiac surgery (31).

As competition for contracted health care becomes progressively more intense and focused, not only on comparisons of the performance of doctors, hospitals, and other health care providers, but also on overall costs, anesthesiologists will be confronted with the responsibility of defining the impact (if any) of anesthetic management on the efficiency of the operating room and the overall cost of recovery after surgery and anesthesia. It is imperative for our specialty to gain a better understanding of whether certain types of anesthetic techniques (such as postoperative epidural analgesia in high risk patients undergoing major vascular, thoracic or abdominal procedures) can shorten ventilator time, decrease ICU stay or reduce the postoperative morbidity which prolongs hospitalization or otherwise increases both direct and indirect costs. This is not an easy or quick process but such an approach can help develop practice guidelines and protocols, and ultimately reduce costs (Figure 1). In the future, if we do not quantitate indirect cost savings when direct cost analysis indicates that a given alternative to patient care is more expensive than another, the government and third-party payers will likely not fund that alternative unless we can demonstrate an outcome benefit compared to a "cheaper" alternative. Without explicit evidence of benefit, anesthesiologists will be at a competitive disadvantage when attempting to introduce costly new technology in an environment where limited resources must be frugally allocated. Viewed another way, if funds are spent on technology which provides minimal benefit in enhancing patient outcome, those funds are not available to purchase more useful technology. Outcome research should not, however, be vigorously pursued primarily because we feel compelled to provide economic justification for our practices, but because it may lead to improvements in the quality of anesthetic care.

Outside of the operating room, anesthesiologists who practice critical care often contribute to escalating health care expenditures. It is estimated that nearly 1/6 of hospital costs (1/12 of the total U.S. health care budget or greater than 1% of the Gross Domestic Product) are generated in the ICU. ICU patients constitute the minority of all surgical patients but consume almost 1/2 of all surgical resources. Costs in the ICU can be reduced by application of three methods: limiting admissions to the critical care area, diminishing charges generated in the ICU, and hastening discharge. The first method of restricting ICU admissions is difficult to apply since in most cases we are still unable to accurately predict nonsurvivors from survivors upon admission to the ICU, despite the development of many severity of illness scoring systems. Diminishing charges in the ICU is currently an easier endeavor. Selective and not routine ordering of so-called "screening" tests is one means of reducing costs. Deletion of standing orders for some tests can make a large impact on cost reduction. For example, in the patient without cardiopulmonary instability, we should discourage the use of standing orders for arterial blood gas analysis (beginning of nursing shifts, after every ventilator change, etc.). Even though the actual cost of a blood gas analysis in a busy laboratory is about $4, charges may vary from $30 to over $100. If even two less blood gas analyses were ordered postoperatively on each patient after CABG surgery, this could reduce annual expenditures in the U.S. by approximately $30 million (about $3 million in actual costs for just two blood samples per CABG patient). The utility of eliminating "small ticket items" can be great when the cumulative number of these items is large.

Just as we have learned that "routine" preoperative testing is inefficient and wasteful of costly resources, we must avoid the routine ordering of postoperative tests, especially when this behavior results from the perceived need to have test results be part of a potential medical-legal "record" rather than of practical patient value. Similar principles should guide the postoperative use of diagnostic technology such as echocardiography, electroencephalography and pulmonary artery catheterization. Such diagnostic technology should be used only if it might change a diagnostic or treatment strategy. Tests with high sensitivity work best for confirming a suspected diagnosis, and those with high specificity are best for excluding a diagnosis. When two technologies have equal diagnostic accuracy we should consider using the one with the lower cost if patient risks are the same. All of this requires familiarity with the cost, sensitivity, and specificity of the various diagnostic and monitoring technologies which we utilize. Published estimates of sensitivity and specificity must not be trusted blindly, since a given test or monitor may be very sensitive and moderately specific in one hospital but moderately sensitive and very specific in another depending on the patient population and how the test or monitor is used. Implementation of practice guidelines based upon these considerations should help achieve substantial and significant reductions in diagnostic testing of hospitalized patients without any demonstrable adverse effect on quality of care as measured by clinical outcome.

By comparison, the most difficult issue in containing ICU costs is not centered on reducing expenditures on diagnostic testing or monitoring, but involves identification of nonsurvivors as early as possible after ICU entry. This requires a dynamic evaluative process which may take 5 days or 5 weeks, but after it is accomplished, there is tremendous potential for cost containment without any change in outcome. All too often we create a state of prolonged dying in the ICU by ordering more and more tests and performing more and more procedures in attempts to "fix something" without changing the outcome of patients who are destined to be nonsurvivors. Physicians as a group, including anesthesiologists who practice critical care, need to change their perspective from contemplating (with patients, families and colleagues) the termination of life support and discontinuation of life-sustaining therapy to considering termination of dying and accepting death as the natural end to human existence. When nonsurvivors are identified we need to avoid the often senseless but expensive prolongation of dying which currently exists in our ICU's. Inappropriate expectations of medical care currently motivate much of the excessive use of diagnostic and therapeutic modalities, especially in the ICU. The course of action dictated by comparing costs with benefits inevitably involves compromise and in the future we must be prepared to adjust our own expectations as well as those of patients and those who fund health care. This can be accomplished only with the education of patients and their families so that inappropriate expectations of medical care can be changed. When this is accomplished, we will likely enter a new era in patient management: intensive home care which will bring hospital level intervention to patients in their homes or as outpatients. Provision of intravenous nutrition, ventilator support, dialysis and management of heart failure (e.g., chronic infusions of inotropes such as dobutamine) at home with avoidance of long-term hospitalization may allow not only greater patient comfort but also potentially contribute to large cost savings, especially in patients who require prolonged support but have irreversible disease processes.

CONCLUSIONS

Intelligent cost containment measures will require greater selectivity in perioperative testing, drug choices, and monitoring (Table 2). This can be done only when we have data to define and then provide only the necessary amount of testing and monitoring for effective patient care and eliminate excessive use of lab testing and high cost drugs and technology unless there is compelling evidence that these more expensive alternatives will be of greater patient benefit. Outcome research is critical to establish what matters and what really works for our patients. Application of disciplined logic must replace the use of standardized protocols. Practice parameters must be used to make informed medical decisions rather than enforce medical decisions and codify the practice of anesthesia. We must not forget the indirect costs or benefits of certain pharmacologic or monitoring paradigms and we must begin to examine the substantial indirect costs of delay in the resumption of normal activities after anesthesia and surgery. In addition, we will need to improve (both allocative as

Table 2. Approaches to achieve value-based anesthesia management.

- focus on costs, not charges
- consider all costs (direct and indirect) for all clinical alternatives
- identify all potential benefits and risks for all clinical alternatives
- evaluate allocative efficiency as well as operational efficiency
- adopt clinical strategies which eliminate ineffective diagnostic and therapeutic procedures (e.g., apply selective discipline in ordering tests and consultations)
- reduce use of high cost strategies whose advantage over lower cost strategies is debatable
- apply available "cost-effectiveness" data to define value of anesthesia services and clinical strategies
- develop clinician generated practice guidelines with an emphasis on real outcomes
- assume a proactive role in operating room, ICU, and facility management
- eliminate administrative waste
- reduce the risk of malpractice litigation that results in excessive use of tests and prophylaxis

well as operational) efficiency of our medical care: reducing length of stay in the ambulatory care unit after hernia surgery will be just as important as reducing the length of stay after CABG surgery. Eliminating administrative waste and increasing flexibility in the administrative aspects of our medical care will be required. Replacing rigid protocols, such as the requirement of a minimal designated time in a phase one recovery area (with protocols that apply physiologic endpoints for discharge criteria), may be the only way to definitively demonstrate the potential impact of drugs such as propofol on overall costs in the ambulatory surgical environment. Anesthesiologists must learn to apply cost-effectiveness analysis to the management of individual patients whenever possible and pursue more outcome research to answer key questions such as whether or when to order preoperative thallium scans or when to use transesophageal echocardiography or a pulmonary artery catheter.

While we want to avoid the uncritical acceptance of new medical technology, we must also accept the fact that advances in medical care are often not possible without introduction of new technologies before they have undergone widespread, vigorous examination. At issue is not the development of new high cost drugs and technologies, but acknowledgment that such cutting-edge developments should not undergo widespread use until we have guidelines on which patients will benefit from their use. Anesthesiologists must, however, resist the temptation to use new technology based upon anecdotal reports of successful patient management, mishap detection, or avoidance of potential morbidity. Use of larger scale clinical evaluations of new anesthetic drugs or monitors before introduction into general practice is only one method which could reduce the widespread use of new, expensive drugs and technology before utility is demonstrated "in the field." The use of continuous ECG monitoring for perioperative ischemia in high risk surgical patients is one example of a dilemma which we will soon face. Data from small numbers of patients suggest that perioperative ischemia is common and serves as a marker of adverse outcome, particularly after major peripheral vascular surgery. Verification of the association of postoperative ischemia with adverse cardiac outcome in larger numbers of patients is mandated and testing the hypothesis that extended postoperative monitoring and aggressive treatment of ischemia reduces actual morbidity will be required. This will likely necessitate large randomized trials to determine whether such endeavors will be clinically useful and cost-effective.

Even if anesthesiologists or other physicians are able to control costs by selectively using expensive drugs and technologies, they will have to be exceptionally proactive to influence health care facility costs and charges which not only impact the health care delivery system but also affect the economic viability of the institutions in which our specialty is practiced. For example, while eliminating the indiscriminate use of expensive drugs and technology, we must also be actively involved in improving the turnaround time between surgical cases and reducing duration of recovery room stay because these interventions will help control direct costs as well as lessen overhead costs. Such improvements in efficiency with institutional cost savings could subsequently be applied not only to indirectly reduce the charges for some technology with high acquisition costs, but have the secondary benefit of making the health care institution where we practice more competitive in today's medical marketplace. Although the government and insurance companies supply the funds to pay for health care, we still currently make the choices of how that money is spent. These choices will be increasingly more important as cost constraints upon every aspect of health care delivery become more stringently imposed. The time has come for our specialty to control escalating costs while fulfilling our classic responsibility to patients and improving the quality of our care in a fiscally responsible way. In doing so, we will establish and validate a value-based practice of anesthesia.

REFERENCES

1. Orkin FK. Moving toward value-based anesthesia care. J Clin Anesth 5:91-98, 1993
2. Eisenberg JM. Clinical economics: a guide to the economic analysis of clinical practices. JAMA 262:2879-2886, 1989
3. Narr BJ, Hansen TR, Warner MA. Preoperative laboratory testing in healthy Mayo patients: Cost effective elimination of tests and unchanged outcomes. Mayo Clinic Proc 66:155-159, 1991
4. Kaplan EB, Sheiner LB, Boeckmann AJ, et al. The usefulness of preoperative laboratory screening. JAMA 253:3576-81, 1985
5. Roizen MF. Preoperative evaluation. In Miller RD: Anesthesia, pp 743-772, New York: Churchill Livingstone, 1990.
6. Meyer P, Thisted R, Roizen MF, et al. Is age a predictor of preoperative test requirements in asymptomatic patients? Anesthesiology 79:A44, 1993 (abstract)
7. Birkmeyer JD, Goodnough LT, AuBuchon JP, et al. The cost-effectiveness of preoperative autologous blood donation for total hip and knee replacement. Transfusion 33:544-551, 1993
8. Birkmeyer JD, AuBuchon JP, Littenberg B, et al. Cost-effectiveness of preoperative autologous blood donation in CABG. Ann Thorac Surg 57:161-168, 1994
9. Lampotang S, Nyland ME, Gravenstein N. The cost of wasted anesthetic gases. (abstract) Anesth Analg 72:S151, 1991
10. Gwinn B. 1993 drug dollar volume leaders in hospital pharmacies. Hospital Pharmacy 29:340-344, 1994

11. Sung YF, Reiss N, Tillette T. The differential cost of anesthesia and recovery with propofol-nitrous oxide anesthesia versus thiopental sodium-isoflurane-nitrous oxide anesthesia. J Clin Anesth 3:391-394, 1991
12. Marais ML, Maher MW, Wetchler BV et al. Reduced demands on recovery room resources with propofol compared to thiopental-isoflurane. Anesth Review 16:29-39, 1989
13. Doze VA, Shafer A, White PF. Propofol-nitrous oxide versus thiopental-isoflurane-nitrous oxide for general anesthesia. Anesthesiology 69:63-71, 1988
14. Smith CE, Patel N, Sidhu T, et al. Does desflurane affect operating room turnover time in an ambulatory care unit? Anesthesiology 81: A37, 1994 (abstract)
15. Greenberg PE, Stiglin LE, Finkelstein SN, Berndt ER. The economic burden of depression in 1990. J Clin Psychiatry 54:405-418, 1993
16. Davidson RA. Does it work or not?—Clinical vs statistical significance. Chest 106:932-934, 1994
17. Johnstone R, Jozefczyk KG. Costs of anesthetic drugs: Experiences with a cost education trial. Anesth Analg 78:766-771, 1994
18. Weiner S, Carter J. Cost containment in the operating room: The role of physician education. (abstract) Anesthesiology 79:A533, 1993
19. Shoemaker W, Appel PL, Kram HB, et al. Prospective trial of supranormal values of survivors as therapeutic goals in high risk surgical patients. Chest 94:1176-1186, 1988
20. Mimoz O, Rauss A, Rekik N, et al. Pulmonary artery catheterization in critically ill patients: A prospective analysis of outcome changes associated with catheter prompted changes in therapy. Crit Care Med 22:573-579, 1994
21. Bashein G, Johnson PW, Davis KB, Ivey TD. Elective CABG without pulmonary artery catheter monitoring. Anesthesiology 63:451-454, 1985
22. Tuman K, McCarthy RJ, Spiess BD, et al. Effect of pulmonary artery catheterization on outcome in patients undergoing coronary artery surgery. Anesthesiology 70:199-206, 1989
23. Spackman TN. A theoretical evaluation of cost-effectiveness of pulmonary artery catheters in patients undergoing coronary artery surgery. J Cardiothorac Vasc Anesth 8:487-489, 1994
24. Iberti T, Fischer EP, Leibowitz AB, et al. A multicenter study of physicians' knowledge of the pulmonary artery catheter. JAMA 264:2928-2932, 1990
25. Moller JT, Johannessen NW, Espersen K, et al. Randomized evaluation of pulse oximetry in 20,802 patients. Anesthesiology 78:445-453, 1993
26. Cooper J, Cullen DJ, Nemeskal AR, et al. Effects of information feedback and pulse oximetry on the incidence of anesthesia complications. Anesthesiology 67:686-694, 1987
27. Eichhorn JH . Prevention of intraoperative anesthesia accidents and related severe injury through safety monitoring. Anesthesiology 70: 572-577, 1989
28. Cullen DJ, Nemeskal AR, Cooper JB, et al. Effect of pulse oximetry, age, and ASA physical status on the frequency of patients admitted unexpectedly to a postoperative intensive care unit and the severity of their anesthesia-related complications. Anesth Analg 74:181-188, 1992

29. Tinker J, Dull DL, Caplan RA, et al. Role of monitoring devices in prevention of anesthetic mishaps: closed claims analysis. Anesthesiology 71:541-546, 1989
30. Mangano DT, Siliciano D, Hollenberg M, et al. Postoperative myocardial ischemia. Therapeutic trials using intensive analgesia following surgery. The Study of Perioperative Ischemia (SPI) Research Group. Anesthesiology 76:342-353, 1992
31. Cheng D, Karski J, Peniston C, et al. A prospective, randomized controlled study of early versus conventional tracheal extubation following CABG surgery: Postoperative complications with ICU and hospital discharge. (abstract) Anesthesiology 81:A145, 1994

TRANSESOPHAGEAL ECHOCARDIOGRAPHY: JUST ANOTHER EXPENSIVE TOY ?

Norbert P. de Bruijn, MD, FACC

INTRODUCTION

Transesophageal echocardiography (TEE) represents one of the more exciting developments in diagnostic cardiology and hemodynamic monitoring of the last decade. Anesthesiologists in the United States were early to recognize its potential use in the perioperative phase and have been instrumental in its development.

The first attempts to assess the heart through this new "window" were made by Frazin et al., who in 1976 described their experience with a single crystal transducer lowered into the esophagus on a coaxial cable. The device was impractical, but a major advance was made in the early 1980s when a phased-array transducer was mounted on a modified gastroscope. This made TEE a practical, high quality cardiac imaging modality. Another advance which contributed to the widespread use of intraoperative TEE was the development of Doppler color flow imaging in the mid 1980s, which opened a whole new array of diagnostic possibilities. Currently, in our practice, it is difficult to imagine cardiac surgery without the application of TEE.

This brief review will touch upon some of the uses of TEE relevant to the (cardiac) anesthesiologist, and make an effort, in this era of managed care, to put its application into perspective with relation to cost.

PERFORMANCE AND SAFETY OF TEE

There is general agreement that TEE should not be used for routine screening and that it should be used only by specially trained physicians (1). The use of TEE by anesthesiologists is generally, but not always, restricted to the use in the operating room and the intensive care unit.

T. H. Stanley and P. L. Bailey (eds.), Anesthesiology and the Cardiovascular Patient, 99–102.

Whether or not antibiotic prophylaxis against bacterial endocarditis should be administered, is usually not an issue in the operating room, because most patients are treated with one or more antibiotics. The question may be of interest in certain cases where TEE is applied in the intensive care setting. Recent evidence suggests that bacteremia rarely occurs during TEE (2); however, in our institution, we generally administered appropriate antibiotic prophylaxis if the risk for endocarditis is present.

When TEE is employed by anesthesiologists who are not well versed in its use for diagnostic purposes, a risk is that a complete examination will not be performed, and that significant cardiac pathology may be overlooked. It is recommended that a complete examination be performed before focusing on the reason for which the study was indicated.

In experienced hands, TEE has been proven to be quite safe. Daniel and coworkers (3) analyzed 10,419 cases in a European multicenter study and found the incidence of unsuccessful probe insertion to be 1.9%. In addition, 0.9% of patients could not tolerate TEE examinations after the probe had been successfully inserted. The mortality rate was 0.01% (one patient died whose esophagus was perforated after TEE insertion due to infiltration of the esophagus by a malignant lung tumor).

Relative contraindications to TEE are the presence of a Zenker's diverticulum, esophageal tumors or stenoses, esophageal perforation and esophageal varices.

INDICATIONS

The main indications for the use of TEE in the operating room are surgery for primary and ischemic valvular disease, surgery for congenital cardiac anomalies and surgery for type I aortic dissections. In addition, there are some evolving indications in which the use of TEE is probably useful but not of proven benefit. The most important of these are its use in cardiac and lung transplantation, and the use of either TEE or pericardial echocardiography for the detection of atheromatous disease in the ascending aorta prior to cannulating the aorta in the hope of preventing plaque rupture and cerebral embolization of atheromatous material.

Other potential indications include are its use in patients with cardiac or extracardiac tumors and to detect sources of embolism in patients with TIAs or CVAs. All patients coming to the operating room with a history of bacteremia should be screened for endocarditis.

TEE can be quite useful as a monitor of ventricular contractility and filling, as well as assist in the detection of regional wall motion abnormalities and myocardial ischemia.

In the intensive setting, TEE is frequently useful in patients with injuries or surgical incisions which limit the application of transthoracic transducers. Important indications include unexplained hypotension or hemodynamic instability, suspicion of endocarditis or aortic disease, disease of native or prosthetic valves, possible tamponade, right-to-left shunting in patients with unexplained hypoxemia and detection of a cardiac source of embolization.

HOW EFFECTIVE IS THE USE OF TEE INTRAOPERATIVELY ?

There is an ongoing discussion in the literature about the effectiveness of TEE in the operating room.

There is at this moment in time little doubt about its use in valve surgery (4). The literature consistently documents that in 8 to 10% of patients undergoing valve surgery (or congenital cardiac surgery) TEE is instrumental in diagnosing a major event which changes the course of surgery and significantly influences patient outcome. Sheikh et al. found that of 123 patients whose valve function was judged to be adequate after cardiopulmonary bypass, 15% had a major postoperative complication and 5% died. In contrast, of 7 patients with moderate residual valve dysfunction, 86% had a major postoperative complication and 43% died. In another prospective study of 246 patients with ischemic mitral regurgitation, the same group found that residual mitral regurgitation at the completion of surgery was a more important predictor of survival than patient age or left ventricular ejection fraction.

In a prospective study of 1000 patients by the Duke pediatric cardiac anesthesia group, length of hospital stay increased 10-fold when surgical outcome was judged unsatisfactory by TEE in the operating room.

There is still a difference of opinion among various authors about the effectiveness of "monitoring" with TEE in the operating room. While several groups have supported its use (5,6) others have questioned its value (7). In our practice we employ TEE solely for monitoring purposes only in very high risk surgical candidates. Capitated care raises considerable concern about the cost-effectiveness of TEE. While there is not much valid data available, it is not difficult to come up with reasonable estimates. In our practice and presuming that TEE is only justified in patients undergoing valve surgery, of which we perform approximately 300 cases a year, the average cost per patient is about $350 (based on 5 year depreciation of the system plus two upgrades, maintenance contracts for echocardiograph and omniplane probe, and administrative expenses). Assuming a considerably longer ICU/hospital stay for patients with major complications, as well as the possibility for reoperation within a short period of time, and using cost numbers available from our pediatric population, we estimate that the additional cost for a major complication is about $125,000. With a major complication rate of 10% for valve surgery, the cost of such complications would be $ 3,750,000 per year. The total additional cost for TEE performed in all valve surgery patients is $105,000, and results in a considerable financial savings. This analysis does not take into account the use of TEE in high risk coronary and other surgical procedures, or its use in the ICU, which would result in at least some significant diagnoses that would reduce costs. Also, not included in this analysis is the cost in terms of patient suffering and mortality or the cost to society in lost working days.

In conclusion, we feel that perioperative transesophageal echocardiography, in spite of its high cost in the form of equipment and training of manpower, results in a major contribution to optimal patient care, not only from an isolated academic standpoint, but also in terms of medical economics.

REFERENCES

1. Pearlman AS, Gardin JM, Freeman WK, et al. Guidelines for physician training in transesophageal echocardiography: recommendations of the American Society of Echocardiography Committee for Physician Training in Echocardiography. J Am Soc Echocardiogr 5:187-94, 1992
2. Nikutta P, Mantey-Stiers F, Becht I, et al. Risk of bacteremia induced by transesophageal echocardiography: analysis of 100 consecutive procedures. J Am Soc Echocardiogr 5:168-72, 1992
3. Daniel WG, Erbel R, Kasper W, et al. Safety of transesophageal echocardiography: a multicenter survey of 10,419 examinations. Circulation 83:817-21, 1991
4. Sheikh KH, de Bruijn NP, Rankin JS, et al. The utility of transesophageal echocardiography and Doppler color flow imaging in patients undergoing cardiac valve surgery. J Am Coll Cardiol 15:363-72, 1990
5. Smith JS, Cahalan MK, Benefiel DJ, et al. Intraoperative detection of myocardial ischemia in high-risk patients: electrocardiography versus two-dimensional transesophageal echocardiography. Circulation 72:1015-21, 1985
6. Gewertz BL, Kremser PC, Zarins CK et al. Transesophageal monitoring of myocardial ischemia during vascular surgery. J Vasc Surg 5:607-13, 1987
7. Eisenberg MJ, London MJ, Leung JM, et al. Monitoring of myocardial ischemia during non-cardiac surgery: a technology assessment of transesophageal echocardiography and 12-lead electrocardiography. JAMA 268:210-16, 1992

PITFALLS IN PULMONARY ARTERY CATHETER DATA INTERPRETATION

Kenneth J. Tuman, MD

MISINTERPRETATION PULMONARY ARTERY CATHETER OF PRESSURE MEASUREMENTS

Estimation of left-sided vascular pressures via catheterization of the right heart requires a static uninterrupted column of blood to be present from the tip of the PA catheter (PAC) to the aortic valve. At the end of diastole, there is no net flow in this common chamber, and if the pulmonary vascular bed distal to the PAC tip is patent, no pressure gradients should exist and the pulmonary wedge pressure (WP) should approximate the mean pulmonary venous (PVP), left atrial (LAP) and left ventricular end diastolic pressures (LVEDP) (Figure 1). Alterations in intrathoracic pressure may markedly affect measurement of the pulmonary wedge pressure. Accurate reflection of pressures in the left side of the heart by the PAC depends upon its placement in a West zone III (PAP and

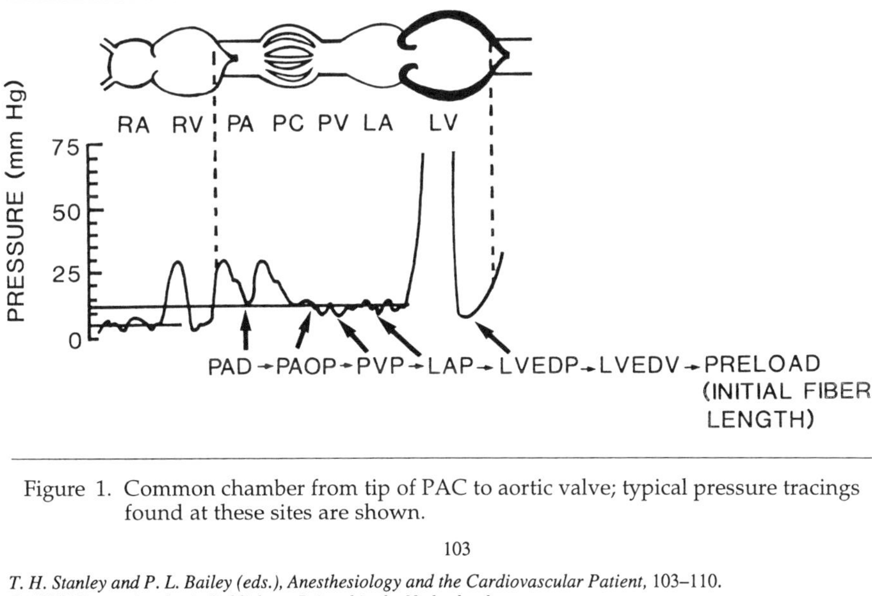

Figure 1. Common chamber from tip of PAC to aortic valve; typical pressure tracings found at these sites are shown.

T. H. Stanley and P. L. Bailey (eds.), Anesthesiology and the Cardiovascular Patient, 103–110.

PVP both exceed alveolar pressure), so that the pulmonary capillaries remain open and allow a patent conduit between the tip of the PAC and the left atrium (LA). If the tip of the PAC is in zone I or zone II, the WP reflects airway pressure rather than mean LAP (Figure 2). Correct zone III placement requires a phasic

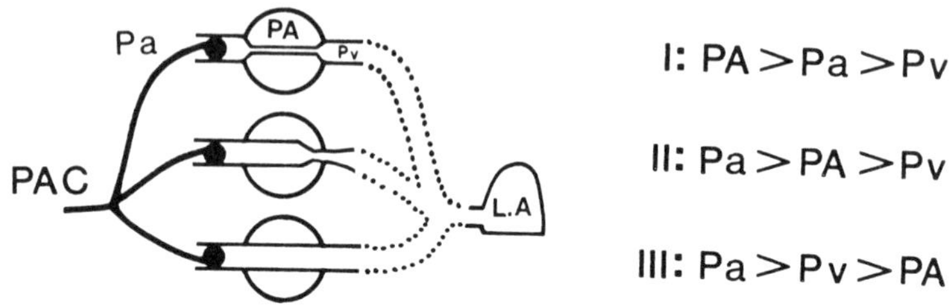

Figure 2. Effect of PAC position on measurement of PAOP in three zones of the lung.

WP tracing with A and V waves which convert to a pulmonary arterial trace with balloon deflation and reappear with inflation. Blood should be easy to aspirate from the distal port of the PAC to exclude lodgment in a vessel without adequate blood flow and the mean WP should be less than the mean PAP (unless large V-waves are present). Finally, in the wedge position arterialized blood can be aspirated, or an increase in mixed venous O_2 saturation to systemic arterial levels or above can be seen if using an oximetric pulmonary artery catheter. However, incomplete arterialization of a wedge position sample may occur if the tip of the PAC is in a low ventilation-perfusion segment of the lung despite being in zone III.

Patients breathing spontaneously without CPAP may change from zone III to zone II during the expiratory phase of ventilation if airway obstruction or bronchospasm causes airway pressure to become markedly positive, whereas mechanically ventilated patients without PEEP may change zone III during exhalation to zone II during inspiration. Because intrathoracic and intrapericardial pressure is closest to atmospheric pressure at the end of exhalation, regardless of the mode of ventilation, intravascular pressures should be measured at this point to minimize the influence of intrathoracic pressure swings. Most time-based electronic sampling of pressure data is nonselective and incorporates respiratory artifact on a digital readout.

Transmural pressure the difference between the pressure inside and that around the blood vessel and must be differentiated from the commonly measured intraluminal pressure usually recorded during clinical care. Increases in mean intrathoracic pressure are generally reflected as increases in intrapericardial pressure and may decrease the effective transmural pressure if the increase in vascular intraluminal pressure is less than the increase in surrounding pleural pressure. When this occurs, intraluminal pressure no longer reflects true filling pressure and this is commonly seen when an increased right atrial pressure (RAP) and WP occur with diminished venous return to the heart during PEEP therapy or with pericardial tamponade. Extravascular pressure may be approximated by measuring intrapleural pressure directly or with an esophageal balloon, although neither method is widely applied clinically. Many formulas have been developed to estimate the effect of PEEP on WP measurement, but these are minimally useful because of wide interpatient variability in pulmonary compliance and the effects of PEEP. Clinical evaluation is more important than absolute intravascular WP in assessing preload in patients when PEEP is applied.

In addition to positive pressure ventilation, PEEP, increased intrathoracic pressure and a non-zone III PAC tip, other conditions result in discrepancies between the WP and LVEDP. When heart rate is increased sufficiently, the LA contracts against a partially closed mitral valve and a small gradient exists between the WP and the LVEDP. The WP may also exceed LVEDP if increases of pulmonary vascular resistance occur, because there may be a functional discontinuity in the common chamber between the PAC tip and the LA at the level of the pulmonary veins. Increases in resistance of the pulmonary venous system to blood flow may cause the WP to exceed the LAP and may occur as a result of sepsis, pulmonary venous occlusive disease, and other conditions.

Obstruction to pulmonary venous drainage may cause WP (and PVP) to exceed LVEDP. Mitral valve obstruction by stenosis, an artificial valve or a LA mass (clot or myxoma) may cause both the LAP and WP to exceed LVEDP. If the pulmonary veins are compressed by a mediastinal neoplastic or fibrotic process, or pulmonary vein thrombosis occurs, PVP and WP will exceed LAP and LVEDP. Compression of the pulmonary venous system may also occur in low-flow states or secondary to increased intrathoracic pressure.

Clinical conditions producing large V-waves in the WP trace also create problems in data interpretation (Figure 3). When V-waves are present in the WP trace, the pressure preceding the large V-wave (after the "a" wave) is a close approximation of LVEDP, and use of the electronic digital mean WP will markedly overestimate LVEDP when a large V-wave is present. Although large

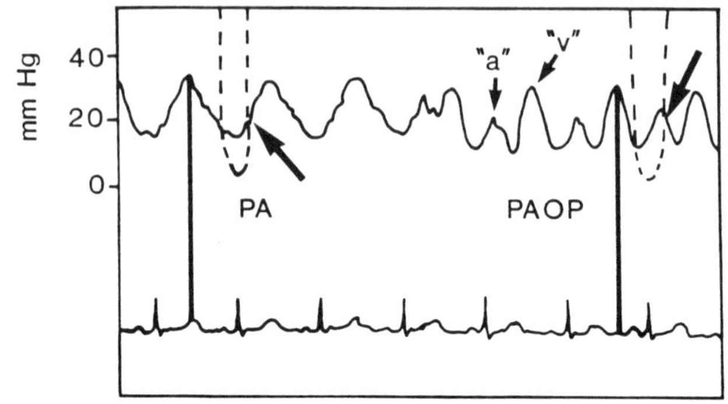

Figure 3. Relationship between electrocardiographic and pulmonary artery (occlusion pressure waveform events. Dashed lines represent LV pressure waveform.

V-waves are typically associated with mitral regurgitation, they also occur with mitral stenosis when there is poor LA compliance, when there is pulmonary venous volume overload as in acute L-to-R shunting, or whenever LA/pulmonary vein compliance decreases with increased WP (such as during myocardial ischemia associated with increased preload).

In contrast to conditions that increase WP relative to LVEDP (Table 1), the WP may underestimate the baseline LVEDP in patients with markedly reduced pulmonary vascular beds, such as after pneumonectomy or significant pulmonary thromboembolism because inflation of the PAC balloon may occlude so much cross-sectional area of the remaining vascular bed that the venous return to the left side of the heart is reduced during the measurement period. Although a noncompliant LA will cause overestimation of the LVEDP when using mean WP, a noncompliant LV may cause the opposite type of discrepancy unless the WP is recorded just after the peak of atrial contraction designated by the A-wave (near the junction of the A and C waves). The discrepancy is largest when the LV is noncompliant, the heart is in slow sinus rhythm, and there is no associated valvular heart disease. In addition, when acute aortic insufficiency exists, regurgitant flow into the LV during diastole causes premature closure of the mitral valve with LAP and WP underestimating the elevated LVEDP.

Although the WP may accurately reflect LVEDP, LAP and PVP, it may be misinterpreted as the hydrostatic pressure determining the rate of fluid filtration from the pulmonary capillaries into the interstitium and air spaces of the lung. However, the WP (or PAOP, pulmonary artery occlusion pressure) is an

Table 1. Conditions Resulting in Discrepancy Between PAOP and LVEDP.

Mean PAOP > LVEDP	
	Positive-pressure ventilation
	PEEP
	Increased intrathoracic pressure
	Non-zone III PAC placement
	Chronic obstructive lung disease
	Tachycardia
	Increased pulmonary vascular resistance
	Mitral valve obstruction (stenosis, myxoma, clot)
	Pulmonary venous compression (tumor, fibrosis)
	Mitral regurgitation
	Left-to-right intracardiac shunt
Mean PAOP < LVEDP	
	Noncompliant left ventricle
	Reduced pulmonary arterial tree (pneumonectomy, pulmonary embolus)

indicator of LAP, not pulmonary capillary pressure (PCP). For blood to flow forward through the lungs, PCP must be higher than WP. Under normal conditions, the vascular gradient across the pulmonary circulation is so small that the WP is very close to PCP. However, when PVR increases, and the majority of the increase in PVR is occurring in the post-capillary vascular bed, then PCP may be much greater than WP. Thus, the WP may underestimate PCP whenever levels of exogenous or endogenous pulmonary vasoconstrictors such as catecholamines, histamine, serotonin or prostaglandins are increased. A method has been described that uses the PAP profile after balloon occlusion of the large pulmonary vessels (precapillary resistance) changing to a slower decline as blood spreads through the cross sectional area of the pulmonary capillaries to the pulmonary veins and the LA (post-capillary resistance). However, respiratory artifact makes it very difficult to estimate PCP with certainty in most critically ill patients.

Although a variety of pathophysiological conditions and ventilatory maneuvers can upset the balance between WP and LVEDP measurements, as well as between intravascular and transmural pressures, even when the WP accurately reflects the LVEDP, there may not be direct correlation of the latter pressure with end-diastolic fiber length which is a more direct measure of preload (the distending force or stretch of the fibers of the LV at end-diastole).

Normally, the relationship between end-diastolic pressure (EDP) and end-diastolic volume (EDV) of the LV is curvilinear. Two variables, ventricular distensibility (compliance) and the transmural distending pressure (LVEDP minus juxtacardiac pressure) determine the EDV (preload). Changes in compliance may result from moving along a single diastolic pressure-volume (P-V) curve or from changes of the inherent stiffness properties of the myocardium, represented by a shift of the P-V curve to the left (lower compliance) or to the right (higher compliance). Thus, an elevated LVEDP or WP may reflect high volume and preload for a ventricle with normal or increased compliance or a low EDV and preload in a ventricle with decreased compliance. An increase in LVEDP may indicate an increase in preload or may reflect a change in the modulus of chamber stiffness with decreased compliance and no change in preload. These phenomena have been shown in both animals and humans to produce significant discrepancies between the WP and LVEDV. Several studies have demonstrated that changes in WP after cardiac surgery do not necessarily correlate with simultaneous changes in LV diastolic cavity size in the same direction. Because the usual Frank-Starling relation is not valid when myocardial compliance changes, the WP may not be an accurate monitor of LV performance. Clinical assessment of patient response to therapy is essential to optimize treatment because the effects of volume infusion, vasodilating agents, ventilatory changes and disease states on LV preload are not entirely predictable when WP alone is measured. However, the net effect can usually be surmised from resultant changes in the measured stroke volume.

PITFALLS IN DETERMINATION OF STROKE VOLUME

The ability to rapidly obtain accurate measurements of cardiac output (CO) in critically ill patients is one of the principle benefits of the PAC. The thermodilution (TD) method is the most widely used means of measuring CO and relies upon the Stewart-Hamilton equation, incorporating the area under the TD curve obtained by plotting the decline in pulmonary artery temperature versus time. A large number of important practical considerations must be satisfied for the appropriate application of the TD method. Thermal stability is a basic requirement for accurate estimation of CO when using either room temperature or cold injectate. Rapid intravenous administration of cold fluids can create large errors in TD-CO measurements unless these determinations are delayed for at least 30 seconds after stopping the rapid volume infusion. In addition, temperature "afterdrop," which can occur after separation from cardiopulmonary bypass with a period of rapid rewarming, can also create significant errors in TD-CO, which may not be recognized unless careful observation is made for baseline temperature stability during and after TD injection.

PITFALLS IN INTERPRETATION OF SYSTEMIC VASCULAR RESISTANCE

The physiologic parameter known as systemic vascular resistance (SVR) is commonly calculated from the relationship: SVR = [MAP-RAP] x 79.9/CO dyne·s·cm^{-5}. The logical basis for this expression arises by analogy from Poiseuille's law for fluid flow within rigid pipes, which states that flow is proportional to the difference between the upstream and downstream pressures. Although CO, stroke volume (SV) and stroke work (SW) are usually indexed to body size, it is not yet common practice to do so for SVR. Because the peripheral arterial tree branches in parallel and is proportional to body size, larger individuals have lower resistance (more vessels in parallel) than smaller individuals although the vascular tone is similarly matched to the CO in individuals with the same MAP, RAP and CO. In addition, most clinicians use RAP as the downstream pressure in SVR calculations, even though there may be a "vascular waterfall" or a critical venous closing pressure producing a venular pressure 22 to 30 mm Hg above RAP. When the RAP is much less than the effective downstream pressure, the simplistic assumption of the equation listed above produces inaccurate estimations of arterial resistance and obscures the assessment of changes of that resistance at different pressures. Because there is no convenient way for clinicians to estimate the effective downstream pressure except under special conditions, the comparison of SVR at widely different pressures should be made with caution.

SUMMARY

If careful attention is paid to the mechanics of pressure measurements, the PAC reliably and reproducibly measures intraluminal vascular pressures. However, considerable clinical judgment is necessary to extrapolate these pressure measurements to estimate preload and to recognize the many artifacts that may negate the relationship between WP, LVEDP and LVEDV. The clinician must also be wary of the pitfalls of interpretation of calculated hemodynamic indices. With careful attention to the above details, the PAC can provide the clinician with extremely useful measures of cardiovascular performance. However, unless clinicians give due consideration to the technical and physiological factors that affect interpretation of PAC data, it will be extremely difficult to demonstrate improved outcome with the use of the PAC even if defined therapeutic hemodynamic regimens can be established. The purpose of this review was to disseminate knowledge of those pitfalls which can prevent such successful application of the PAC.

REFERENCES

1. Tuman KJ, Carroll GC, Ivankovich AD. Pitfalls in interpretation of pulmonary artery catheter data. J Cardiothorac Anesth 3:625-641, 1989
2. Iberti TJ, Fischer EP, Leibowitz AB, et al. A multicenter study of physician's knowledge of the pulmonary artery catheter. JAMA 264:2928-2932, 1990
3. Bazaral M, Petre J, Novoa R. Errors in thermodilution cardiac output measurements caused by rapid pulmonary artery temperature decreases after cardiopulmonary bypass. Anesthesiology 77:31-37, 1992
4. Raper R, Sibbald W. Misled by the wedge? Chest 89:427-434, 1986.
5. Sharkey SW. Beyond the wedge: Clinical physiology and the Swan-Ganz catheter. Am J Medicine 83:111-122,1987

THE INTERACTION OF COAGULATION AND INFLAMMATION

Bruce D. Spiess, MD

INTRODUCTION

Coagulation function has often been viewed by clinicians as a protein mediated process cascading from one reaction to the next with an eventual outcome of solid clot. This view has been fostered by medical school teaching that has focused upon the coagulation cascades. The effects of platelet numbers and platelet function may be less well understood and monitored. The complexity of coagulation and its many nuances can be daunting.

All too often, a work-up for a coagulopathy consists of several screening tests for the intrinsic cascade (activated partial thromboplastin time—aPTT), the extrinsic cascade (partial thromboplastin time—PT) and a platelet count. Is it any wonder that these few tests have little predictive value for perioperative hemorrhage, particularly in cardiopulmonary bypass? (1)

A different way to conceptualize coagulation may be more appropriate. Coagulation occurs at the interface of blood and endothelium. Blood is actively maintained in a liquid state (2-4). This is accomplished by endothelial cells, neutrophils and circulating plasma protein inhibitors (antithrombin III and 2 antitrypsin). Endothelial cells are coated with proteoglycan that forms a non-wettable or replant surface for plasma proteins. Hepar in is incorporated into the proteoglycan and it can interact with circulating antithrombin III. Endothelial cells mediate vascular tone by synthesis of nitric oxide. Nitric oxide (endothelial relaxant factor—EDRF) is not only a vasodilator, but also a potent localized platelet inhibitor and neutrophil inhibitor (6). Prostaglandins produced by the endothelial cells inhibit platelet aggregation. Also, the endothelial cells possess the protein S, C thrombomodulin system which acts as a potent antithrombin (4). When endothelial damage occurs, a very localized reaction occurs that may lead to eventual thrombus formation.

The entire coagulation process should be viewed as a four-step sinusoidal wave (Figure 1) (5). Endothelial cell dysfunction or tissue damage exposes or decreases the barrier of anticoagulation. Sub-endothelial collagen may be exposed and/or von Willebrand's factor is released from nearby endothelial

T. H. Stanley and P. L. Bailey (eds.), Anesthesiology and the Cardiovascular Patient, 111–121.

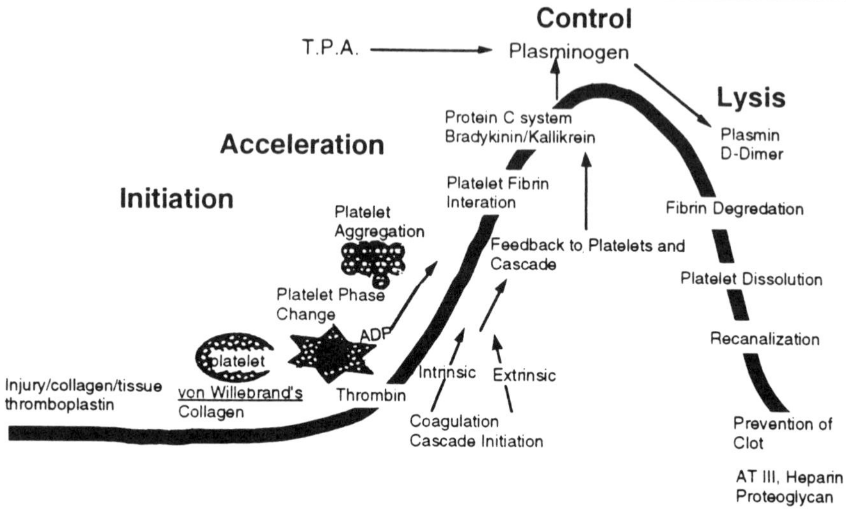

Figure 1: The sine wave of coagulation occurs at the microenvironment of vascular injury. It represents a continuum of reactions from initiation to eventual clot lysis. From Spiess (5) with permission.

cells as well as from damaged cells. von Willebrand's factor forms the glue by which platelets adhere to the site of injury. The release of von Willebrand's factor and the binding of the first few platelets forms what can be termed the initiation phase of coagulation. Once a small number of platelets are bound to the site of injury, they are further activated by a number of mechanisms including: changes in eicosanoid concentration, collagen activation, von Willebrand's factor activation and tissue thromboplastin release. The acceleration phase occurs as platelets release the contents of their alpha and dense granules (serotonin, epinephrine, thrombin, fibrinogen, ADP, thromboxane). These contain vasoactive compounds and agents that activate and attract other platelets, further fueling the speed and extent of the acceleration phase. The coagulation cascades interact at this point and the serine proteases sequentially act. Enzymes probably come on and off platelet surfaces flowing in from the plasma, being activated and transferring their products to the next enzyme. The macromolecular complex of factor X, calcium, factor V and factor VIII must be attached to the surface of a platelet for coagulation to behave normally *in vivo*. Once this macromolecular complex has formed, then prothrombin is cleaved into thrombin.

Thrombin is a key element in all of coagulation and probably inflammation. Once formed, it further accelerates the growing platelet plug as well as triggers the formation of solid fibrin from fibrinogen. Fibrin has six binding sites of a specific amino acid sequence for platelets and, therefore, each molecule can link a number of platelets into a cement-like structure which we know as solid clot. Once acceleration has been triggered, control is also well underway. Thrombin and other activation products trigger the local formation and activation of thrombomodulin (4). Protein S and C in turn are activated and protein C acts as a potent inhibitor of further thrombin formation (4). Thrombin, and also activated factors XI and XII, trigger a series of events that leads to plasmin formation. Plasmin further controls the runaway reaction of clot acceleration by degrading fibrinogen and fibrin. Eventually it prevails to create clot lysis and platelet disaggregation. The sine wave of coagulation activity (initialization, acceleration, control and lysis) occurs at a local site of tissue injury or at larger regions if systemic toxic effects occur (sepsis, shock, chemotherapy, etc.).

A contemporary view of coagulation should, therefore, not only include the sine wave of activity at the site of endothelial dysfunction but realize that coagulation is only one part of a triangular interaction between itself the endothelial lining and the inflammatory response (Figure 2). It is this paper's intention to examine some of the relationships that occur within the coagulation system that both activate and inhibit the inflammatory response. Also movement occurs in the reciprocal direction such that inflammation can up- and downregulate a number of coagulation reactions. No longer should we conceptualize coagulation as a limited event whose purpose is to halt bleeding. Rather, a more encompassing approach to coagulation as a mediator, amplifier and controller of the inflammatory response appears correct.

PROTEIN CASCADE INTERACTIONS

Activation of the protein cascades appears to have a modest or secondary link to the inflammatory response. Contact activation of the intrinsic cascade leads to immediate production of factor XIIa, which proceeds rapidly to change factor XI to XIa. Both XIIa and XIa then activate a host of reactions. Prekallikrein is converted to the vasoactive agents kallikrein and bradykinin (7). These in turn secondarily can activate the classic complement pathway with its ultimate output being C_3a. Kallikrein and factor XIIa as well as other mediators are activators of single chain urokinase plasminogen activator (scu-PA) (8). This plasma fibrinolytic protein is less effective than other fibrinolytic proteins but it does have importance. It, in turn, can further activate the more active compound tissue plasminogen activator (t-PA). Scu-PA may be more important outside of the vascular compartment in promoting proteolysis and enhancing

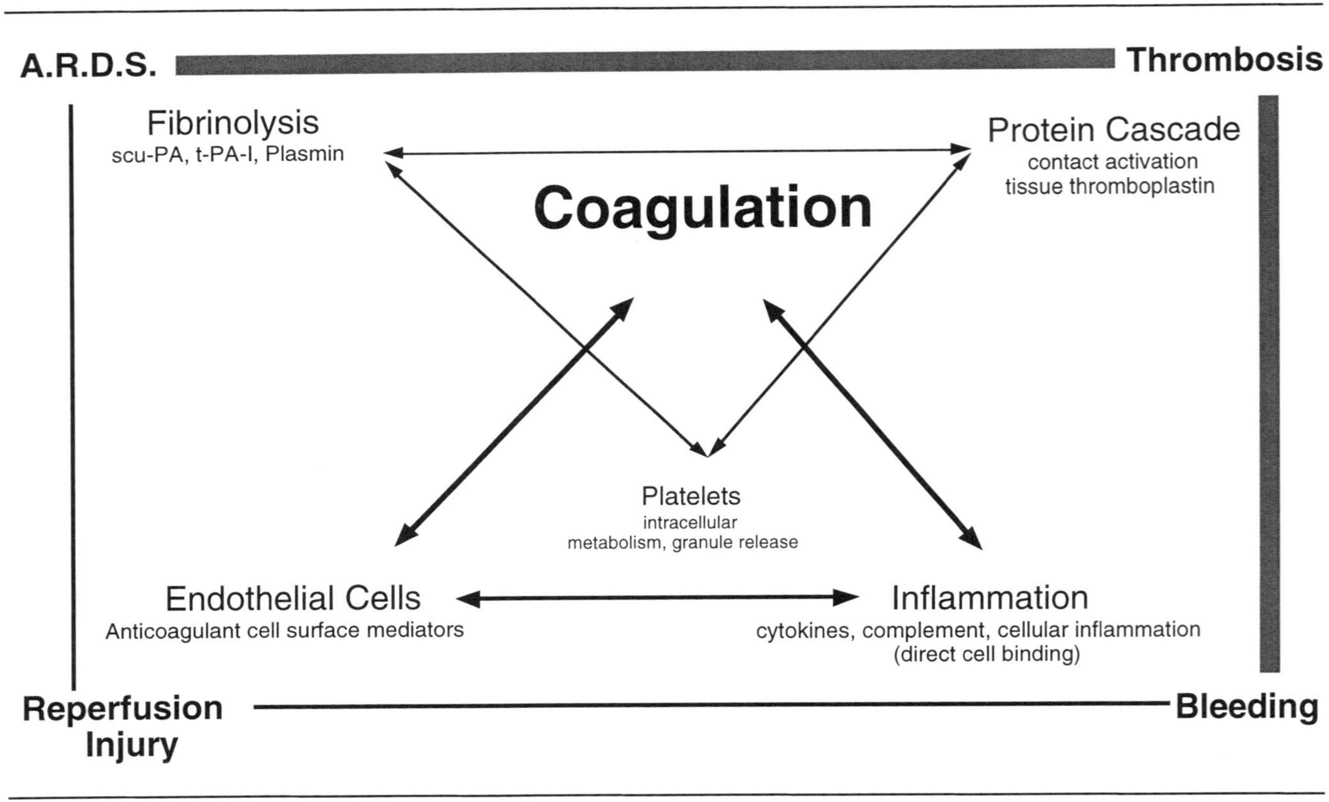

Figure 2. The interactions of coagulation endothelial cell function and inflammation.

cell migration and inflammation (8). Factor XIa enhances the release of plasminogen activator inhibitor-1 (PAI-1) (9). PAI-1 is contained in platelets and endothelial cells. When released it directly binds to t-PA and inhibits plasmin formation. The interaction between the fibrinolytic system and the inflammatory system is extensive and will be reviewed shortly.

Once the inflammatory system is induced there may be release of cytokines (10). These proteins act as messengers or binding sites which definitely up-regulate a number of inflammatory responses (11-14). Tissue thromboplastin release is enhanced when endothelium is challenged with interleukin-1 (IL-1) or tumor necrosis factor (TNF) (15). Tissue thromboplastin activates the extrinsic cascade and of course proceeds to the solid clot formation through the common pathway. However, there are some cross reactions which can activate the intrinsic cascade, predominately factor IX. The presence of these cytokines also decreases the activity of thrombomodulin. Therefore, the activation of protein coagulation activates inflammation and, once activated, inflammation may provide further feedback to stimulate more coagulation. PAI-1 activity is increased and t-PA activity is decreased by cytokines (16). This might appear to be a self-perpetuating feedback loop; however, the fibrinolytic system also has input.

FIBRINOLYSIS AND INFLAMMATION

Fibrinolysis is a fascinating subsystem of coagulation that has extensive interactions with the inflammatory system. It is now being widely investigated with many implications. Tissue plasminogen activator is a much more powerful activator of plasmin than is scu-PA. Plasmin hydrolyses both fibrinogen and fibrin. It is, therefore, responsible for the dissolution of formed clots. Also, if platelets are aggregating and clot is forming, an early excessive response of t-PA will lead to the disaggregation of platelet aggregates. Plasmin may be a platelet inhibitor at normothermia (17). This may be caused by secondary breakdown products of fibrin. However, it is interesting that with hypothermia, plasmin may be a platelet aggregator (18).

Endothelial cells have the highest concentration of t-PA, although it is contained in many cell types (19). If endothelial cells are exposed to thrombin in tissue culture they empty themselves of their t-PA contents (20). T-PA is cleared from the blood by the liver and by the active binding to t-PA's inhibitor PAI-1. For t-PA to have its effects it must overcome circulating levels of PAI-1. PAI-1 is also produced in endothelial cells and hepatocytes but over 80% of the blood levels are released from platelets (21,22). PAI-1 is pro-thrombotic, causing those effects by stopping the early disaggregation effects of t-PA. If platelets are allowed to interact and the platelet plug matures, thrombogenic effects will be enhanced. Increased PAI-1 levels are seen in pregnancy, eclampsia/pre-eclampsia, deep venous thrombosis, pulmonary embolism, unstable angina, and acute myocardial infarction (23-27). PAI-1 levels increase after routine surgery and trauma.

Thrombin stimulated release of t-PA from endothelium is lost with endothelial cell dysfunction or death (28,29). Ischemia, blood stasis, distention of the vasculature or direct trauma from a missile (i.e., bullet) all cause decreases in the production of t-PA (28). There are influences in the diurnal rhythm upon the fibrinolytic cycle (30). PAI-1 is increased through the night and is highest early in the morning. The reverse effect occurs in the afternoon and early evening as t-PA increases during the afternoon. In surgery, minor operations and major operations cause an increase in t-PA, although the magnitude is greater in more extensive operations. Fibrinolysis is almost universally stimulated during cardiopulmonary bypass (CPB) with the highest levels of t-PA activity occurring within 10 minutes after going onto cardiopulmonary bypass (31). The cause of the sudden rise in t-PA on CPB is still not known. Is it mediated by thrombin, histamine, or inflammatory mediators? It is very important to discern total t-PA activity from t-PA antigen. Antigen may be highest after the infusion of protamine but by that time PAI-1 is rising and therefore the activity of t-PA is waning. Although a number of studies have focused upon mean changes in this enzyme it is important to note that there is a very large variability within the population that undergoes CPB. Some patients appear to be non-responders and have little or no response of t-PA to CPB (32). Another group, in contrast, are profound releasors of t-PA. PAI-1 response does not seem to be related to t-PA response and some are small or normal responders whereas a small number of patients have very high releases of PAI-1. To date it is not known whether those patients who have the highest response in t-PA are at risk for excessive coagulopathy and if those with profound release of PAI-1 have increased thrombotic risks such as early postoperative ischemia or graft thrombosis.

Although t-PA and PAI-1 have their greatest effects in the area of their greatest concentration, the site of endothelial or platelet release, they are carried throughout the blood and are also found in lymphatic drainage as well (33). What effects these enzymes have within the lymph system is unclear. The inflammatory system has effects upon the release of both t-PA and PAI-1. Histamine and heparin both can cause the release of t-PA from endothelium (34). Heparin is utilized as the anticoagulant for almost all CPB cases. It does cause some element of histamine release. Interleukin-1 and TNF decrease the overall fibrinolytic function by increasing the release of PAI-1 from endothelium. It is less clear whether these cytokines increase the release of PAI-1 from platelets. Endotoxin also increases the release of PAI-1 and increases the release of platelet aggregating factor from endothelial tissue.

PLATELET AND INFLAMMATORY CELLULAR INTERACTIONS

Platelets are of key importance in the cellular coagulation process. Their activation and aggregation causes the primary plug formation that creates initial control of bleeding. Platelets interact with each other by releasing ADP, thromboxane, and other compounds. They undergo a change. They form pseudopods and a change in the makeup of receptor sites on their surfaces enhance the intracellular communications. The platelet aggregate and early clot has cell types other than just platelets involved. These cell lines are sometimes passively and others actively involved. As fibrin is formed, erythrocytes are enmeshed in the clot. Erythrocytes, although not actively attracted to the clot, are not just passive members in the clot process. Indeed, when entrapped they do release large amounts of adenosine diphosphate which further feeds the acceleration phase of coagulation (36). Nitric oxide is absorbed and deactivated by hemoglobin. Therefore, it is conceivable that in areas of growing clot the erythrocytes function in the destruction of the platelet and neutrophil inhibiting compound, nitric oxide. In patients with moderate anemia, the bleeding time may be mildly prolonged and this is thought to be due to decreased erythrocyte release of ADP

Intracellular metabolism is a unique process that involves production of a compound in one cell type. That first compound has no effect or diluted effect in the first cell type. However, when that compound is exported from the first cell it may be further processed in a second cell wherein it either has an action or can be exported for further changes. Erythrocytes participate in intracellular metabolism. Erythrocytes enhance eicosanoid transformation from platelet exported phospholipids. Platelet released arachidonic acid may be further hydrolyzed in erythrocytes and exported to activated neutrophils. Activated neutrophils in turn use the partially changed arachidonate to generate leukotriene B4.

Platelets and neutrophils have a number of interactions. When platelet and neutrophil suspensions combined together are activated with thrombin or collagen, relatively small amounts of serotonin are released from the platelets (35). This is in contrast to the effect of the same activation on platelet suspensions alone. It could therefore be concluded that neutrophils, in contrast to erythrocytes, depress the activation of platelets. The mechanism by which this inhibition occurs is not completely elucidated. There may be effects of neutrophil produced endothelial relaxant factor/nitric oxide as well as other possible mechanisms. The neutrophils used in these studies were nonactivated. However, other research laboratories have shown that neutrophils can actually increase platelet reactivity (37). Perhaps these neutrophils were treated in a different manner and were activated or up-regulated with production of cytokines.

Platelets, when activated, release the contents of their alpha granules. This causes the externalization of an alpha granule protein known as glycoprotein 140 (GMP-140) (38). GMP-140 creates an active site for binding of platelets to monocytes and neutrophils (39,40). Platelet monocyte and neutrophil platelet interactions occur fairly rapidly after CPB is begun. The monocytes appear to have a greater affinity for platelets as compared to the neutrophils. Lymphocytes and platelets decrease their binding during CPB. CD11b (known as complement receptor 3) is increased on the surface of monocytes and neutrophils during cardiopulmonary bypass. Monocyte CD11b increases quickly whereas neutrophil CD11b increase requires considerably longer time (39,40).

What are the effects of these platelet leukocyte interactions? Pulmonary sequestration of platelet leukocyte combinations may produce localized vascular reactivity and inflammation. It is unclear what intra-cellular communications the platelets and leukocytes are undergoing. It would seem that not only do these events occur in the blood stream at large but also within the matrix of a more solid clot. Neutrophils are enmeshed in the clot early; however, monocytes actively move into a solid clot later.

CD11b has been investigated as an important mediator of reperfusion injury. Blockage of CD11b in a number of animal studies has shown improvement or prevention of such injury (41,42). Since CD11b also binds complement its link with the inflammatory response seems certain. However this one surface receptor may have multiple roles. CD11b is a receptor also for factor X and fibrinogen (43). Does it perform similar functions to the glycoprotein IIb/IIIa site on platelets? Much work is yet to be done but the presence of this cell surface receptor that binds platelets, complement and coagulation proteins strengthens a hypothesis that reperfusion injury not only has inflammatory mediators but also involves coagulation events.

SUMMARY

There are clear interactions on all levels between coagulation and the inflammatory system. Proteins when activated both enhance and inhibit each system. The cellular components form direct intercellular linkages when activated. Cellular communicators by compounds may effect both platelets and inflammatory cells. The complexity of activators and inhibitors within coagulation makes it quite difficult to reach conclusions about the overall effect of any single event. What is important is that there are unique checks and balances within the systems of inflammation and coagulation. Importantly these checks and balances extend between systems such that cross activation and inhibition exists. As research continues into coagulopathy generation, inflammatory response, reperfusion injury, myocardial dysfunction, transient ischemia, and thrombosis, it should be remembered that coagulation and inflammation are not distinct separate entities but are seamless continuums of a total homeostatic system.

REFERENCES

1. Essell JH, Martin TJ, Salinas J, et al. Comparison of thromboelastography to bleeding time and standard coagulation tests in patients after cardiopulmonary bypass. J Cardiothorac Vasc Anesth 7:410-415, 1993
2. Gertler JP, Abbott WM. Prothrombotic and fibrinolytic function of normal and perturbed endothelium. J Surg Res 52:89-95, 1992
3. Eisenberg PR, ed. Endothelial cell mediators of thrombosis and fibrinolysis. Coronary Artery Disease. 2:129-166, 1991
4. Esmon CT. The roles of protein C and thrombomodulin in the regulation of blood coagulation. J Biol Chem 264:4743-4746, 1989
5. Spiess BD. Perioperative coagulation concerns: function, monitoring and therapy. Clinical Anesthesia Updates 4:1-16, 1993
6. Mollace V, Salvemini D, Sessa WC, Vane JR. Inhibition of human platelet aggregation by endothelium-derived relaxing factor, sodium nitroprusside or iloprost is potentiated by captopril and reduced thiols. J Pharmacol Exp Ther 258:820-823, 1991
7. Lucore CL. Regulation of fibrinolysis by vascular endothelium. Coronary Artery Disease 2:157-166, 1991
8. Laiho M, Keski-Oja J. Growth factors in the regulation of pericellular proteolysis: a review. Cancer Res 49:2533-2553, 1989
9. Van Hinsbergh VW, Binnema D, Scheffer MA, et al. Production of plasminogen activators and inhibitor by serially propagated endothelial cells from adult human blood vessels. Arteriosclerosis 7:389-400, 1987
10. Butler J, Rocker GM, Westaby S. Inflammatory responses to cardiopulmonary bypass. Ann Thorac Surg 55:552-559, 1993
11. Jansen NJ, VanOeveren W, Gu YJ, et al. Endotoxin release and tumor necrosis factor formation during cardiopulmonary bypass. Ann Thorac Surg 54:744-748, 1992
12. Gu YJ, VanOeveren W, Boonstra PW, et al. Leukocyte activation with increased expression of CR3 receptors during cardiopulmonary bypass. Ann Thorac Surg 53:839-843, 1992

13. Menasché P, Peynet J, Larivière J, et al. Does normothermia during cardiopulmonary bypass increase neutrophil-endothelium interactions? Circulation 90:II275-279, 1994
14. Hynes RO. Integrins: versatility, modulation and signaling in cell adhesion. Cell 69:11-25, 1992
15. Scarpati EM, Sadler JE. Regulation of endothelial cell coagulant properties. Modulation of tissue factor, plasminogen activator inhibitors, and thrombomodulin by phorol 12 myristate 13 acetate and tumor necrosis factor. J Biol Chem 264:20705-20713, 1989
16. Schleef RR, Bevilacqua MP, Sawdey M, et al. Cytokine activation of vascular endothelium. J Biol Chem 263:5797-5803, 1988
17. Gouin I, Lecompte T, Morel MC. In-vitro effect of plasmin on human platelet function in plasma. Inhibition of aggregation caused by fibrinogenolysis. Circulation 85:935-941, 1992
18. Kowalski E, Kopec M, Wegrzynowicz Z. Influence of fibrinogen degradation products (FDP) on platelet aggregation, adhesiveness and viscous metamorphosis. Thromb Diatr Haemorr 10:406, 1963
19. VanHinsbergh VW. Regulation of the synthesis and secretion of plasminogen activators by endothelial cells. Haemostasis 18:307-327, 1988
20. Hanss M, Collen D. Secretion of tissue-type plasminogen activator and plasminogen activator inhibitor by cultured human endothelial cells: modulation by thrombin, endotoxin and histamine. J Lab Clin Med 109:97-104, 1987
21. Erickson L, Ginsberg MH, Loskutoff DJ. An inhibitor of plasminogen activator in platelets. Haemostasis 14:65, 1984
22. Kruithof EK, Nicolosa G, Bachmann F. Plasminogen activator inhibitor 1: development of radioimmunoassay and observations on its plasma concentration during venous occlusion after platelet aggregation. Blood 70:1645-1653, 1987
23. Kluft C, Verheijen JH, Jie AF, et al. The postoperative fibrinolytic shutdown: a rapidly reverting acute phase pattern for the fast-acting inhibitor of tissue type plasminogen activator after trauma. Scand J Clin Lab Invest 45:605-610, 1985
24. Hamsten A, Walldius G, Szamosi A, et al. Plasminogen activator inhibitor in plasma: risk factor for recurrent myocardial infarction. Lancet 2:3-9, 1987
25. Margaglione M, DiMinno G, Grandone E, et al. Abnormally high circulation levels of tissue plasminogen activator and plasminogen activator inhibitor -1 in patients with a history of ischemic stroke. Arterioscler Thromb 14:1741-1745, 1994
26. Cortellaro M, Cofrancesco E, Boschetti C, et al. Increased fibrin turnover and high PAI-1 activity as predictors of ischemic events in atherosclerotic patients. Arterioscl Thromb 13:1412-1417, 1993
27. Eriksson B, Eriksson E, Gyzander E, et al. Deep vein thrombosis after total hip replacement—relationship to the fibrinolytic system. Acta Orthop Scand 60:159-163, 1989
28. Larsson J, Risberg B. Fibrinolytic activity in human legs in tourniquet ischemia. Thromb Res 11:817-825, 1977

29. Mellbring G, Dahlgren S, Reiz S, et al. Fibrinolytic activity in plasma and deep vein thrombosis after major abdominal surgery. Thromb Res 32:575-584, 1983
30. Andreotti F, Davies GJ, Hackett D, et al. Major circadian fluctuations in fibrinolytic factors and possible relevance to time of onset of myocardial infarction, sudden cardiac death and stroke. Am J Cardiol 62:635-637, 1988
31. Tanaka K, Takao M, Yaka I, et al. Alterations in coagulation and fibrinolysis associated with cardiopulmonary bypass during open heart surgery. J Cardiothorac Anesth 3:181-188, 1989
32. Chandler WL, Fitch JCK, Wall MH, et al. Individual variations in the fibrinolytic response during and after cardiopulmonary bypass. J Thromb Hemost (submitted) 1995.
33. Andreasson S, Smith L, Aasen AO, et al. Local pulmonary activation of proteolytic enzymes after Escherichia-coli-induced lung injury in sheep. Eur Surg Res 20:289-297, 1988
34. Saksela O, Moscatelli D, Rifkin DB. The opposing effects of basic fibroblast growth factor and transforming growth factor beta on the regulation of plasminogen activator activity in capillary endothelial cells. J Cell Biol 105:957-963, 1987
35. Marcus AJ. Thrombosis and inflammation as multicellular processes: pathophysiologic significance of transcellular metabolism. Blood 76:1903-1907, 1990
36. Santos MT, Valles J, Marcus AJ, et al. Enhancement of platelet reactivity and modulation of eicosanoid production by intact erythrocytes. J Clin Invest 87:571-580, 1991
37. Del Maschio A, Evangelista V, Rajtar G, et al. Platelet activation by polymorphonuclear leukocytes exposed to chemotactic agents. Am J Physiol 258:870-879, 1990
38. Nurden AT, Caen JP. Specific roles for platelet surface glycoproteins in platelet function. Nature 255:720-722, 1975
39. Rinder CS, Bonan JL, Rinder HM, et al. Cardiopulmonary bypass induces leukocyte platelet adhesion. Blood 79:1201-1205, 1992
40. Rinder CS, Gaal D, Student LA, Smith BR. Platelet-leukocyte activation and modulation of adhesion receptors in pediatric patients with congenital heart disease undergoing cardiopulmonary bypass. J Thorac Cardiovasc Surg 107:280-288, 1994
41. Simpson PJ, Todd RF III, Fantone JC, et al. Reduction of experimental canine myocardial reperfusion injury by a monoclonal antibody (anti-Mol, anti-CD11b) that inhibits leukocyte adhesion. J Clin Invest 81:624-629, 1988
42. Wallis WJ, Beatty PG, Ochs HD, Harlan JM. Human monocyte adherence to cultured vascular endothelium: monoclonal antibody-defined mechanisms. J Immunol 135:2323-2330, 1985
43. Wright SD, Weitz JI, Huang AJ, et al. Complement receptor type three (CD11b/CD18) of human polymorphonuclear leukocytes recognizes fibrinogen. Proc Natl Acad Sci 85:7734-7738, 1988.

NEW CONCEPTS IN ANTICOAGULATION AND REVERSAL

Jerrold H. Levy, MD

NEW CONCEPTS IN ANTICOAGULATION AND REVERSAL

Introduction

One of our most unusual clinical practices is to anticoagulate patients with heparin, an extract from bovine lung or porcine intestine, and reverse the heparin with protamine, a histone and a arginine rich polypeptide extracted from salmon sperm. Perhaps our practice of medicine is more medieval than we wish to realize. Furthermore, most clinicians managing patients during cardiac surgery have minimal understanding of the problems associated with anticoagulation and its reversal. Although cardiologists are evaluating different thrombin and platelet inhibitors to prevent graft reocclusion during angioplasty, there are few advances in the field of anticoagulation and reversal for cardiac surgical patients that are available for clinicians. This review will discuss the perspectives in anticoagulation and reversal, and novel agents on the horizon for heparin reversal.

Heparin

Heparin represents the only available intravenous anticoagulant available to prevent clotting during cardiac or vascular surgery (1). Although the Malaysian pit viper derivative, Ancrod, has been used to facilitate cardiopulmonary bypass (CPB), it prevents clotting by defibrinogenating the patient and creating a coagulopathic state (2). Heparin is isolated from either porcine intestine or from beef lung where it is bound to histamine and stored in mast cell granules. When heparin is isolated, the purification leads to a heterogeneous mixture of molecules often referred to as unfractionated heparin. Heparin is an acidic polysaccharide with side groups, either sulfates or N-acetyl groups, attached to individual sugar groups. The sulfate groups are extremely impor-

T. H. Stanley and P. L. Bailey (eds.), Anesthesiology and the Cardiovascular Patient, 123–129.

tant for the anticoagulant activity of heparin. Several other steps in the coagulation cascade, including clotting factor X, are also inhibited to a lesser degree by antithrombin III, and then also by heparin (AT III) (1).

Anticoagulation with heparin depends on the presence of adequate amounts of circulating AT III. The advantage of this is that heparin anticoagulation can be reversed immediately by removing heparin from AT III with protamine. AT III levels decrease in patients who receive preoperative heparin, but also fall significantly during cardiopulmonary bypass (3,4). There are now purified concentrates of AT III available for patients with altered heparin dose responses or with known AT III deficiency states. These concentrates have been heat treated to remove potential viral contaminants.

Heparin also binds to a number of other blood and endothelial proteins including high molecular weight kininogen, von Willebrand factor, plasminogen, fibronectin, lipoproteins and platelet and endothelial receptors (1). Each of these may potentially influence the ability of heparin to act as an anticoagulant, and may, along with AT III levels, affect heparin dose requirements in patients.

Heparin can also produce platelet dysfunction following acute and/or constant administration, especially with high dose administration during cardiac surgery. One of the most important considerations in patients receiving heparin for 7-10 days is that thrombocytopenia can occur (5).

Low Molecular Weight Heparin

Standard heparin fractions (unfractionated heparin) used in clinical practice consist of multiple negatively charged, glycosaminoglycans that range from 3,000 to 30,000 daltons with an average molecular weight of approximately 15,000. Low molecular weight heparins (LMWH) are components of unfractionated heparin with an average size of 5000 daltons. LMWH's major mechanism of antithrombotic action is inhibition of factor Xa inhibition, with less adverse effects on platelets. In addition, LMWH has a higher and more predictable bioavailability (100% compared to 30% for unfractionated heparin) and a longer biologic half life (4-7 hr). The plasma clearance is mainly by renal filtration. Monitoring the effects of LMWH use requires anti-Xa activity tests because coagulation tests that examine the intrinsic clotting cascade, including the activated clotting time (ACT) and activated partial thromboplastin time, are relatively insensitive to LMWH, and protamine may not consistently reverse the anticoagulant activity. LMWH preparations have not been widely used for extracorporeal circulation (6).

Heparin Reversal

Unfractionated heparin has a relatively short half life and is not routinely reversed in patients following cardiac catheterization. However, anticoagulation is routinely reversed following cardiac surgery to reestablish hemostatic mechanisms in patients who have bleeding defects due to multiple hemostatic abnormalities. Protamine can immediately reverse the anticoagulation effect of unfractionated heparin by nonspecific polyionic-polycationic (acid-base) interactions. There are different methods to determine the amount of protamine to be administered, but using 1.3 mg protamine for every 100 units of unfractionated heparin administered is effective. Although protamine has the potential to function as an anticoagulant, this effect is only seen when large excessive doses have been administered (7). More importantly, protamine, a polypeptide isolated from fish sperm, does have the potential to produce anaphylactic reactions, and therefore must be administered slowly. The incidence of anaphylaxis appears to be higher in certain patient groups, including diabetics who have received protamine containing insulin preparations like NPH. We have reported the incidence of anaphylaxis to protamine in NPH insulin dependent diabetics to be 0.6-2% compared to 0.06% in most other patients (9-11). Other patient groups may be at an increased risk for adverse reactions to protamine, including patients with a prior vasectomy or previous fish allergy, however, our data does not support this contention (11).

Monitoring Anticoagulation

Partial thromboplastin times are used to monitor low levels of heparinization preoperatively, but are inaccurate measures of anticoagulation when higher heparin concentrations are used (i.e., cardiac surgery). The gold standard for monitoring anticoagulation during CPB is the activated clotting time (ACT) (12). The ACT provides a direct measure of anticoagulation. When blood is allowed to encounter a negatively charged surface, such as kaolin (Hemotec) or diatomaceous earth (Hemochrom), platelets provide the tissue thromboplastin and the intrinsic pathway of blood coagulation is activated. The ACT measures the functional ability of heparin to inhibit the intrinsic pathway. Although clinicians routinely use the ACT to assess the degree of anticoagulation during cardiopulmonary bypass, there is no correlation between plasma heparin levels and the ACT (13). ACT levels assumed adequate for cardiopulmonary bypass do not completely inhibit thrombin formation (14).

More recently, additional monitors have been developed to measure heparin levels during cardiopulmonary bypass. Heparin-protamine titrations can determine the amount of circulating heparin in the presence of anticoagulation. Although the data supporting the use of these systems during CPB is still forthcoming, many clinicians use heparin-protamine titrations to guide additional heparin administration and reversal, or as an adjunct to ACT monitoring. In addition, the heparin-protamine titration can be used to determine the exact amount of protamine required to reverse heparin.

However, when patients are heparinized in the presence of circulating aprotinin, the ACT is greatly prolonged, making ACT-determinations, as measurements of circulating heparin levels, inaccurate (12), Heparin-protamine titrations to measure heparin levels can be used to determine anticoagulation levels in the presence of circulating aprotinin. Alternately, fixed dose heparin administration with the use of kaolin based ACT systems represent another method of monitoring patients during aprotinin therapy, administering doses of 100 U/kg every hour during CPB.

Novel Methods For Reversing Anticoagulation

New methods for reversing anticoagulation are under current investigation that are based on different principals and offer unique mechanisms for reversing systemic heparinization. Heparin binding filters, recombinant platelet factor 4, and heparinase are the new methods under current investigation as potential protamine replacements (15-22) (Table 1).

Table 1. Potential alternatives for heparin neutralization.

Hexadimethrine
Heparin binding filters
Heparinase
Recombinant platelet factor 4

Recombinant Platelet Factor 4

Platelet factor 4 (PF4) is a basic protein with a molecular weight of approximately 7,800 daltons that is normally stored in the alpha granules of platelets. PF4 can neutralize the anticoagulant effects of vascular heparins. A recombinant form of PF4 (rPF4) has been synthesized and studied in vitro, in animals, and in humans for heparin reversal.

We have studied the ability of rPF4 to neutralize anticoagulated blood in cardiac surgical patients with heparin levels ranging from 2.7-4.1 units/ml. We found that an rPF4 reversal ratio of 3.0:1 was the minimum dose required for heparin reversal, which is different than the ratio of 2.0:1 previously reported (7,16). However, when thromboelastography was attempted with ratios less than 3.0:1, coagulation did not occur. Our current clinical studies have supported this dose. Recombinant PF4 did not interfere with platelet-fibrinogen interaction or differences in clot lysis compared to protamine when reversing heparin as determined by thromboelastography.

The advantage of recombinant PF4 is its lack of adverse hemodynamic effects in both experimental models and preliminary human studies (17,19). Although preliminary reports in the sheep model have suggested PF4 produces pulmonary hypertension (18), data from human studies of heparin reversal with PF4 following cardiac catheterization have not supported this finding (19). Sheep have different inflammatory cell populations that may predispose them to acute pulmonary vasoconstriction.

Heparinase

Heparinase, an enzyme isolated from *Flavobacterium heparinum*, metabolizes heparin-like carbohydrates by cleaving alpha-glycosidic linkages to produce fragments without anticoagulant activity (20). Heparinase is currently under development and has been successfully used for in vitro studies and in in vitro preparations (20-22). Animal investigations currently in progress will determine its effectiveness as an injectable heparin neutralizing agent and its side effects. We reported the concentration-response relationship between heparinase I concentrations and heparin neutralization in residual blood obtained from the extracorporeal circuit immediately after cardiac surgery in patients (21). Heparinase I at concentrations >0.054 IU/ml successfully decreased heparin concentrations of 3.3 ± 0.3 (mean±SEM) U/ml (n=12), and maximally reduced the ACT. However, in vitro data suggests neutralization takes 5 minutes as compared to an ionic neutralizing agent that produces immediate reversal.

In canine studies, heparinase neutralized heparin as effectively as did protamine (21). Both heparinase I, at all doses, and protamine neutralized heparin-induced increases in ACT within 5 to 10 minutes. In this animal model, Heparinase I at all doses did not affect hemodynamics when compared to its vehicle alone. However, protamine caused severe systemic hypotension and pulmonary hypertension. Because heparinase comes from bacteria, injection into humans may produce potential sensitization for repeat exposure.

REFERENCES

1. Salzman EW, Hirsh J, Marder VJ. Clinical use of heparin. In: Colman RW HJ Marder VJ, Salzman EW, ed. Hemostasis and Thrombosis: Basic Principles and Clinical Practice. 3rd ed. Philadelphia: J.B. Lippincott 1584-1591, 1994
2. Teasdale SJ, Zulys VJ, Mycyk T. Ancrod anticoagulation for cardiopulmonary bypass in heparin-induced thrombocytopenia and thrombosis. Ann Thorac Surg 48:712-723, 1989
3. Cloyd GM, D'Ambra MN, Akins CW. Diminished anticoagulant response to heparin in patients undergoing coronary artery bypass grafting. J Thorac Cardiovasc Surg 94:535-8, 1987
4. Zaidan JR, Johnson S, Brynes R, Monroe S, Guffin AV. Rate of protamine administration: its effect on heparin reversal and antithrombin recovery after coronary artery surgery. Anesth Analg 65:377-380, 1986
5. Anderson GP. Insights into heparin-induced thrombocytopenia. Br J Haematol 80:504-508, 1992
6. Hemker HC, Beguin S. Low molecular weight heparins: an introduction. Haemostasis 20(S):74-80, 1991
7. Levy JH, Cormack JG, Morales A. Heparin neutralization by recombinant platelet factor 4 and protamine. Anesth Analg 81:35-37, 1995
9. Stewart WJ, McSweeney SM, Kellett MR, Faxon DP, Ryan TJ. Increased risk of severe protamine reactions in NPH insulindependent diabetics undergoing cardiac catheterization. Circulation 70:788-792, 1984
10. Levy JH, Zaidan JR, Faraj BA. Prospective evaluation of risk of protamine reactions in NPH insulin-dependent diabetics. Anesth Analg 65:739-742, 1986
11. Levy JH, Schwieger IM, Zaidan JR, Faraj BA, Weintraub WS. Evaluation of patients at risk for protamine reactions. J Thorac Cardiovasc Surg 98:200-204, 1989
12. Wang JS, Lin CY, Hung WT, Karp RB. Monitoring of heparin-induced anticoagulation with kaolin activated clotting time in cardiac surgical patients treated with aprotinin. Anesthesiology 77:1080-1084, 1992
13. Culliford AT, Gitel SN, Starr N, et al. Lack of correlation between activated clotting time and plasma heparin during cardiopulmonary bypass. Ann Surg 193:105-11, 1981
14. Slaughter TF, LeBleu TH, Douglas JM, Leslie JB, Parker JK, Greenberg CS. Characterization of prothrombin activation during cardiac surgery by hemostatic molecular markers. Anesthesiology 80:520-526, 1994
15. Montalescot G, Zapol WM, Carvalho A, Robinson DR, Torres A, Lowenstein E. Neutralization of low molecular weight heparin by polybrene prevents thromboxane release and severe pulmonary hypertension in awake sheep. Circulation 82:1754-1764, 1990

16. Williams RD, D'Ambra MN, Maione TE, Lynch KE, Keene DF. Recombinant platelet factor 4 reversal of heparin in human cardiopulmonary bypass blood. J Thorac Cardiovasc Surg 108:975-83, 1994
17. Cook JJ, Niewiarowski S, Yan Z, Schaffer L, Lu W, Stewart GJ, Mosser DM, Myers JA, Maione TF. Platelet factor 4 efficiently reverses heparin anticoagulation in the rat without adverse effects of heparin-protamine complexes. Circulation 85:1102-1109, 1992
18. Kurrek MM, Winkler M, Robinson DR, Zapol WM. Platelet factor 4 injection produces acute pulmonary hypertension in the awake lamb. Anesthesiology 82:183-7, 1995
19. Dehmer GJ, Fisher M, Tate DA, Teo S, Bonnem EM. Reversal of heparin anticoagulation by recombinant platelet factor 4 in humans. Circulation 91:2188-2194, 1995
20. Hoving P, Linker A. The enzymatic degradation of heparin and heparitin sulfate. iii. Purification of a heparitinase and a heparinase from flavobacterium. J Biol Chem 245:6170, 1970
21. Michelsen LG, Kikura M, Lee MK, Szlam F, Levy JH. Heparinase as an alternative for reversing heparin anticoagulation. In Review
22. Zimmermann J, Lee K, Lambert C, Bier C. Efficacy and pharmacokinetics of heparinase, a novel and improved heparin-reversal agent, in rabbits. Catheterization and Cardiovascular Diag 32:88, 1994

PERFLUOROCARBON EMULSIONS: ONE APPROACH TO INTRAVENOUS ARTIFICIAL RESPIRATORY GAS TRANSPORT

Bruce D. Spiess, MD

INTRODUCTION

The viral infectious risks of allogeneic transfusion have recently been reduced (1). This is due to changes in viral marker testing along with surrogate risk testing using a number of biochemical tests. These data have been widely heralded with comments that the blood supply is now the safest it has ever been. This may be true; however, these data are reported from one study only and a wide range of risks associated with blood transfusion exist that will not be changed by reducing viral transmission. These risks include ABO and Rh incompatibility, graft versus host disease, volume overload, and immunosuppression leading to increased secondary infection or solid tumor recurrence. Therefore, even though viral transmission is less troublesome today than it was 5 years ago, allogeneic blood transfusion carries significant risks. For many years physicians have searched for ways to circumvent those risks. The development of safe, more efficacious, and cost effective oxygen transport medias are being investigated.

Two principal approaches to the production of a "blood substitute" are being pursued: hemoglobin preparations and perfluorocarbon chemicals. Hemoglobin preparations have evolved from simple free hemoglobin, removed from erythrocytes, to polymerized hemoglobin preparations. Attempts have also been made to repackage hemoglobin in artificial lipid matrices, so that ABO-Rh typing is unnecessary. Today, a number of companies are investigating multiple different formulations in both animal models and human. This chapter will not discuss these "blood substitutes."

The lay press has coined the term "artificial blood" in reference to a group of chemicals that have enhanced solubility for oxygen. Blood, as a complex living fluid organ has thousands of functions and the transport of oxygen is only one very vital function. Therefore, "artificial blood" is a misnomer, but one that has stuck. Perfluorocarbon compounds (PFC) differ from hemoglobin

T. H. Stanley and P. L. Bailey (eds.), Anesthesiology and the Cardiovascular Patient, 131–142.

preparations in a number of ways. PFC acts as effective plasma expanders with limited gas transport capabilities. In a number of gas transport aspects, PFC does out perform human blood.

EARLY DEVELOPMENT

Carbon fluoride chemistry was an area of intense research in the 1950's and 1960's. The development of non-stick cooking pan coatings is an event known to most of us. During experimentation in developing these compounds it was noted that liquid PFC dissolves far greater quantities of some non-polar gases than do aqueous liquids at equal temperatures and pressures (2).

The effects of fluorination of an organic compound can be seen with the simple benzene ring. If it has six fluorides substituted for hydrogens, hexafluorobenzene is formed. Hexafluorobenzene has powerful anesthetic properties and little, if any, increased respiratory gas solubility. The addition of six more fluorides to saturate all the double bonds leads to the formation of perfluorocyclohexane. Anesthetic properties are lost and oxygen is at least twice as soluble as it is in benzene alone (3).

The carbon fluoride bond is a high energy bond (120 kcal/mole). It is difficult for biologic systems to break that bond, especially if all carbon atoms are completely occupied by fluorides. Therefore, once completely substituted with fluorides most compounds loose biologic activity, and therefore, the release of fluoride is negligible.

PFC liquids are passive gas transporters. This is in contrast to hemoglobin which actively binds oxygen to the iron in the heme moiety (Figure 1). The sigmoidal curve of the oxy-hemoglobin dissociation curve is very well understood by clinicians. The effects of pH, temperature and the concentration of 2,3-diphosphoglycerate influence the relative binding and release of oxygen from hemoglobin. Gas transport by PFC is based on enhanced solubility. That enhanced solubility is related to the physics of the molecules involved, making them less polar. The physical forces governing the uptake and release of oxygen (nitrogen or carbon dioxide) from a PFC, are the partial pressure gradients for that gas. Many PFCs in their pure liquid form can dissolve (carry) and completely release up to 50-60 volume percent of oxygen (Table 1) (4). Plasma or crystalloid solutions can carry a maximum of three volume percent if equilibrated with 100%

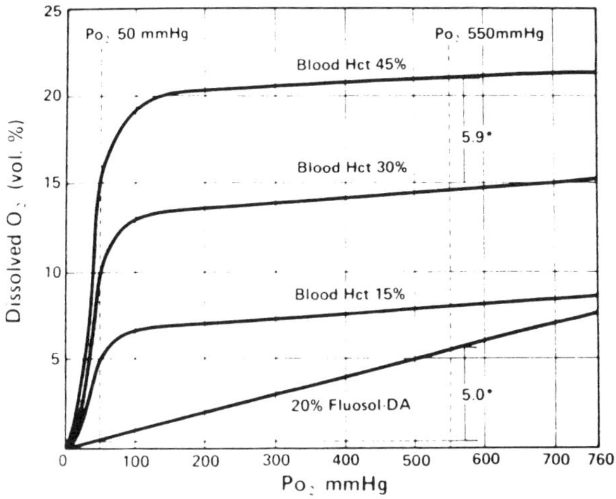

Figure 1. Oxygen content and release from hemoglobin versus Fluosol-DA(20%). Reprinted with permission from Suyama T, Yokoyama K, Naito R (10).

Table 1. Oxygen solubility of various perfluorochemicals. Reprinted with permission from Geyer RP (4).

Compound	O_2 solubility:ml O_2/100 ml of compound
Perfluorodihexyl ether	55.42
Perfluorodibutyl sulfur tertrafluroide	48.02
Perfluorotriisobutylamine	44.37
Perfluoro-(N-ethylmorpholine)	50.10
Perfluroro-N,N-dipropylmethylamine	52.60
Perfluorotriethylamine	53.86
Perfluoro-N-methylpiperidine	41.33
Perfluoro-N-methylmorpholine	37.57
Perfluoro-N,N-dimethyl-N-hexylamine	51.51
Perfluoro-N-butylmorpholine	59.59
Perfluoro-4(N,N -dimethyl-2-aminoethyl)-morpholine	45.07
Perfluoropentyl ether	49.67

oxygen at atmospheric pressure and 37°C (5). Whole blood, in contrast, with a normal hemoglobin and hematocrit, can carry up to 21 volume percent. The O_2 carrying capacity of any PFC emulsion is determined by fluorocrit, PaO_2 and the solubility of O_2 in the PFC.

$$(O_2)\ PFC = \text{solubility}\ O_2\ PFC \times PO_2 \times \text{fluorocrit}$$

Fluorocrit can be determined utilizing a routine centrifuge for doing spin hematocrits. The fluorocarbon emulsion will separate out at the bottom of the capillary tube as a white layer.

In 1966 it was first demonstrated that a PFC liquid could be utilized to supply oxygen in organ perfusion models (6). L.C. Clark, at the University of Alabama, created an uproar in the lay press when he published his work on the survival of mice actually breathing oxygenated perfluorochemicals (7). Goldfish, mice, rats and several cats were submerged in different liquid environments. Mice were placed in silicone oils (polymethylsiloxanes) having oxygen solubilities approximately 1.5 times the oxygen content in whole blood. Mice were able to survive in these low viscosity oils but only at reduced temperatures (18°C). All mice succumbed within 10 minutes after being taken out of the silicone oil. Goldfish could survive for weeks under silicone oil bubbled with oxygen. Immersion in perfluorocarbons (perfluorobutyltetrahydrofurans) was much more satisfactory. An oxygen electrode affixed to a mouse's brain prior to immersion showed the same level of oxygenation following immersion as when the animal was breathing room air. After removal from the PFC, the mice survived for weeks (7). Cats breathing PFC upon return to room air breathing all succumbed to massive pulmonary edema.

Vapor pressure of PFC is a key important criteria for making a particular compound biocompatible. Rats injected intraperitoneally with perfluorotetrahydrofuran died with massive abdominal distention as liquid PFC vaporized (8). The same phenomenon has occurred with multiple PFCs. It appears that there is a critical value for vapor pressure of approximately 40 mm Hg (3). Vapor pressures of 50 mm Hg or greater cause death in mammals with massive gas emboli.

Elimination of PFC is probably dependent upon vapor pressure. It is thought that PFCs are not soluble at all in water and, therefore, there is no renal filtration. Vaporization through the lungs and the skin may form the major route of egress. Low vapor pressure compounds are not cleared and have prolonged half-lives. A very low vapor pressure PFC may stay in an experimental animal for the animal's entire life-span (3). Perfluorodecalin is rapidly eliminated through the skin and lungs. Its half-life for circulation is 24 hours and whole body is 8.9 days (8).

Perfluorocarbons that meet the correct vapor pressure criteria do not form stable emulsions and are immiscible with plasma. Therefore, emulsions of the PFCs must be created to allow them to be mixed with plasma. A commercially available emulsifying agent, polyoxyethelene, is readily available and has been laboratory tested (9). Perfluorotripropylamine forms a stable emulsion with polyoxyethelene but because of vapor pressure it has a slow elimination time. In combination with perfluorodecalin the elimination becomes quite reasonable (10). This formulation is now commercially produced by The Green Cross Corporation, Osaka, Japan, under the name Fluosol-DA(20%).

FLUOSOL-DA(20%)

The composition of Fluosol-DA(20%) is shown in Table 2. It is a 20% weight-to-volume emulsion and actually a 10% volume-to-volume PFC to inactive agent solution. The PFC emulsion has seven parts perfluorodecalin to three parts perfluorotripropylamine with both pluronic F-68 and egg yolk phospholipids as stabilizers/emulsifiers. The emulsion is not stable at room temperature for transport but must be frozen, thawed and sonicated to get it in the correct emulsion state for infusion (11). It has 410 milliosmoles for osmolarity and 390 mm H_2O for oncotic pressure. In the final emulsion the particle size is considerably smaller than an erythrocyte (0.1 micron) (12). The

Table 2. The composition of Fluosol-DA(20%). Modified from Mitsuno T, et al. (19).

Perfluorodecalin	14.0 gm/100 ml
Perfluorotripropylamine	6.0 gm/100 ml
Pluronic F-68	2.7 gm/100 ml
Yolk phospholipids	400.0 gm/100 ml
Glycerol	800.0 gm/100 ml
Sodium chloride	600.0 gm/100 ml
Potassium chloride	34.0 gm/100 ml
Magnesium chloride	20.0 gm/100 ml
Calcium chloride	28.0 gm/100 ml
Sodium bicarbonate	210.0 gm/100 ml
Glucose	180.0 gm/100 ml
Hydroxyethyl starch	3.0 gm/100 ml
pH	7.4
Osmolality	410.0 mOsm
Oncotic pressure	380-395 mm H_2O

difference in particle size may have striking importance in the eventual clinical utilization and side effects of these PFC emulsions. Surface area for gas exchange is massively increased by the size differential.

The oxygen dissociation curve for Fluosol-DA(20%) as compared to whole blood and plasma at different oxygen tensions is similar to that shown in Figure 1 (10). Oxygen dissolved in this and all other PFCs changes linearly in accordance with Henry's law. Uptake and release is completely reversible and as stated earlier, there is no oxygen hemoglobin dissociation curve. The maximum amount of oxygen dissolved in Fluosol-DA(20%) at 760 Torr at 37°C is approximately 7 volume percent. That is about 33% of that carried by fully oxygenated whole blood. Pure PFC may carry up to 60 volume percent but the emulsion is only 10% v/v. Clearly, all the oxygen carried by whole blood is not available for metabolic needs. The usual metabolic oxygen demand is approximately 5 volume percent and therefore it is theoretically conceivable with full exchange transfusion that Fluosol-DA(20%) could meet the body oxygen requirements (10). Patients cannot oxygenate their blood with 760 mm Hg because of intrapulmonary shunt, carbon dioxide transfer in the alveolus and water pressure; therefore, the best that could be reasonably expected is an equilibration with 550 Torr of oxygen.

Animal studies with exchange transfusion of Fluosol-DA(20%) have shown excellent tissue oxygen delivery and organ function. Animals given PFCs could survive for days with up to 90% of their residual hemoglobin poisoned with carbon monoxide (11). In other studies animals have been exchange transfused to as low as 1% hematocrit and had adequate respiratory gas exchange to sustain life (12-14). In animal models of acute myocardial and cerebral ischemia, Fluosol has demonstrated significant capability in preventing tissue damage (15,16). One report of intraluminal instillation of oxygenated PFC in gut ischemia has shown preservation of the mucosa (17). Also reports of improved efficacy of a cardioplegia solution containing PFC in an isolated heart model have been published (18).

Early human work from Japan included a series of 186 patients given PFC for oxygen transport. The majority of the patients were experiencing surgical hemorrhage and for one reason or another had refused blood products. No major cardiovascular biochemical or anatomical abnormalities occurred in this early study (19). Total oxygen supplied by the PFC was thought to be approximately 1.2 to 1.3 volume percent. In an early study with seven patients in the United States who had ongoing hemorrhage, Fluosol did demonstrate some contribution to total oxygen supply (20). The patients were required to have high inspired concentrations of oxygen and the total fluorocrit got as high as 3%. With those two factors the total oxygen content contributed by the PFC was only .8%. That may seem to be a rather small percentage of total oxygen carrying capacity but the authors point out that in critically ill patients, of those who have end-organs at risk for ischemia it is conceivable that that level of oxygenation may make some survival difference. One case report notes the successful use of Fluosol-DA(20%) in a Jehovah's Witness patient who required a Whipple pancreatoduodenectomy. Such a procedure is expected to result in significant blood loss. The patient began the procedure with only 5 gm/dl of hemoglobin and did quite well after the infusion of the PFC (21). These reports of success with PFC have been overshadowed by concern regarding the potential side effects from the emulsifying agent. Complement release, hypotension and white cell depression have been implicated (22-23). Also, uptake by the reticuloendothelial system with hepatic sequestration of the PFC coupled with marginal oxygen carrying contributions stalled the development of these early PFC emulsions. At the present time Fluosol-DA(20%) has won FDA approval for only one indication. That is, its use as a distal perfusate in coronary angioplasty interventions to prevent or treat distal myocardial ischemia (24,25). The preparation of the emulsion has also proven cumbersome with it requiring frozen storage, thawing, sonication and equilibration with an oxygen carbon dioxide mixture. Therefore, that indication has not led to widescale utilization.

SECOND GENERATION PFC

Two companies are now producing and testing second generation PFC emulsions: HemaGen PFC, St. Louis, Missouri; and Alliance, San Diego, California. Both are using proprietary formulations of PFCs that are different than those in Fluosol-DA(20%) and the total concentration of the new formulations includes the usage of different emulsifying agents. The total available PFC is up to 40% v/v in these new formulations. Therefore, the second generation emulsions can carry up to 4 times as much oxygen as that seen with Fluosol. In the PFC equilibrated with 100% oxygen, prior to infusion this translates into 17 to 25 volume percent of oxygen available (26). In animal experiments with intravenous infusions of up to 20 cc/kg this may provide levels of oxygen far in excess of the 0.8 volume percent found in humans with Fluosol.

Both second generation emulsions are now undergoing early FDA drug testing. The utilization of one of the PFCs in volunteers undergoing small amounts of blood loss for elective surgery has shown it to be well tolerated (27). From the abstracts available to date it is difficult to judge the effectiveness of oxygen delivery. However, one study reported PFC usage in seven patients losing more than 1000 cc blood (28). These patients were monitored with pulmonary artery catheters and arterial lines. During progressive hemorrhage hemoglobin concentration dropped yet mixed venous oxygen saturation was stable or slightly (statistically significant) increased. Unfortunately, this early report did not permit calculation of the total oxygen carried by PFC.

OTHER GAS TRANSPORT USAGES

PFC, unlike whole blood or plasma, has enhanced capacity for transport of gases other than oxygen. All non-polar gases are soluble in PFC. Of particular interest is nitrogen. In pure PFC, nitrogen may be up to 10,000 times as soluble as it is in plasma. Nitrogen, being the major constituent gas of air, can cause problems in a number of surgeries. These include micro-air embolic events in cardiopulmonary bypass, and larger air emboli in neurosurgery, orthopedics and some gynecological procedures (29-33).

A number of animal studies have been performed demonstrating that PFC, if given as a pretreatment, can prevent the harmful sequelae of venous air embolism (34). Data from studies of the formulations of PFC show that nitrogen absorption is one of the possible mechanisms by which protection may be afforded (35). Protection from intracoronary air embolism has been suggested in one canine model and cerebral protection has been demonstrated in rabbits and other animal models (36-38). Decompression sickness is caused by insoluble gas embolism within either central nervous tissue or the blood stream. Several small rodent studies have shown that PFC can treat decompression sickness if the animals also breathe 100% oxygen (39,40).

Further work with new PFC emulsions that are 40% v/v also are producing positive data. In dogs ventilated with xenon and subsequently given PFC, it was noted that the muscle clearance of xenon, an insoluble gas, was increased by a factor of greater than 2 (41). Accelerated wash out of nitrogen from tissue would be expected to be many-fold that of xenon due to its solubility ratios (41). In swine models of massive cerebral air embolism during cardiopulmonary bypass there have been demonstrations of major brain preservation in animals where PFC has been added to the bypass machine (42).

UNIQUE APPLICATIONS

The carbon fluoride bonds make PFC emulsions unique. By proper tuning of the radio frequency of a nuclear magnetic resonance scanner, certain

PFC emulsions can be utilized as NMR dyes. Indeed, they may first reach FDA approval for use as intravenous contrast agents (43,44). Also, the installation of PFC into the respiratory bronchial tree has again become an experimental activity. Historically, this was where PFCs had their first dramatic public enthusiasm. Recent work with liquid PFC ventilation in neonatal sheep and some models of adult respiratory distress are at least promising (45). There is a suggestion that filling of the tracheobronchial tree with a newly constructed piston liquid ventilator may not be necessary. Merely filling the functional residual capacity with PFC may be enough to enhance gas transport across lungs that would otherwise have extensive physiologic shunt (46). Other areas of research are in the use of PFCs to enhance the delivery or efficacy of certain chemotherapeutic agents. An elevated oxygen tension may increase the killing capacity of chemotherapeutic agents and simultaneous administration of a PFC and chemotherapy agent may result in a synergistic effect (47). One group has also reported on the construction of a new type of oxygenator for extracorporeal oxygenation that utilizes a blood PFC interface to transmit oxygen (47).

SUMMARY

The PFC emulsions have had a developmental history of promise that is as yet unfulfilled. Today, second generation PFC emulsions are poised with the right gas carrying capabilities to be able to make significant contributions to oxygen transport and delivery. The vision of a stable, safe, easily transportable intravenous fluid, with universal rapid application, is not yet at hand. However, we appear to be a great deal closer than in the mid 1980's. If these 40% v/v emulsions prove safe then an entirely new realm of therapeutic options will become available. Not only will uses for trauma and acute blood loss replacement become a reality, but extremes of euvolemic hemodilution may become possible. The use of these compounds for prevention of stroke, ischemic organ salvage and prevention of air embolism or decompression sickness are particularly exciting. It is clear from the recent developments in PFC technology that some product will come to market in the not-to-distant future. How such a PFC will be utilized, as compared to hemoglobin preparations, is yet to be determined, but the two concepts are quite different. Each will have its own specific indications.

REFERENCES

1. Donahue JG, Munoz A, Ness PM, et al: The declining risk of post-transfusion hepatitis C-virus infection. N Engl J Med 327:369-373, 1992

2. O'Brien RN: Diffusion coefficients of respiratory gases in a perfluorocarbon liquid. Science 217:153-155, 1982
3. Clark LC: Emulsions of perfluoronated solvents for intravenous gas transport. Fed Proc 34:1468-1477, 1981
4. Geyer RP: Perfluoronated blood replacement preparations. Excerpta Medica International Congress Series 486: 1978
5. Maugh TH: Blood substitute passes its first test. Science 206:205, 1981
6. Gollan F, Clark LC: Organ perfusion with fluorocarbon fluid. Physiologist 9:191, 1966
7. Clark LC, Gollan F: Survival of mammals breathing organic liquids equilibrated with oxygen at atmospheric pressure. Science 152:1755-1757, 1966
8. Lapin R, Freidman A, Levine E: The preoperative use of Fluosol-DA(20%) in major abdominal surgery. J Abd Surg 22:15, 1980
9. Geyer RP: Bloodless rats through the use of artificial blood substitutes. Fed Proc 34:1449-1505, 1975
10. Suyama T, Yokoyama K, Naito R: Development of a perfluorochemical whole blood substitute Fluosol-DA(20%): An overview of clinical studies with 185 patients. Prog Clin Biol Res 55:609-628, 1981
11. Sloviter HA, Petkovic M, OGoshi S, Yamada H: Dispersed fluorochemicals as substitutes for erythrocytes in intact animals. J Appl Physiol 2:666-668, 1969
12. Clark LC, Jr, Becanttini F, Kaplan S: The physiological effects of artificial blood made from inert organic oxygen solvents. Ala J Med Sci 9:16-29, 1972
13. Gould SA, Rosen AL, Sehgal LR, et al: How good are fluorocarbon emulsions as O_2 carriers? Surg Forum 32:299-301, 1981
14. Geyer RP: Fluorocarbon-polyol artificial blood substitutes. N Engl J Med 289:1077-1082, 1973
15. Glogar DH, Kloner RA, Muller J, et al: Fluorocarbons reduce myocardial ischemia damage after coronary occlusion. Science 211:1439-1441, 1981
16. Peerless SJ, Ishikawa R, Hunter IG, Peerless MJ: Protective effect of Fluosol-DA in acute cerebral ischemia. Stroke 193:206-209, 1981
17. Oldham KT, Giuce KS, Gourley WK, Lobe TE: Treatments of intestinal ischemia with oxygenated intraluminal perfluorocarbons. Am J Surg 153:291-294, 1987
18. Toyohira H, Taira A, Arikawa K, et al: Isolated heart perfusion with FC-43: An experimental study. Excerpta Medica International Congress Series 486: 1978
19. Mitsuno T, Ohyanagi H, Naito R: Clinical studies of a perfluorochemical whole blood substitute (Fluosol-DA): Summary of 186 cases. Ann Surg 195:60-69, 1982
20. Tremper KK: The preoperative treatment of severely anemic patients with a perfluorochemical oxygen-transport fluid Fluosol-DA. N Engl J Med 307:277-283, 1982
21. Atabek U, Spence RK, Pello M, et al: Pancreaticoduodenectomy without homologous blood transfusions in an anemic Jehovah's Witness. Arch Surg 127:349-351, 1992

22. Draffehn J, Reichelt H: The toxicity of surface-active substances for emulsifying perfluorocarbon compounds as components of blood substitute preparations. Pharmazie 46:271-272, 1991
23. Lane TA, Lamkin GE: Increased infection mortality and decreased neutrophil migration due to a component of an artificial blood substitute. Blood 68:351-354, 1986
24. Kerins DM: Role of the perfluorocarbon Fluosol-DA in coronary angioplasty. Am J Med Sci 307:218-221, 1994
25. Young LH, Jaffe CC, Revkin JH: Metabolic and functional effects of perfluorocarbon distal perfusion during coronary angioplasty. Am J Cardiol 15:986-990, 1990
26. Goodin TH, Kaufman RJ, Richard TJ, Grossbard EB: The use of perfluorochemical oxygen carriers in surgical hemodilution. In press
27. Cernaianu AC, Spence RK, Vassilidze TV, et al: A safety study of a perfluorochemical emulsion, oxygent™, in anesthetized surgical patients. Anesthesiology 81:A397, 1994
28. Wahr JA, Trowborst A, Spence RK: A pilot study of the efficacy of an oxygen carrying emulsion, oxygent™, in patients undergoing surgical blood loss. Anesthesiology 81:A313, 1994
29. Gronert G, Messick J, Cucciara R, et al: Paradoxical air embolism from a probe - patent foramen ovale. Anesthesiology 50:548-549, 1979
30. Oka Y, Inoue T, Hong Y, et al: Retained intracardiac air. Transesophageal echocardiography for definition of incidence and monitoring removal by improved techniques. J Thorac Cardiovasc Surg 91:329-338, 1986
31. Butler B, Hills B: Transpulmonary passage of venous air emboli. J Appl Physiol 59:543-547, 1985
32. Justice C, Leach J, Edwards WS: The harmful effects in treatment of coronary air embolism during heart surgery. Ann Thorac Surg 14:45-53, 1972
33. Perkins-Pearson N, Marshall W, Bedford R: Atrial pressures in the seated position. Anesthesiology 57:493-497, 1982
34. Spiess BD, McCarthy R, Piotrowski D, Ivankovich AD: Protection from venous air embolism with fluorocarbon emulsion FC-43. J Surg Res 41:439-444, 1986
35. Tuman KJ, Spiess BD, McCarthy RJ, et al: Cardiorespiratory effects of venous air embolism in dogs receiving a perfluorocarbon emulsion. J Neurosurg 65:238-244, 1986
36. Spiess BD, Braverman B, Woronowicz AW, Ivankovich AD: Protection from cerebral air emboli with perfluorocarbons in rabbits. Stroke 17:1146-1149, 1986
37. Menasch'e P, Pinard E, Desroches AM, et al: Fluorocarbons: A potential treatment of cerebral air emboli in open heart surgery. Ann Thorac Surg 40:494-497, 1985
38. Spiess BD, McCarthy RJ, Tuman KJ, Ivankovich AD: Protection from coronary air embolism by a perfluorocarbon emulsion (FC-43). J Cardiothorac Anesth 1:210-215, 1987

39. Cassuto Y, Nunnely SA, Fahri LE: Inert gas washout in rats: enhancement by fluorocarbon infusion. Aerosp Med 45:12-14, 1974
40. Spiess BD, McCarthy RJ, Tuman KJ: Treatment of decompression sickness with a perfluorocarbon emulsion (FC-43). Undersea Biomed Res 15:31-37, 1988
41. Novotny JA, Bridgewater BJ, Himm JF, Homer LD: Quantifying the effect of intravascular perfluorocarbon on xenon elimination from canine muscle. J Appl Physiol 74:1356-1360, 1993
42. Spiess BD, Cochran RP, Kunzelman K, et al: Cerebral protection from massive air embolism with a perfluorocarbon emulsion prime addition for cardiopulmonary bypass. Anesthesiology 81:A692, 1994
43. Boernert P, Dreher W, Schneider W: 19F chemical shift imaging in perfluorocarbons. NMR Biomed 2:278-283, 1989
44. Mason RP, Antich PP, Babcock EE, et al: Perfluorocarbon imaging in vivo. A 19F MRI study in tumor-bearing mice. Mag Res Imag 7:475-485, 1989
45. Curtis SE, Fuhrman BP, Howland DF, et al: Cardiac output during liquid (perfluorocarbon) breathing in newborn piglets. Crit Care Med 19:225-230, 1991
46. Leach CL, Fuhrman BP, Morin FC 3rd, Roth MG. Perfluorocarbon-associated gas exchange (partial liquid ventilation) in respiratory distress syndrome: A prospective, randomized, controlled study. Crit Care Med 21:1270-1278, 1993
47. Coleman CN, Bump EA, Kramer RA. Chemical modifiers of cancer treatment. J Clin Oncol 6:709-733, 1988

PRINCIPLES OF HEMODYNAMIC MANAGEMENT*

Robert N. Sladen, MB, MRCP(UK), FRCP(C)

CARDIAC FUNCTION AND FAILURE

Measurement of cardiac output provides a global index of oxygen delivery, if arterial oxygen content is optimal. However, one or two caveats apply. Abnormal distribution of peripheral blood flow, such as occurs in sepsis (distributive shock), leads to inadequate oxygen supply to affected tissues despite a quantitatively normal cardiac output. Regional blood flow alterations that may occur in shock are not reflected in the simple mathematical calculation of DO_2. Nevertheless, a decrease in total cardiac output leads to a decrease in DO_2, so a consideration of factors that affect cardiac output are germane to any discussion of shock.

Cardiac output is the product of stroke volume (SV) and heart rate (HR). The most important clinical determinants of cardiac function are heart rate and rhythm, preload, afterload, and contractility. Contractility and heart rate are intrinsic myocardial properties; preload and afterload depend on both myocardial and peripheral vascular function. Indeed, cardiac function is coupled intimately to the vascular system: the heart pumps blood into the circulation, which determines the quantity of blood returned and the impedance to flow. Clearly, both intrinsic myocardial performance and the vascular status determine cardiac output, and both may be altered in the vascular surgery patient.

Preload

The Frank-Starling hypothesis evolved in separate laboratories to support the concept that increased diastolic ventricular distention (preload) causes a cor-

*Extracted, with permission, from: Sladen RN, Doherty D. Low Output States in the Postoperative Period. In: Kaplan J (ed.). Vascular Anesthesia. Churchill Livingstone, New York, pp 603-642, 1991.

T. H. Stanley and P. L. Bailey (eds.), Anesthesiology and the Cardiovascular Patient, 143–174.

responding increase in ventricular output (1,2). The relationship between a given index of preload (e.g., left ventricular end-diastolic volume) and output (e.g., stroke volume index) is described by a left ventricular function curve. Alterations in left ventricular contractility, compliance, or afterload shift the curve to the left or the right and alter the output response to a given preload. Myocardial depression and failure shifts the curve rightwards and downwards, so that for a given preload, output is decreased. In the failing heart, the curve becomes flattened, so that increases in preload result in pulmonary congestion and edema rather than increases in output.

Traditional clinical correlates of preload derived by invasive hemodynamic monitoring use pressure indices such as central venous pressure (CVP), left atrial pressure (LAP), and pulmonary artery occlusion pressure (PAOP). The usefulness of pressure indices of preload depends on the ventricular diastolic pressure-volume relationship, i.e., ventricular diastolic compliance. With increased ventricular compliance (e.g., in mitral regurgitation), large changes in end-diastolic volume are associated with small changes in end-diastolic pressure. Thus, LAP or PAOP provide unreliable correlates with ventricular preload. With decreased ventricular compliance (e.g., ventricular hypertrophy), small changes in end-diastolic volume are associated with large changes in end-diastolic pressure. LAP or PAOP provide sensitive indicators of preload alteration. Instantaneous increases in compliance (e.g., acute myocardial ischemia) reflect increases in ventricular stiffness rather than increased preload *per se*. The smaller, thinner right ventricle is substantially more compliant than the left ventricles, so that even in normal patients the CVP is an insensitive index of left ventricular filling; this disparity is exacerbated by left ventricular stiffness and failure. The introduction of two-dimensional transesophageal echocardiography (TEE) affords direct estimation of left ventricular end-diastolic volume in the OR and ICU. This, correlated with simultaneously measured pressures, has increased our understanding of dynamic pressure-volume relationships in low cardiac output syndromes.

During hypovolemia, left ventricular filling pressures are maintained by increased vasomotor tone and enhanced blood return to the heart—a passive response to altered vascular function. Indeed, this is an important compensatory mechanism in low cardiac output states. Intense venoconstriction may actually elevate venous pressures despite hypovolemia, giving a false impression of intravascular volume—with dramatic consequences when venoconstriction is abolished by sedation or anesthesia. With myocardial depression, left ventricular filling pressures increase despite normovolemia—an active response to altered myocardial function. Both scenarios demonstrate the coupling of vascular and myocardial function.

Afterload

Ventricular afterload is generally defined as the intramyocardial systolic wall tension, or "wall stress". It is directly related to the impedance to ventricular outflow, and a very important determinant of the pressure work of the ventricle. The La Place relationship, which is used to describe surface tension in a sphere, relates the components of afterload, as follows:

$$\text{Wall tension} = P\,r\,/\,2\,t$$

where P = pressure generated in the myocardium during systole (especially during isovolumic contraction), r = intracavitory radius, and t = ventricular wall thickness.

The response to an acute increase in afterload (systolic pressure work) is an acute increase in preload (diastolic filling), which maintains cardiac output. After several beats, ventricular performance tends to improve, perhaps reflecting recovery from subendocardial ischemia (Anrep effect) (3). Further increases in afterload cause compensation until the limit of preload reserve is reached, after which cardiac failure and pulmonary edema occur. Chronic increases in myocardial afterload (e.g., in aortic stenosis) results in concentric hypertrophy of the left ventricle. That this is an appropriate compensatory mechanism is understood by again examining the La Place relationship: the decrease in intracavitory radius and increase in ventricular wall thickness modify the increases in wall tension caused by increased intramyocardial systolic wall pressure.

An ischemic or scarred left ventricle (and a normal right ventricle) operates close to its limit of preload reserve, and is exquisitely sensitive to increases in afterload. The more impaired the left ventricle, the less it responds to inotropic stimulation and the more dependent it becomes on the therapeutic reduction of afterload by vasodilator therapy.

Systolic wall tension may be calculated by analyzing the area under a ventricular pressure tracing (systolic pressure-time index, SPTI), and approximated by a peripheral arterial tracing. In the absence of mechanical outflow obstruction, the most important determinant of ventricular afterload is peripheral resistance (R), derived by Ohm's Law of the circulation:

$$BP = CO \times R$$
$$R = BP / CO$$

Rather artificial pressure gradients are used to derive systemic and pulmonary vascular resistances (SVR, PVR):

$$SVR = (MAP - CVP / CO) \times 80 \quad dyne{\cdot}sec{\cdot}cm^{-5}$$

$$PVR = (MPAP - PAOP / CO) \times 80 \quad dyne{\cdot}sec{\cdot}cm^{-5}$$

where MAP = mean arterial pressure, CVP = central venous pressure, MPAP = mean pulmonary artery pressure, PAOP = pulmonary artery occlusion pressure, and CO = cardiac output. The factor of 80 converts from Wood units to SI units. "Normal" SVR is in the range of 800 to 1500 dyne·sec·cm^{-5}, and "normal" PVR is 50 to 150 dyne·sec·cm^{-5}.

A number of caveats apply to the clinical use of calculated vascular resistance. Thermodilution cardiac output estimation carries an inherent variability of 10 to 15%; in the calculation of vascular resistance this error is magnified by a factor of 80. Measured CVP probably bears little relationship to the systemic arterial pressure gradient, which should ideally be represented by mean arterial pressure minus precapillary arteriolar pressure. Small errors in PAOP measurement cause large errors in the estimation of PVR. Although the alteration in SVR with changes in blood pressure and cardiac output is relatively linear, the pulmonary circulation is much more complex and PVR is not inversely related to cardiac output at equal pulmonary artery pressures. The "normal" range of vascular resistance depends on the "normal" range of cardiac output. Since this is dependent on body size, *cardiac index* should be used to derive a *vascular resistance index* to define normality. For example, a 100 kg patient should have a higher resting cardiac output than a 50 kg patient. Thus "normal" SVR for a large patient tends toward 800, and that for a small patient toward 1500 dyne·sec·cm^{-5}, with identical hemodynamic states. Nonetheless non-indexed SVR and PVR are clinically useful to examine alterations in hemodynamic status when the patient is used as his/her own control.

Vascular resistance varies inversely with the arterial radius to the fourth power, i.e., small decreases in radius cause large increases in resistance. However, blood viscosity (affected by blood temperature and hematocrit) is also an important determinant of vascular resistance. Finally, in the presence of ven tricular outflow tract obstruction (e.g., aortic stenosis, idiopathic subaortic stenosis) systemic vascular resistance is completely dissociated from intramyocardial systolic pressure and is a meaningless indicator of myocardial afterload.

Contractility

Contractility may be described as the intrinsic myocardial force of contraction developed at a given resting myocardial fiber length. It is usually expressed in terms of change in fiber length per unit time (velocity of fiber shortening, dl/dt) or change in ventricular pressure per unit time (dp/dt). The contractile state can be theoretically defined by the velocity of fiber shortening at zero afterload, i.e., where velocity would be maximal (V_{max}).

Cardiac output generated at a given contractile state depends on loading conditions, i.e., preload and afterload effects—but changes in preload and afterload do not alter the intrinsic contractile state: V_{max} is unchanged. A decrease in cardiac output under the same loading conditions represents a decrease in the contractile state (negative inotropic effect), and vice versa (positive inotropic effect). Clinical measurement of contractility requires elaborate and invasive monitoring (e.g., a left ventricular catheter to measure dp/dt). Instead, the contractile state is *inferred* by ventricular function curves.

Heart Rate

Heart rate determines cardiac output at any given stroke volume. It is also the most important clinical determinant of myocardial oxygen balance. Increase in heart rate occurs at the expense of diastolic time, i.e., during maximal coronary perfusion to the left ventricle. If heart rate is too slow, cardiac output may be inadequate despite maximal increases in stroke volume and enhanced coronary perfusion time. If heart rate is too fast, the shortened diastolic time prevents adequate ventricular filling and coronary perfusion, so that cardiac output decreases and myocardial oxygen imbalance results. The latter effect is enhanced by the increase in myocardial oxygen consumption caused by tachycardia, because of increased systolic work per minute. In addition, contractile force increases with increased contractile frequency; this is known as the staircase or *Treppe* phenomenon, or Bowditch effect, and is calcium dependent (4.5). (This effect is actually more apparent in the anesthetized animal or depressed heart than in an intact, conscious individual).

Increased heart rate is an essential compensatory mechanism (and important clinical sign) when stroke volume is decreased by hypovolemia or myocardial ischemia. Bradycardia induced by sinus node disease or negatively chronotropic drugs exacerbates low cardiac output. However, compared with other mechanisms of increasing cardiac output (preload augmentation, afterload reduction, positive inotropism), increased heart rate is the most expensive in terms of myocardial oxygen balance. In the presence of myocardial ischemia and low cardiac output, it remains a clinical dilemma as to what increase in heart rate will take advantage of the Treppe phenomenon without exacerbating ischemia.

PRINCIPLES OF HEMODYNAMIC MANAGEMENT

Regardless of the etiology of the low cardiac output syndrome, an effective approach to hemodynamic management must follow a logical, orderly sequence based on accurate clinical and hemodynamic data.

1. Stabilize Heart Rhythm And Rate

Disturbances of heart rhythm and rate are very often secondary to hypovolemia, myocardial ischemia, or metabolic derangements, and may be refractory to therapy until the underlying disorder is corrected. Indeed, tachycardia and tachyarrhythmias are important clinical markers of the severity of illness. Spontaneous resolution or a sustained response to therapy generally indicates that the patient's overall condition is improving, and *vice versa*. On the other hand, bradycardia and bradyarrhythmias more commonly reflect underlying conduction system disease or drug toxicity. As long as the heart rhythm and rate are unstable, it will be very difficult to achieve a meaningful hemodynamic assessment and optimize the other determinants of cardiac function.

Sinus Tachycardia

Sinus tachycardia is an appropriate reflex physiologic response to low stroke volume, whether it is due to hypovolemia or cardiac failure. Excessive tachycardia (>120 beats/min) may be due to pain, acute myocardial ischemia, hypoxemia, or hypercarbia, which should be identified and aggressively treated. In compensated low output states, attempts to slow sinus tachycardia with beta blockers are likely to cause acute hemodynamic decompensation. Instead, the underlying cause of shock must be treated.

The most immediate indicator of an improvement in stroke volume in response to fluid, inotropic, or vasodilator therapy is a decrease in the rate of sinus tachycardia. For example, two serial measurements of cardiac output may both be 5.0 l/min; and a superficial assessment might suggest no change in hemodynamic status. However, if the heart rate with the first is 120 beats/min and with the second 90 beats/min, the implication is a substantial improvement in myocardial function (calculated stroke volume increases by 33%, i.e., from 42 ml/beat to 56 ml/beat).

Heart rates of >160 beats/min are more likely to be due to supraventricular tachyarrhythmias.

Supraventricular Tachyarrhythmias

These include atrial tachycardia, atrial flutter and atrial fibrillation.

The etiology of supraventricular tachyarrhythmias is multifactorial. Amongst the most important is high circulating endogenous catecholamines, which is an implicit component of the low cardiac output state. Other factors which increase catecholamines include pain, acidosis, hypoxemia and hypercarbia. Arrhythmia threshold is decreased by hypokalemia, hypomagnesemia or hypercalcemia. In this milieu supraventricular tachyarrhythmias are more likely to occur as a dose-related side effect of any inotropic agent. Direct mechanical stimulation of the right atrium by the tip of a deeply placed central venous catheter is obvious in retrospect, but may be missed unless sought.

Therapeutic interventions may be transiently successful, but are unlikely to cause sustained resolution until most if not all of the above factors are corrected.

Patients with chronic atrial fibrillation represent a special challenge. First, there is usually some form of underlying heart disease (valvular, ischemic or hypertensive). Second, their cardiovascular reserve is compromised by the lack of an atrial kick, and they will develop a low cardiac output syndrome with a lesser insult. Conversion to sinus rhythm is usually impossible. Although increases in ventricular response rate occur with hypovolemia or other causes of increased sympathetic tone, they are irregular and unpredictable, and may further compromise ventricular filling in a diseased heart. On the other hand, increased endogenous and exogenous catecholamines may render it impossible to slow fast ventricular response rates; attempts at pushing digoxin invariably result in toxicity.

In patients with severe obstructive lung disease undergoing major vascular surgery, multifocal atrial tachycardia (MAT) is an important and often poorly treatable contributor to hemodynamic instability in the perioperative period. It is a rapid, chaotic atrial arrhythmia often difficult to distinguish from atrial fibrillation. It is usually refractory to digoxin and responds best to verapamil or esmolol, whose negative inotropic effects to all intents and purpose contraindicate their use in low cardiac output states.

Sinus Bradycardia and Conduction Problems

Although sinus bradycardia is usually defined as a heart rate less than 60 beats/min, in the presence of the other manifestations of a low cardiac output syndrome, a heart rate less than 90 beats/min is quite inappropriate and suggests some underlying conduction disease. This is particularly likely if a slow heart rate has been noted both before and during surgery. The most common cause is sinus node fibrosis due to aging or ischemic heart disease. A previous history of palpitations or syncope is suggestive of a sick sinus syndrome; this diagnosis is likely if there are intermittent supraventricular tachyarrhythmias, either spontaneously or with chronotropic therapy. Preoperative therapy with long-acting beta blockers, notably nadolol, but also occasionally atenolol, can cause sinus bradycardia extending into the postoperative period. Sinus bradycardia also occurs with severe hypothermia (central temperature less than 33°C) which can occur with massive blood transfusion.

Acute onset of bradycardia or bradyarrhythmias may occur with digitalis toxicity or acute inferior myocardial ischemia or infarction. Digitalis-induced conduction problems are enhanced by acute hyperkalemia and metabolic acidosis, which are common in low output shock, and include wandering atrial pacemaker, junctional rhythm, second-degree heart block (Mobitz type I, Wenckebach phenomenon) and complete heart block. However, conduction block may coexist with tachyarrhythmias (e.g., paroxysmal atrial tachycardia with block).

For brief episodes of bradycardia or heart block, intravenous anticholinergic agents such as atropine 0.5 mg or glycopyrrolate 0.2 mg may be sufficient to overcome vagal tone. However, repeated doses may result in a central anticholinergic syndrome. "Pharmacological pacing" with isoproterenol (2 mg in 250 ml D5W, start at 0.01 μg/kg/min) can be useful for sinus bradycardia because its chronotropic effect is so potent; the heart rate can be carefully titrated to a more physiologic rate. However, if the sinus node is resistant to isoproterenol, increasing dosage results in increasing peripheral vasodilation. In patients with a true sick sinus syndrome, isoproterenol can precipitate tachyarrhythmias.

Electrical pacing is the safest, most reliable method of treating bradyarrhythmias. In particular, if a combination of conduction disease and irritability exists (digitalis toxicity, sick sinus syndrome), it allows treatment of the tachyarrhythmias while supporting the possibility of complete heart block. A transvenous pacemaker can usually be placed via the right internal jugular approach without difficulty, and capture achieved by monitoring the P wave on an electrocardiogram attached to the pacing wire, with or without the help of fluoroscopy. There is always a concern that a pacing wire may entangle a pulmonary artery catheter already in place, but in the authors' experience, this has not represented a problem.

An alternative approach is to utilize a pulmonary artery catheter with integrated pacing capability. A number of products are now available that allow the passage of a pacing wire via a right ventricular port. Ventricular capture is usually obtained and maintained reliably. A new catheter which also provides an atrial pacing wire has recently been introduced. This has the distinct advantage of allowing atrial and/or atrioventricular sequential pacing, which is a great advantage in low cardiac output states because provision of an atrial kick can increase cardiac output by up to 40%. An earlier type, the so-called multipurpose catheter, which has the atrial and ventricular wires fused to the catheter itself, does not provide reliable pacing. A drawback of all these pulmonary artery catheters is that it may be impossible to achieve balloon occlusion of the pulmonary artery and pace simultaneously. They also preclude the use of continuous monitoring of mixed venous oxygen saturation, which may be extremely helpful in managing low cardiac output states.

Finally, if access for transvenous pacing is difficult or impossible, an external pacemaker (usually integrated with a defibrillator unit) can provide life-saving temporary ventricular pacing (6). Because there is a tendency to pace large muscle groups ("pace the entire patient"), the patient should be kept sedated, if possible.

Ventricular Arrhythmias

Ventricular ectopy and tachycardia share the same etiologic factors as supraventricular tachyarrhythmias. However, one the most important and ominous signs of acute myocardial ischemia is the onset of increasing ventricular irritability. In cardiogenic shock, recurrent ventricular arrhythmias may become increasingly refractory to therapy and are often the cause of death. Signs that suggest "malignant" ventricular ectopic activity (i.e., likely to progress to ventricular tachycardia) include multifocal ectopics, ventricular bigeminy or trigeminy, or "R on T" phenomenon (ectopic beat starts during preceding T wave).

2. *Optimize Preload*

Identify Optimal Preload

Optimal preload is not that filling pressure which happens to fall within the normal range (4 to 12 mmHg), but that which provides the most effective cardiac function under prevailing conditions of contractility and afterload.

In hypovolemic shock, optimal preload is obtained when cardiac function is sufficiently enhanced to restore vital organ perfusion. This includes improvement in mental status and cutaneous perfusion; a cardiac index greater than 2.2 $l/min/m^2$ and mixed venous oxygen saturation (SvO_2) greater than 65%; adequate stroke volume (i.e., heart rate less than 120 beats/min); stable blood pressure, and urine flow greater than 1.0 ml/kg/hr.

In cardiogenic shock, optimal preload is obtained when cardiac function is sufficiently enhanced to maintain the above indices but with a lessening of pulmonary congestion and edema, at least to a level that is readily managed by relatively low levels of inspired oxygen fraction (F_IO_2) and positive end-expiratory pressure (PEEP).

Restore Deficient Preload

In hypovolemic shock the most fundamental step in management is to restore deficient cardiac preload. Optimal filling pressure is achieved by a series of fluid challenges (see below), each followed by a careful hemodynamic profile to assess the effect on heart rate, blood pressure, filling pressures, cardiac output, stroke volume, calculated SVR, and urine flow. An effective response is indicated by an improvement in these parameters as the filling pressure is increased. Aggressive fluid administration should be continued until either hemodynamic stability is achieved, cardiac output no longer increases with each challenge (i.e., the "flat part" of the Starling curve has been reached) or there is evidence of pulmonary dysfunction caused by increasing extravascular lung water, suggested by new onset of rales, lung stiffness, and worsening intrapulmonary shunt. At this point if the patient is still unstable, inotropic support should be added to enhance contractility and decrease the filling pressure required for a given stroke volume.

Blood transfusion

The hematocrit is an extremely misleading index of red cell volume with acute hemorrhage; indeed, with severe fluid sequestration and hemoconcentration, the hematocrit may be *increased* despite major blood loss. Packed RBCs should be given on the basis of estimated blood losses even if the hematocrit appears normal, particularly if it starts to decrease with infusion of nonblood fluids. There is no clear agreement as to the ideal hematocrit. However, it seems reasonable to achieve an hematocrit of at least 30% to obtain adequate oxygen delivery without compromising capillary perfusion; in patients with active myocardial ischemia or severe pulmonary dysfunction it would not be unreasonable to achieve 34%.

Crystalloid versus colloid

Controversy has existed for decades regarding the relative advantages and drawbacks of crystalloid versus colloid solutions in the treatment of shock. No one has been able to show a significant difference in outcome. In this authors' opinion, as long as continued and aggressive efforts are made to restore and expand the intravascular volume, it doesn't really matter which fluid is used!

Advantages attributed to colloid solutions (e.g., 25% or 5% human albumin, 5% purified plasma derivative, 6% hetastarch, 10% pentastarch) which justify their increased cost are based on their ability to rapidly expand the intravascular volume to a greater degree than their actual volume by their osmotic effect on drawing extravascular fluid into the plasma space (7). Human blood derivatives (albumin, plasma protein fraction) are heat treated to remove any possibility of disease transmission. However, colloid solutions do not rehydrate the extracellular volume, which may be depleted. If they did diffuse out of the plasma in the presence of a capillary leak syndrome, they could draw fluid with them and exacerbate interstitial (especially pulmonary) edema. Large volumes of plasma expanders hasten the onset of dilutional coagulopathy; in addition, hetastarch coats platelets and impairs their aggregation. In the mid-1970's there were several reports of paradoxic hypotension associated with the rapid administration of plasma protein fraction, attributed to the presence of Hageman-factor fragments (prekallikrein activator) and the formation of bradykinin (8), although this does not appear to have been a problem in recent years.

Crystalloids (0.9% saline, lactated Ringer's solution) have the advantage of being cheap, readily available, and associated with a virtually zero possibility of adverse reaction. They readily diffuse into the interstitial space so that plasma expansion and preload augmentation is not as rapid nor as striking as that achieved by colloids; however, in the longer term their ability to rehydrate the extracellular fluid may offset this. In a capillary leak syndrome they do not increase interstitial osmotic pressure and are more readily removed by diffusion back into the intravascular space than colloids when the Starling equilibrium is restored. The main disadvantage of crystalloids is that in hemorrhagic shock much larger volumes of fluid (up to four times) are required for an equivalent increase in preload, leading to at times extraordinarily large increases in total body water and weight gain(9). Large amounts of normal saline (154 mEq chloride per liter) may lead to a hyperchloremic metabolic acidosis; lactated Ringer's contains 28 mEq/liter of lactate (which can buffer hydrogen ion but later manifest as a metabolic alkalosis) and 3 mEq/liter calcium (which could cause clot formation if mixed with citrated blood).

There is evidence that the judicious use of hypertonic (3% to 7.5%) saline ("hot saline") can provide greater hemodynamic response and improved outcome in experimental hemorrhagic shock with less increase in total body water, extravascular lung water and intracranial pressure than standard crystalloid solutions (10,11). However, its use in an uncontrolled hemorrhage model actually resulted in increased bleeding (perhaps due to rapid volume expansion) and mortality (12). Clinical studies in humans are required before its use can be advocated for hemorrhagic shock after aortic aneurysm surgery.

Decrease Excessive Preload

In states of severe myocardial depression with flattening of the Frank-Starling left ventricular function curve, the administration of fluid to maintain blood pressure readily results in excessive preload. This has a number of adverse effects. High cardiac filling pressures are transmitted through the pulmonary circulation, causing pulmonary congestion and edema, increased intrapulmonary shunt and hypoxemia, and predisposing to atelectasis and pneumonia. Acute respiratory failure occurs quickly. Excessive preload directly increases end-diastolic intracavitory radius, and thereby intramyocardial systolic wall stress, afterload, and myocardial oxygen consumption. Elevated left ventricular diastolic pressure compresses the subendocardium and worsens its perfusion. A vicious cycle of myocardial ischemia, hypoxemia and acute cardiac failure develops.

Diuretic therapy

Loop diuretics. Attempts to increase urine flow with loop diuretics (e.g., furosemide, ethacrynic acid) are unlikely to be successful as long as hemodynamic instability persists. This is because renal venoconstriction is intense and renal blood flow diminished in low cardiac output states. In animal studies the administration of furosemide increases renal cortical blood flow, and when given with low-dose dopamine, protects against ischemic renal injury; however, the diuretic effect needs to be in place *before* the onset of ischemia to be beneficial (13). Rapid intravenous administration of loop diuretics is associated with venodilation, which may cause abrupt hypotension. Lucas et al. in attempting to convert oliguric to nonoliguric acute renal failure with furosemide, found that it increased urine flow and osmolar and sodium clearance, but produced no change in glomerular filtration rate, renal blood flow, or distribution of intrarenal perfusion. In addition, 20% of the critically ill patients in whom furosemide was used had a dramatic decrease in blood pressure two to ten hours later (14).

In sum, loop diuretic response is difficult to predict, and a short-lived but brisk increase in urine flow may decrease intravascular volume excessively, requiring additional fluid administration and defeating the object of therapy. Instead, lung function should be supported by mechanical ventilation and PEEP, and diuretic therapy should be reserved for the stage of hemodynamic recovery, when dramatic fluid mobilization may be very well tolerated. Continuous infusion of furosemide (2.5-15 mg/hr) may be very useful in providing a smooth, rather than intermittent, diuresis which can be fairly precisely controlled by adjusting the infusion rate; it is also likely to be more effective than bolus furosemide in patients with diminished glomerular filtration rate (15,16,17).

Dopamine. Dopamine in the "low-dose" range (0.5-2.0 μg/kg/min) has a predominant action on dopaminergic (DA_1) receptors located on vascular smooth muscle cells in the renal and splanchnic vasculature and on renal tubular cells, causing vasodilation, increased renal blood flow and glomerular filtration rate, and saluresis (18,19). Additional vasodilation is caused by activation of DA_2 receptors on sympathetic nerve terminals, by inhibiting adenylate cyclase and norepinephrine release.

Low-dose dopamine is much more likely to cause a sustained increase in urinary flow than the loop diuretics, while conferring some renal protection (indeed, it may also have a salutary effect in modifying splanchnic ischemia induced by low cardiac output). In addition, there is some animal evidence that low-dose dopamine maintains renal blood flow in the face of norepinephrine-induced vasoconstriction (20). For this reason, it is our practice to use a continuous infusion of 1-2 μg/kg/min dopamine whenever more potent inotropic or vasopressor agents are administered (see below). Even low-dose dopamine may have a substantial chronotropic or arrhythmogenic effect in some patients, which may limit its use (21). Rarely, its vasodilator effect exacerbates hypotension.

Venodilator therapy

Nitroglycerin (NTG). NTG is a rapidly acting vasodilator agent with a predominant effect on the venous side of the circulation. However, it must be carefully titrated through its low-dose range (0.5-1.5 μg/kg/min), because with increasing dosage it causes arteriolar dilation and systemic hypotension. Its primary benefit is to improve myocardial oxygen balance, which it does by several mechanisms: direct coronary artery vasodilation, preferential dilation of epicardial (conductance) arterioles, and (at low dosage) decrease in left ventricular end-diastolic pressure without a decrease in aortic diastolic pressure. The net effect is to decrease heart size, improve the transmyocardial gradient of coronary perfusion, and increase blood flow into areas of ischemic myocardium. Excessive reduction in preload may result in decreased cardiac output (22).

The major limitation to the use of NTG is systemic hypotension and reflex tachycardia, which negates its benefit on myocardial oxygen balance. In the presence of acute myocardial ischemia without cardiac failure, coronary perfusion pressure may be maintained and reflex tachycardia avoided by the simultaneous infusion of phenylephrine. However, the adverse effects of α-adrenergic systemic vasoconstriction on cardiac afterload negates the beneficial effect of NTG when PAOP exceeds 15 mmHg (23,24)'. In addition, although NTG may decrease pulmonary congestion by reducing left ventricular filling pressures, oxygenation may actually worsen as hypoxic pulmonary vasoconstriction is overcome and intrapulmonary shunting increases (this is a potentially adverse effect of all vasodilator agents).

Inotropic support

Inotropic support can decrease excessive preload by shifting the left ventricular Frank-Starling function curve upwards and to the left, i.e., a given stroke volume is achieved at a lower filling pressure. Required preload is further decreased if inotropic support is combined with arterial vasodilation and afterload reduction ("inodilation"). However, increased myocardial oxygen consumption caused by increased contractility and heart rate may negate the benefit provided by preload reduction. These approaches are discussed below.

3. *Enhance Contractility*

Normalize pH and Electrolyte Milieu

An important early step in improving the inotropic state of the myocardium is to correct metabolic acidosis. When pH is less than 7.25, myocardial response to catecholamines is depressed, and with prolonged duration of shock, the left ventricular function curve becomes progressively shifted down and to the right. Mechanical minute ventilation (V_E) should be increased to provide respiratory compensation as long as it does not embarrass the circulation. Sodium bicarbonate, usually given in 50 mEq aliquots (50 ml of 8% $NaHCO_3$) should be administered not by any preassigned formula but guided by repeated estimation of arterial blood gases (ABGs), with the goal of achieving a pH of equal or greater than 7.25. In states of severe lactic acidosis, it may be necessary to provide a continuous $NaHCO_3$ infusion, but this should be discontinued as soon as the pH is consistently above 7.25. Serial estimation of serum lactate levels (normal, less than 2.0 mEq/liter) may be helpful in assessing the response to therapy and improvement or deterioration at the microcirculatory level.

Calcium ion is essential for normal contractility of cardiac and smooth muscle (see below). Ionized hypocalcemia (normal, 1-1.25 mM/l or 4.1-5.1 mg/dl) occurs during very rapid administration of citrated blood, i.e., during resuscitation in hemorrhagic shock. If hypocalcemia is suspected or measured, 10% calcium chloride (which provides 13.4 mEq Ca^{2+} per gram) can be given slowly I.V., up to 10-20 mg/kg. This may have the effect of markedly enhancing the response to catecholamines; blood pressure increases because of increased contractility and peripheral vasoconstriction. Administration of calcium exacerbates the arrhythmogenic effect of hypokalemia, and both the therapeutic and toxic effects of digoxin.

Hyperkalemia may be caused by muscle ischemia, acute renal insufficiency, excessive administration of potassium supplements, or use of α-adrenergic agents (phenylephrine). Not only does potassium in excess threaten cardiac conduction (asystolic arrest being the primary fear), but it also exerts a negative inotropic effect. A serum potassium level greater than 6.0 mEq/l should be aggressively treated with calcium chloride, hyperventilation, sodium bicarbonate or insulin and glucose.

Select Appropriate Inotropic Agent

Mechanisms of cardiac inotropy

The contractile state of cardiac muscle depends on the number of cross bridges formed between actin and myosin. Tropomyosin inhibits this interaction. Calcium ion associates with troponin, and the complex formed alters tropomyosin, allowing actin and myosin to interact. The more calcium available, the greater the force of contraction. Dissociation of calcium from troponin-C reverses the process and relaxation occurs.

Membrane depolarization is caused by sodium influx through fast sodium channels, followed by calcium influx through slow calcium channels. The influx of calcium stimulates further release of calcium from the sarcoplasmic reticulum (25). The ubiquitous intracellular second messenger, cyclic adenosine monophosphate (cAMP), is formed from ATP by membrane-bound adenylate cyclase, and controls intracellular calcium concentration. Adenylate cyclase activity and cAMP production is stimulated by catecholamine activation of β-adrenergic receptors. Cyclic AMP activates cAMP-dependent protein kinases that facilitate calcium influx by phosphorylating slow calcium channels (26). Degradation of cAMP is accomplished specifically by phosphodiesterase III.

Inotropic agents act at any point in the above processes to increase free intracellular calcium, enhance the sensitivity of contractile elements to calcium, or both. [α-adrenergic receptors, coupled to the polyphosphoinositide second messenger system, also mediate increased myocardial contraction—slower and more sustained—when stimulated (27).]

Sympathomimetic amines (catecholamines)

β-phenylethylamine, a benzene ring with an ethylamine side chain, constitutes the structural basis for all sympathomimetic amines. Substitutions of hydroxyl groups at the 3 and 4 positions of the benzene ring (catecholamines), or the alpha and beta carbons of the ethylamine side chain distinguish the compounds.

Inotropic effect depends on cardiac β_1 adrenergic stimulation. However, this is inevitably accompanied by greater or lesser chronotropic, dromotropic and bathmotropic effects, resulting in (unwanted) tachycardia, accelerated cardiac conduction and/or tachyarrhythmias. Although a few sympathomimetic agents have pure β-adrenergic activity, most agents have mixed effects. Peripheral action may be predominantly vasodilator (i.e., β_2 adrenergic effect: isoproterenol, dobutamine) or vasoconstrictor (i.e., α_1 adrenergic effect: norepinephrine, high-dose dopamine). Salutary effects of the latter may occur not simply by increased myocardial contractility, but rather as a result of potent venoconstrictor effects and enhanced preload (an effect that could be achieved by less dramatic interventions) (28). The catecholamines listed below are presented in order of frequency of use at our institutions.

Dopamine hydrochloride. Dopamine, the metabolic precursor of norepinephrine and epinephrine, acts directly on α-, β- and dopaminergic receptors, but about 50% of its action is indirect, mediated through the release of norepinephrine from nerve terminals (29). It is therefore less effective when norepinephrine stores are depleted, as in chronic cardiomyopathy or severe myocardial dysfunction.

Dopamine's major advantage is that in the low-dose range (0.5-2.0 μg/kg/min) it selectively acts on dopaminergic receptors in the renal and splanchnic beds (see above). Low-dose dopamine infusion may be used as a diuretic, or to protect the kidneys from renal vasoconstrictor effects of more potent vasopressor drugs. In the dose range of 3 to 10 μg/kg/min dopamine has a predominantly β_1 adrenergic action on cardiac contractility, but some dopaminergic action remains. For this reason it has remained the first-line agent to provide moderate inotropic support for the last two decades. In this range there is a low incidence of tachyarrhythmias or myocardial ischemia.

Dopamine maintains blood pressure through peripheral α_1 adrenergic vasoconstrictor activity even in the presence of moderate hypovolemia, and allows independent titration of SVR (and thereby afterload) by vasodilators such as sodium nitroprusside. Above a dosage of 10 μg/kg/minute, its α-adrenergic and chronotropic effects become increasingly prominent, resulting in cutaneous and splanchnic vasoconstriction, oliguria and tachyarrhythmias, and it offers little advantage over the potent α-adrenergic effects of norepinephrine [in fact, plasma norepinephrine levels increase progressively as dopamine dose is increased]. Dopamine has also been shown to increase diaphragmatic blood flow and strength in patients with chronic obstructive lung disease, which may be of additional benefit in this population of patients being treated for low cardiac output (30).

Epinephrine. Epinephrine infusion is usually indicated when the inotropic effect of dopamine is inadequate despite a dose of 7 to 10 μg/kg/min. Epinephrine is a direct-acting catecholamine, with very potent cardiac β_1 adrenergic activity. Its peripheral receptor effects are mixed, with β_2 mediated vasodilation on muscular arterioles, and an α_1 vasoconstrictor effect on the cutaneous and splanchnic beds. As the dose of epinephrine is increased, receptor effects range from predominantly β- (25-50 ng/kg/min), combined α- and β-, and ultimately predominant α-adrenergic (75-100 ng/kg/min) (31). The net effect on SVR therefore depends on the dose.

Low doses of epinephrine may result in *decreased* blood pressure because of β_2 mediated vasodilation and increased muscle blood flow. Epinephrine's predominant effect, however, is both positive inotropic and chronotropic action on the heart, resulting in increased cardiac output, cardiac automaticity, and systolic blood pressure. At the higher dose range it causes profound venoconstriction and increased preload, and decreases flow through the vessels of the skin, mucosa, and kidney. Tachycardia, tachyarrhythmias and splanchnic and peripheral vasoconstriction (oliguria, metabolic acidosis, limb ischemia) become prominent. Stimulation of glycogenolysis not infrequently results in hyperglycemia; lactic acidosis may be worsened by the excessive formation of pyruvate.

Epinephrine is extremely useful in providing inotropic support in states of myocardial depression following CPB. The simultaneous administration of 5 mg/kg boluses of calcium chloride increases blood pressure, but does not appear to enhance epinephrine's inotropic effect in this situation (32). However, when the inotropic action of epinephrine is combined with afterload reduction, provided by either a pure vasodilator such as sodium nitroprusside or a phosphodiesterase inhibitor such as amrinone, the enhancement of stroke volume is greater than if either agent used alone (33).

Dobutamine. Dobutamine, a synthetic derivative of isoproterenol, exists in a 50:50 racemic mixture of two optical isomers: the (-) enantiomer (predominantly α_1 adrenergic) and the (+) enantiomer (β_1 and β_2 adrenergic); however in the racemic mixture the β-adrenergic activity predominates (34). It shares isoproterenol's property of virtually pure β-adrenergic action, but lacks its profound chronotropic activity. Dobutamine enhances myocardial performance by combining a positive inotropic effect with afterload reduction. It also causes pulmonary vasodilation and right ventricular afterload reduction. Unlike dopamine, it does not depend on release of norepinephrine, act on the dopaminergic receptor, or increase vascular tone.

It is useful in patients with longstanding congestive heart failure, cardiomyopathy or right ventricular dysfunction with pulmonary hypertension. In severe pulmonary hypertension, however, increase in cardiac output may be at the expense of increased right ventricular stroke work. There is some evidence that dobutamine may enhance coronary artery flow in ischemic myocardium, compared with dopamine (35). For the above reasons, there are many who advocate dobutamine as a first-line inotropic agent in place of dopamine. However, it should be kept in mind that, unlike dopamine, any increase in renal or splanchnic blood flow is due only to an increase in overall cardiac output. Its potent vasodilator activity can provoke hypotension in hypovolemic patients. Dobutamine has a reputation of lacking chronotropic effects, but that is in comparison with isoproterenol, not dopamine. Indeed, its chronotropic and arrhythmogenic effects become quite prominent at the higher dose range, and, in our experience, are certainly no less troublesome than those associated with dopamine.

Norepinephrine. Norepinephrine is structurally similar to epinephrine (it lacks a methyl radical; *n*-*o*hne-*r*adikal is "n without a radical" in German). It is also a very potent β_1 agonist, but its peripheral actions differ in that it has extremely potent α-, and relatively weak β_2-adrenergic activity. Consequently, vascular resistance (and hence preload and afterload) of both the left and right heart is increased, as is systolic and diastolic blood pressure. Therefore, despite increased cardiac contractility, cardiac output may be little changed, or reflexly decreased. Norepinephrine is indicated in states of severe reduction of SVR which jeopardize coronary perfusion pressure, e.g., septic shock, or to maintain perfusion pressure in combination with amrinone (see below). Its use in high doses for protracted periods will induce severe renal and splanchnic ischemia (and may result in acute renal failure or ischemic bowel syndrome).

Isoproterenol. Isoproterenol is a very potent synthetic catecholamine that acts exclusively on the β-adrenergic receptors. Its pronounced chronotropic effect elicits an increase in heart rate at the lowest of doses, and always precedes demonstrable inotropic effect. Although it is a potent inotropic agent its use as such is severely limited by its predisposition toward tachycardia and tachyarrhythmias. Its powerful β_2 adrenergic activity has been taken advantage of in its use as a bronchodilator (which has been curtailed because of its cardiac effects); the marked reduction in SVR causes hypotension unless the cardiac output increases accordingly. Isoproterenol has been used with some success in the treatment of severe pulmonary hypertension, but again its usefulness is limited by tachycardia. In recent years, isoproterenol has been confined to use in low doses as a chronotropic agent, to provide "pharmacologic pacing" in sinus bradycardia or other conduction defects.

Dopexamine hydrochloride. Dopexamine is an investigational synthetic catecholamine presently undergoing extensive clinical trials in Europe. It has a unique pharmacologic profile: sixty times the β_2 adrenergic effect of dopamine, one third its dopaminergic (DA_1) effect, and relatively weak β_1 adrenergic (i.e., inotropic) activity (36). Dopexamine increases cardiac output primarily by reducing afterload (and hence decreasing metabolic oxygen demand), and has been shown to enhance renal blood flow. It exhibits less tachyphylaxis and more profound afterload reduction than dobutamine (37). Like dopamine, it is capable of releasing norepinephrine, but appears to have much less arrhythmogenic potential. Its place in the pharmacopoeia of catecholamines awaits further clinical experience.

Phosphodiesterase inhibitors

Intracellular cAMP controls intracellular calcium concentration, cardiac muscle contractility, and smooth muscle relaxation. Its levels can be directly increased by catecholamine-induced β-adrenergic stimulation, or, alternatively, by inhibition of its breakdown by phosphodiesterase. There are three known types of phosphodiesterase. Phosphodiesterase I and II facilitate the breakdown of cyclic guanine monophosphate (cGMP) and non-specific cyclic nuclear phosphate, respectively. Phosphodiesterase III selectively breaks down cAMP. Theophylline and the methylxanthines are non-selective phosphodiesterase inhibitors; their benefit in increasing contractility is outweighed by toxic side-effects (nausea, vomiting, tachyarrhythmias, seizures). On the other hand, selective phosphodiesterase III inhibitors have clinically useful inotropic activity.

Amrinone. Amrinone, a bipyridine derivative, is a selective phosphodiesterase III inhibitor, and acts independently of the β-adrenergic receptor. It is a non-adrenergic inotropic agent with potent vasodilator effects which reduce both SVR and PVR, with marked reduction in both left and right ventricular afterload (38). The combination of afterload reduction with a milder chronotropic effect suggests that amrinone may have a beneficial effect on myocardial oxygen balance compared with the catecholamines, and would be indicated in myocardial depression associated with ischemia. However, this benefit may be negated if amrinone's potent vasodilator effect causes hypotension. Maintenance of adequate coronary perfusion pressure usually requires the simultaneous administration of a vasoconstrictor agent such as norepinephrine or phenylephrine. Amrinone appears to be particularly useful in the treatment of right ventricular dysfunction associated with elevated pulmonary artery pressures. In patients who have developed tachyphylaxis to catecholamines because of down-regulation of beta receptors, the addition of amrinone can provide an enhanced inotropic response. In fact, the combination of amrinone with any of the catecholamines (dopamine, epinephrine, norepinephrine) further increases intracellular cAMP and augments the inotropic response.

The pharmacokinetic profile of amrinone differs from that of the catecholamines in that a loading dose is required, but is similar to many agents used in anesthesia. Amrinone has a short redistribution half-life ($t_{1/2}$-*alpha)* of one to two minutes, and a long elimination half-life *($t_{1/2}$-beta)* of 2 to 6 hours. About 25% is excreted unchanged by the kidney. Amrinone infusion must be prepared in normal saline (*not* dextrose) and protected from light to prevent degradation. A loading dose of sufficient magnitude to sustain therapeutic plasma levels (2-9 µg/ml) until they are achieved by the maintenance infusion is of the order of 1.5 to 3.0 mg/kg (39,40). It should be given *slowly* over 15 to 20 minutes to minimize hypotension, while a maintenance infusion of 10 to 15 µg/kg/min is started. [If the risk vs. benefit of amrinone needs to be evaluated before committing to a long-term infusion, a small loading dose (0.75-1.0 mg/kg) can be given: it will last five to fifteen minutes, after which a decision can be made about further therapy]. After prolonged infusion is stopped, levels fall slowly ("auto-wean"), especially in the presence of renal or hepatic dysfunction. Platelet dysfunction and ventricular arrhythmias, seen with chronic administration, do not appear to be a problem with short-term use in the ICU.

Milrinone. Milrinone is about fifteen times as potent as amrinone, but has a very similar pharmacologic profile. The usual loading dose is 50 µg/kg, followed by a maintenance infusion of between 0.375 and 0.75 $\mu g \cdot kg^{-1} \cdot min^{-1}$. A recent multicenter European study on patients with low cardiac index after CPB (less than 2.5 $L \cdot min^{-1} \cdot M^{-2}$) demonstrated that milrinone provided significant and sustained inodilation, although two patients developed rapid atrial fibrillation shortly after the loading dose (41). In the oral form milrinone has less potential to cause thrombocytopenia than amrinone.

Enoximone and piroximone. Two other phosphodiesterase III inhibitors, enoximone and piroximone, which are imidazoline derivatives but have similar vasodilator and inotropic properties to amrinone, are presently undergoing clinical trials in low cardiac output states (42,43).

Cardiac glycosides

The digitalis glycosides exert their inotropic effect by increasing intracellular calcium concentration. Inhibition of sodium-potassium ATPase by these compounds results in the accumulation of intracellular sodium. As sodium accumulates, it is replaced by calcium as a result of compensatory augmentation of a sodium-calcium exchange.

Digoxin's inotropic effect is relatively trivial compared with the catecholamines, however, it is the only inotropic agent with a *negative* chronotropic, dromotropic and bathmotropic effect. Prophylactic administration for its antiarrhythmic effect is controversial because of its narrow therapeutic window (especially in the face of rapid alterations in pH and serum potassium), but it should be given at the first sign of atrial ectopy or supraventricular irritability.

Enhancement of adenylate cyclase and other non-adrenergic mechanisms

At present, agents acting to provide inotropic activity by stimulation of adenylate cyclase independently of the adrenergic receptor system are of historical or investigational interest only. Compounds capable of acting distally to the adrenergic receptor may prove useful in catecholamine insensitive patients, and this may be a fruitful area of development in the coming decade.

Glucagon, a single chain pancreatic polypeptide with a molecular weight of 3500 dalton, exerts its metabolic effects throughout the body by stimulating the synthesis of cAMP. Initial interest in the inotropic potential of this compound has waned because of its profound gastrointestinal side effects and lack of potency (44). Similarly, specific H_2 agonists, which have significant inotropic effect on myocardial cell receptors, are unlikely to be of clinical use because of widespread side effects (45). *Forskolin,* a plant derivative that acts on the catalytic subunit of adenylate cyclase, has been used in humans in congestive heart failure with significant inotropic and vasodilator effect; but its chronotropic effect is unacceptable (46). *Dibutyryl-cAMP* is a phosphodiesterase-resistant cAMP analogue which, administered intravenously to patients in congestive heart failure, reduces both SVR and pulmonary artery pressures, while significantly increasing cardiac output (47). It is unclear how much positive inotropic effect played in this salutary effect as compared to simple afterload reduction.

4. *Normalize Systemic Vascular Resistance (SVR)*

Reduce Excessive Afterload (Vasodilator Therapy)

Reduction of excessive myocardial afterload enhances cardiac function by decreasing impedance to ventricular outflow, thereby reducing pressure work in favor of volume work. The net effect is increased stroke volume, decreased heart size and improved myocardial oxygen balance. The more impaired and ischemic the ventricle, the less responsive it is to inotropic support and the more dependent it becomes on reduction of excessive afterload for maintenance of function. Inotropic agents with vasodilator properties (dobutamine, amrinone) can provide effective afterload reduction ("inodilation"), but there are distinct advantages in titrating afterload independently with a rapidly acting vasodilator drug such as sodium nitroprusside.

Vasodilator agents may be classified by their mode of action, but it is also important to consider whether their effect is predominantly on the venous system (i.e., preload reduction), arterial system (i.e., afterload reduction) or both. Vasodilator therapy cannot provide benefit if the patient is still hypovolemic or hypotensive—it will simply precipitate acute hypotension.

Direct Vasodilators

Sodium nitroprusside (SNP)

Sodium nitroprusside has a unique chemical structure in that acts as a donor of nitric oxide (NO)—which has a direct, potent vasodilator action on vascular smooth muscle—loosely bound to a ferrous ion (Fe^{2+}) with five cyanide molecules. The dissociation of the compound and its cyanide on entry into the bloodstream confers its very rapid clinical onset and offset of action, but also the potential for cyanide toxicity. Cyanide binds preferentially to ferric ion (Fe^{3+}), so that an important pathway for detoxification is the simultaneous oxidation of hemoglobin (Fe^{2+}) to methemoglobin (Fe^{3+}), which forms cyanmethemoglobin. The remaining cyanide is absorbed into red cells where it binds with thiosulfate under the influence of rhodanase to form thiocyanate, which is excreted in the urine. Excessive cyanide irreversibly binds with the ferric ion of cytochrome oxidase, poisoning the cytoplasmic electron transport chain and causing anoxic cellular hypoxia. Early toxicity is revealed by rapid rise in SvO_2 and metabolic (lactic) acidosis. Cyanide toxicity is entirely related to the rate of administration; fatal overdose of SNP has been reported when infusion rates of 15 to 40 μg/kg/min were given. Limitation of dosage to less than 8 μg/kg/min avoids this danger and has allowed SNP to become established as widely used intravenous vasodilator agent.

Afterload reduction with SNP is indicated when, despite stabilization of heart rate, augmentation of inadequate preload, and inotropic support, there is a persistent low cardiac output state (CI less than 2 $l/min/m^2$) associated with an elevated SVR (greater than 1500 $dyne{\cdot}sec{\cdot}cm^{-5}$). Since SVR is a calculated variable, the MAP is used as a continuous parameter to guide therapy. After baseline hemodynamic data, an infusion of SNP is started slowly (e.g., 0.2 μg/kg/min) with the goal of providing slight reduction in MAP, e.g., from 85 mmHg to 75 mmHg. SNP is easily titratable, with an onset and offset of action of less than two minutes. The desired effect is an increase in cardiac output with a decrease in SVR. A sharp decrease in blood pressure caused by a very small dose of SNP indicates intravascular hypovolemia.

The vasodilator effect of SNP is balanced between the arterial and venous systems. Preload reduction is achieved simultaneously, i.e., PAOP will decrease after the institution of SNP therapy. To achieve the full benefit of afterload reduction from SNP, the PAOP should be restored to its previous level by a fluid challenge (250-500 ml of crystalloid or the osmotic equivalent of colloid). Afterload reduction is continued using serial increments in SNP dosage, with fluid challenges to restore preload, until the desired cardiac output is achieved. The main limitation is hypotension: an SNP dose of greater than 2 μg/kg/min is seldom required or tolerated when used for afterload reduction.

The most common adverse effects of SNP therapy are abrupt hypotension, reflex tachycardia and myocardial ischemia. Arterial vasodilation decreases aortic diastolic pressure and coronary perfusion pressure. SNP promotes intracoronary steal by dilating both conductance and impedance arteries, shunting blood away from ischemic areas. Hypoxemia due to inhibition of hypoxic pulmonary vasoconstrictor responses is a potential problem in the non-ventilated patient. Cyanide toxicity is a non-issue as long as infusion rates are kept low (see above), but thiocyanate (a neurotoxin) may accumulate with prolonged infusions in patients with renal dysfunction.

Nitroglycerin (NTG). The benefits of nitroglycerin in reduction of preload have already been discussed. However, preload and afterload effects are integrated into the cardiac cycle. Reduction of excessive preload by NTG can decrease heart size and intraventricular radius at the end of diastole, which in turn reduces afterload during the following systolic contraction. Myocardial oxygen consumption is decreased. Because its venodilator effects predominate, use of NTG seldom causes an increase in cardiac output, and if preload reduction is excessive, cardiac output will decrease.

Hydralazine. Hydralazine acts predominantly on the systemic arterial circulation, and in patients with low cardiac output, high SVR states it provides specific afterload reduction, without reduction of preload. This allows a greater reduction in SVR and increase in cardiac output than is achieved by a non-specific vasodilator such as SNP, without hypotension, and without the requirement for fluid challenges to restore the preload (48). Reflex tachycardia, a hallmark of its use in the treatment of systemic hypertension, is not seen because the stroke volume increases as SVR decreases. Effective dosage is much smaller than that used in hypertension, i.e., 2.5 to 7.5 mg IV, given every 4 hours. The pharmacokinetics are unpredictable based on weight, because patients may genetically be rapid or slow acetylators of the drug. Onset of effect is usually 20 min after initial injection, and serial hemodynamic measurements are required for dose adjustment. Hydralazine is taken up into storage depots in the arterial muscularis, and dosage requirements gradually decrease over 24 to 48 hours, to every 6 to 8 hours. Conversion from the IV to oral route requires a 5- to 10-fold increase in dosage (e.g., 25 mg po q8hr) because of first-pass clearance by the liver.

Because of its slow, rather unpredictable onset and duration of action, hydralazine is not suitable for the initial management of the low cardiac output state, but rather provides a means of continuing afterload reduction in patients who have demonstrated dependence on SNP for longer than 12-24 hours. Hydralazine worsens coronary perfusion pressure by decreasing aortic diastolic pressure without decreasing left ventricular diastolic pressure. Its use should be avoided in the presence of myocardial ischemia.

Calcium channel blockers

Nifedipine. Nifedipine is a calcium channel blocker with predominantly vasodilator effects on the coronary, pulmonary and systemic circulations; it has very little negative inotropic or negative dromotropic action. As such it has been used to reduce afterload and improve systolic function in patients with CHF (49). However, excessive vasodilation, hypotension, reflex tachycardia and exacerbation of myocardial ischemia have been reported with the use of nifedipine after myocardial infarction. Hypotensive insults to other organs, including the kidney, have also been reported (50). Nifedipine is relatively water-insoluble and light-sensitive, and its parenteral use is restricted to sublingual administration of the aspirated contents of a capsule—so that its effects are rather unpredictable and difficult to titrate. Diltiazem and verapamil, which have negative inotropic and dromotropic effects, are unlikely to exacerbate myocardial ischemia, but are not indicated in low cardiac output states unless they are associated with obstructive cardiomyopathy or supraventricular arrhythmias.

Nicardipine. Nicardipine is an analog of nifedipine with similar actions, but it is water-soluble and light-insensitive, allowing its administration by direct intravenous injection or infusion (51). It has been used extensively in Japan and will be released in the USA in the near future. Because of its relatively slow onset and offset of action, it is unlikely to replace SNP in acutely unstable patients, but may be of benefit in states of persistently elevated SVR (where it might be more suitable than hydralazine).

Alpha-adrenergic antagonists

Phentolamine. Phentolamine is of historical interest because it was one of the first vasodilator agents used to provide afterload reduction in low cardiac output states. However, it is a non-selective α-adrenergic antagonist, i.e., it also blocks presynaptic α-2 receptor mediated inhibition of endogenous norepinephrine release, resulting in undesirable reflex tachycardia.

Prazosin. Prazosin provides selective α_1 receptor blockade, i.e., reflex norepinephrine release is suppressed by the unblocked α_2 receptor, so that reflex tachycardia is not a problem. Its action on the circulation is balanced, like SNP, so that administration decreases both preload and afterload by combined arterial and venous vasodilation (52). Tachyphylaxis, hypotension and lack of an intravenous formulation (in the USA), and limit prazosin's use in acute low cardiac output syndrome.

Angiotensin converting enzyme (ACE) inhibitors

Captopril and enalapril. Captopril and its analog enalapril are oral and intravenous ACE inhibitors which dilate both the arterial and venous components of the circulation. The effects of administration of both agents are quite similar, eliciting increases in stroke volume and cardiac output as a result of preload and afterload reduction. While it has been extensively used in the therapy of chronic congestive heart failure, captopril administration (25 mg IV q 6 hr) affords clinical improvement in acute heart failure and cardiogenic shock as well (53,54). ACE inhibitors have a number of additional potential benefits, including the reduction of the norepinephrine response to submaximal exercise, prevention of the formation of myocardial depressant factor (MDF), reduction in ventricular arrhythmias, and enhanced free radical scavenging (55-58).

The most important adverse effect of ACE inhibition is hypotension (especially in the presence of hypovolemia), resulting in reduced glomerular filtration rate and potassium excretion (59). Abrupt and dramatic deterioration in renal function may occur because compensatory angiotensin-induced efferent arteriolar constriction is blocked, so that glomerular filtration pressure declines *pari passu* with decreased renal blood flow and perfusion pressure. Although this effect can be attenuated by dose reduction, it frequently limits the application of ACE inhibition in the immediate perioperative period, when renal blood flow is borderline and renal insufficiency is so common.

Inodilator therapy

Agents which combine the properties of inotropic activity with vasodilation, i.e., inodilators, potentially simplify hemodynamic management because they obviate titration of a vasopressor with a vasodilator such as SNP. Because they decrease SVR and PVR, they decrease heart size, wall stress and cardiac work, making them attractive agents in the therapy of cardiogenic shock (60). Isoproterenol, the progenitor inodilator, has excessive chronotropic activity which contraindicates its use in states of myocardial ischemia. Dopamine has vasodilator activity due to its dopaminergic and β_2 adrenergic action in the lower dose range only (probably less than 5 μg/kg/min); above this range, its α_1 adrenergic action causes increasing vasoconstriction. Dobutamine and amrinone are currently available inotropic agents with potent vasodilator activity which provides the advantage of simultaneous afterload reduction (inodilation). Additional vasodilation with SNP is seldom indicated or tolerated, because of hypotension. In our experience, inodilation is particularly helpful when right ventricular dysfunction is prominent. This is because the right ventricle is exquisitely sensitive to increases in its afterload, and these agents are effective in decreasing elevated PVR.

Restore inadequate SVR (vasopressor therapy)

Occasionally systemic vasoconstrictor responses to hypovolemia and/or low cardiac output are ineffectual or absent. This may be due to autonomic neuropathy (diabetes, chronic renal failure), arteriovenous shunts (liver failure), endotoxemia (splanchnic ischemia) or drugs (long-acting vasodilators, such as ACE inhibitors, calcium blockers). Restoration of adequate SVR is especially important in the presence of myocardial ischemia, in order to maintain adequate coronary perfusion pressure. However, use of vasopressor agents must be very carefully titrated to achieve the most effective balance between perfusion and flow. Excessive vasoconstriction induces splanchnic, renal and peripheral ischemia, exacerbates cellular hypoxia (with increased lactic acidosis and DIC) and if myocardial afterload is increased too much, acute cardiac decompensation and pulmonary edema.

Vasopressor agents should be used alone only if life-threatening hypotension persists despite all efforts to restore blood pressure by the use of aggressive fluid administration and inotropic support, and if calculated SVR is inappropriately low (e.g., less than 1000 $dyne \cdot sec \cdot cm^{-5}$). The therapeutic goal should be to maintain a MAP of about 60 mmHg (to ensure adequate coronary perfusion pressure), while continuing other means to restore blood pressure.

On the other hand, the combination of a vasopressor agent with a vasodilator or inodilator drug may be an effective means of maintaining systemic and coronary perfusion pressures while obtaining the benefits of the vasodilation on the coronary or systemic circulations. Examples would be the combination of phenylephrine with nitroglycerin (sustained coronary perfusion pressure with coronary vasodilation), or the use of norepinephrine or epinephrine with amrinone (sustained systemic pressure with pulmonary vasodilation, as well as potentiation of inotropic effect).

Phenylephrine. Phenylephrine is a non-catecholamine α_1 adrenergic agonist that provides peripheral vasoconstriction without inotropy or reflex tachycardia (in fact, reflex slowing may occur). Effective circulating blood volume is diverted towards the heart and the brain, which lack potent α_1 vasoconstrictor responses. Phenylephrine is therefore indicated for temporary therapy when hypotension and tachycardia threaten myocardial oxygen balance. $Alpha_1$ mediated coronary vasoconstriction does occur, but appears to enhance rather than hurt epicardial blood flow. $Alpha_1$ inotropic receptors also exist, but this response appears clinically unimportant in the acute phase. Small bolus doses (50-100 μg) may be given and repeated as necessary, while other steps are being taken to restore blood pressure and cardiac output; if necessary, a continuous infusion can be started.

Norepinephrine. Norepinephrine causes intense α_1 mediated peripheral vasoconstriction, but it also has considerable β_1 adrenergic activity. It therefore has the advantage of providing inotropic stimulation which may more than compensate for increased afterload, so that cardiac output is increased. However, tachycardia and tachyarrhythmias may occur, and the marked increase in pressure work of the ventricles adversely affects myocardial oxygen balance. Norepinephrine is therefore indicated in the temporary management of hypovolemic rather than cardiogenic shock, especially when endotoxin-mediated splanchnic vasodilation is prominent.

REFERENCES

1. Frank O: Zur Dynamik des Herzmuskels. Z Biol 32:370-447, 1895
2. Patterson SW, Starling EH: On the mechanical factors which determine the output of the ventricles. J Physiol 48:357-379, 1914
3. Berne RM, Levy MN: Regulation of the heartbeat. In: Berne RM, Levy MN (ed): Physiology, 2nd Ed. CV Mosby Co, St. Louis, 1988. p463
4. Sands SD, Winegard S: Treppe and total calcium content of the frog ventricle. Am J Physiol. 218:908-10, 1970

5. Bodenheimer MM, Banka VS, Helfant RH: Effect of heart rate on zonal tension and ischemia following coronary occlusion: optimal rate for Treppe versus ischemia. Cardiovasc Res. 10:336-40, 1976
6. Zoll PM, Zoll RH, Falk RH, Clinton JE, Eitel DR, Antman EM. External noninvasive temporary cardiac pacing: clinical trials, Circulation 71:937-944, 1985
7. Hankeln K, Rädel C, Beez M, Laniewski P, Bohmert F. Comparison of hydroxyethyl starch and lactated Ringer's solution on hemodynamics and oxygen transport of critically ill patients in prospective crossover studies. Crit Care Med 17:133-135, 1989
8. Alving BM, Hojima Y, Pisano JJ, Mason BL, Buckingham RE, Mozen MM, Finlayson JS. Hypotension associated with prekallikrein activator (Hageman-factor fragments) in plasma protein fraction. New Engl J Med 299:66-70, 1978
9. Hein L-G, Albrecht M, Dworschak M, Frey L, Brückner UB. Long-term observation following traumatic-hemorrhagic shock in the dog: a comparison of crystalloid vs. colloidal fluids. Circ Shock 26:353-364, 1988
10. Nakayama S, Sibley L, Gunther RA, Holcroft JW, Kramer GC. Small-volume resuscitation with hypertonic saline (2,400 mOsm/liter) during hemorrhagic shock. Circ Shock 13:149-159, 1984
11. Chudnofsky CR, Dronen SC, Syverud SA, Zink BJ, Hedges JR. Intravenous fluid therapy in the prehospital management of hemorrhagic shock: improved outcome with hypertonic saline/6% dextran 70 in a swine model. Am J Emerg Med 7:357-363, 1989
12. Gross D, Landau EH, Klin B, Krausz MM. Treatment of uncontrolled hemorrhagic shock with hypertonic saline solution. Surg Gynec Obstet 170:106-112, 1990
13. Lindner A, Cutler RE, Goodman WG. Synergism of dopamine plus furosemide in preventing acute renal failure in the dog. Kidney Int 16:158-166, 1979.
14. Lucas CE, Zito JG, Carter KM, Cortez A, Stebner FC. Questionable value of furosemide in preventing renal failure. Surgery 82:314-320, 1977
15. Lawson DH, Gray JMB, Henry DA, Tilstone WJ. Continuous infusion of frusemide in refractory oedema. BMJ 2:476, 1978
16. Copeland JG, Campbell DW, Plachtka JR, Salamon NW, Larson DF. Diuresis with continuous infusion of furosemide after cardiac surgery. Amer J Surg 146:796-799, 1983
17. Krasna MJ, Scott GE, Scholz PM, Spotnitz AJ, Mackenzie JW, Penn F. Postoperative enhancement of urinary output in patients with acute renal failure using continuous furosemide therapy. Chest 89:294-295, 1986
18. Schwartz LB, Bissell MG, Murphy M, Gewertz BL. Renal effects of dopamine in vascular surgical patients. J Vasc Surg 8:367-374, 1988
19. Murphy MB. The therapeutic role of drugs acting on cardiovascular dopamine receptors. J Cardiothoracic Anesth 4:23-26, 1990
20. Schaer GL, Fink MP, Parrillo JE. Norepinephrine alone versus norepinephrine plus low-dose dopamine: enhanced renal blood flow with combination pressor therapy. Crit Care Med 13:492-496, 1985

21. Chiolero R, Borgeta A and Fisher A. Postoperative arrhythmias and risk factors after open heart surgery. Thorac Cardiovasc Surgeon 1991;39:81-84
22. Stratton MA. Use of nitrates in patients with acute myocardial infarction. Clin Pharm 3:32-39, 1984
23. Borer JS, Redwood DR, Levitt B, et al. Reduction in myocardial ischemia with nitroglycerin or nitroglycerin plus phenylephrine administered during acute myocardial infarction. N Engl J Med 293:1008-1012, 1975
24. Epstein SE, Borer JS, Kent KM, Redwood DR, Goldstein RE, Levitt B. Protection of ischemic myocardium by nitroglycerin: experimental and clinical results. Circulation 53, Suppl 1:191-198, 1976
25. Fabioto A: Calcium-induced release of calcium from the cardiac sarcoplasmic reticulum. Am J Physiol. 245:C1-4, 1983
26. Colucci WS, Wright RF, Braunwald E: New positive inotropic agents in the treatment of congestive heart failure: mechanisms of action of recent clinical developments: (first of two parts). N Eng J Med. 314:290-99, 1986
27. Bruckner R, Meyer W, Mugge A, Schmitz W, Scholz H: Alpha-adrenoreceptor-mediated positive inotropic effect of norepinephrine in isolated human ventricular myocardium. Eur J Pharm. 99-345-7, 1984
28. Sharpey-Schafer EP, Ginsburg J: Humoral agents and venous tone. Effects of catecholamines, 5 - hydroxytryptamine, histamine and nitrites. Lancet. 2:1337, 1962
29. Goldberg LI: The dopamine vascular receptor: New areas for biochemical pharmacologists. Biochem Pharmacol. 24:651,1975
30. Aubier M, Murciano D, Menu Y, Boczkowski J: Dopamine effects on diaphragmatic strength during acute respiratory failure in chronic obstructive pulmonary disease. Ann Int Med. 110:17-23, 1989
31. Freyschuss U, Hjemdahl P, Juhlin-Dannfelt A, Linde B: Cardiovascular and metabolic responses to low dose adrenaline infusion: an invasive study in humans. Clin Sci 70:199-206, 1986
32. Royster RL, Butterworth JF, Prielipp RC, et al. A randomized, blinded, placebo-controlled evaluation of calcium chloride and epinephrine for inotropic support after emergence from cardiopulmonary bypass. Anesth Analg 74: 3-13, 1992
33. Royster RL, Butterworth JFt, Prielipp RC, et al. Combined inotropic effects of amrinone and epinephrine after cardiopulmonary bypass in humans. Anesth Analg 77(4): 662-72, 1993
34. Majerus TC, Dasta JF, Bauman JL, Danziger LH, Ruffolo RR. Dobutamine; ten years later. Pharmacotherapy 9:245-259, 1989
35. Fowler MB, Alderman EL, Oesterle SN et al. Dobutamine and dopamine after cardiac surgery: greater augmentation of myocardial blood flow with dobutamine. Circulation 70:1103-1111, 1984
36. Smith GW, O'Connor SE: A symposium: Focus on heart failure -Current experiences in basic research and clinical studies on dopexamine hydrochloride (Dopacard ®): An introduction to the pharmacologic properties of Dopacard (dopexamine hydrochloride). Am J Card. 62:9C-17C, 1988

37. Baumann G, Felix SB, Filcek S: Congestive heart failure: usefulness of dopexamine hydrochloride versus dobutamine in chronic congestive heart failure and effects on hemodynamics and urine output. Am J Card. 65:748-54, 1990
38. Baim D: Effects of amrinone on myocardial energetics in severe congestive heart failure. Am J Cardiol. 56:16B, 1985
39. Bailey JM, Levy JH, Rogers HG, et al. Pharmacokinetics of amrinone during cardiac surgery. Anesthesiology 75: 961-968, 1991
40. Levy JH, Ramsay J, Bailey JM: Pharmacokinetics and pharmacodynamics of phosphodiesterase-III inhibitors. J Cardiothoracic Anesth 4, Suppl 5: 7-11, 1990
41. Feneck RO and the European Multicentre Milrinone Trial Group: Intravenous milrinone following cardiac surgery: I. Effects of bolus infusion followed by variable dose maintenance infusion. J Cardiothoracic Vasc Anesth 6: 554-562, 1992
42. Boldt J, Moosdorf R, Hempelmann G. Enoximone treatment of impaired myocardial function during cardiac surgery: combined effects with epinephrine. J Cardiothoracic Anesth 4:462-468, 1990
43. Axelrod RJ, De Marco T, Dae M, Botvinick EH, Chaterjee K. Hemodynamic and clinical evaluation of piroximone, a new inotrope-vasodilator agent, in severe congestive heart failure. J Am Coll Cardiol 9:1124-1130, 1987
44. Lvoff R, Wilcken D: Glucagon in heart failure and in cardiogenic shock: experience in 50 patients. Circulation. 45:534-42, 1972
45. Baumann G, Felix B, Riess G, Loher U, Ludwig L, Blomer H: Effective stimulation of cardiac contractility and myocardial metabolism by impromidine and dimaprit--two new H2-agonist compounds--in the surviving catecholamine -insensitive myocardium after coronary occlusion. J Cardiovasc Pharmacol. 4:542-53, 1982
46. Linderer T, Biamino G, Bruggeman T, Pweslin K, Schroder R: Hemodynamic effects of forskolin, a new drug with combined inotropic and vasodilating properties. J Am Coll Cardiol. 3:562, 1984
47. Matsue S, Murakami E, Takekoshi N, Emoto J, Matoba M: Hemodynamic effects of dibutyryl cyclic AMP in congestive heart failure. Am J Cardiol. 51:1364-8, 1983
48. Sladen RN, Rosenthal MH. Specific afterload reduction with parenteral hydralazine following cardiac surgery. J Thorac Cardiovas Surg 78:195-202, 1979
49. Reicher-Reiss H: Calcium antagonists in heart failure. Eur Heart J 9 Suppl H:101-4, 1988
50. Eicher J, Morelon P, Chalopin J, Tanter Y, Louis P, Rifle G: Acute renal failure during nifedipine therapy in a patient with congestive heart failure. Crit Care Med. 16:1163-4, 1988
51. Turlapaty P, Vary R, Kaplan JA. Nicardipine, a new intravenous calcium antagonist: a review of its pharmacology, pharmacokinetics, and perioperative applications. J Cardiothoracic Anesth 3:344-355, 1989

52. Miller R, Awan N, Maxwell KS, et al: Sustained reduction of cardiac impedance and preload in congestive heart failure with the antihypertensive vasodilator, prazosin. N Eng J Med 297:303, 1977
53. Flynn K, Coughlan MG, Phelan DM, Luke D, Neligan M, Wood AE: Letters to the editor: Intravenous captopril in acute heart failure. Lancet. 1(8578):173-74, 1988
54. Lipkin D, Frenneaux M, Maseri A: Letters to the Editor: Beneficial effect of captopril in cardiogenic shock. Lancet. 2(8554):327, 1987
55. Corbalan R, Jalil J, Chamorro G, Casanegra P, Valenzuela P: Effects of captopril versus milrinone therapy in modulating the adrenergic nervous system response to exercise in congestive heart failure. Am J Cardiol. 65:644-9, 1990
56. Trachete G, Lefer AM: Mechanism of the protective effect of angiotensin-converting enzyme inhibition in hemorrhagic shock. Proc Soc Exp Biol Med. 162:54-7, 1979
57. Cleland J, Dargle H, Hodsman G, et. al. Captopril in heart failure. A double blind controlled trial. Br Heart J. 52:530-5, 1984
58. Lefer AM: The pathophysiologic role of myocardial depressant factor as a mediator of circulatory shock. Klin-Wochenschr. 60:713-716, 1982
59. Dzau VJ. Renal effects of angiotensin-converting enzyme inhibition in cardiac failure. Am J Kidney Dis 10(Suppl 1):74-80, 1987
60. Kaplan JA, Guffin AV. The inodilators: an expanding role in the perioperative period. J Cardiothoracic Anesth 4:27-31, 1990

MYOCARDIAL STUNNING: AN OVERVIEW[*]

Dennis T. Mangano, PhD, MD

ABSTRACT Over the past two decades, we have challenged the belief that transient ischemia is benign with little functional sequelae following resolution of ischemia. The phenomenon of prolonged postischemic contractile dysfunction, or of myocardial stunning, has been developed and is under investigation using multiple experimental and clinical models. Classifications of myocardial stunning have been suggested and include single and multiple reversible ischemic episodes, partially reversible episodes, and global ischemia. More challenging is the understanding of the mechanisms of myocardial stunning, including free radical protection, excitation-contraction uncoupling, altered calcium flux, microvascular dysfunction, and impaired energy production and use. Finally, advances have been made in the clinical arena, including development of new more sensitive technologies to detect dysfunction, and development of potentially important therapies, including free radical scavengers, adenosine-regulating agents, and calcium channel blockers. In this brief overview, we focus on myocardial stunning, including a historical perspective of coronary occlusion, and definition, classification, and clinical implications of myocardial stunning. (J Card Surg 8[Suppl]:204-213, 1993)

EVOLVING CONCEPT OF ISCHEMIA

Research in myocardial ischemia and coronary occlusion dates nearly 300 years and has led to the development of many new concepts regarding the etiology, pathophysiology, diagnosis, and treatment of myocardial ischemia and infarction. Older concepts have been challenged; newer concepts have evolved. Over the past decade, advances in research have furthered our understanding of myocardial ischemia and the important relationship between ischemia and contractile function. It now is clear from the work of Heyndrickx (1,2), Braunwald (3,4), Bolli (5), Kloner (6), and others that myocardial ischemia is not an all-or-

[*]Reproduced with permission from JOURNAL OF CARDIAC SURGERY, Vol. 8 (Suppl), No. 2, March 1993. Copyright 1993 by Futura Publishing Company, Inc. Armonk, NY, U.S.A.

T. H. Stanley and P. L. Bailey (eds.), Anesthesiology and the Cardiovascular Patient, 175–193.

none process. No longer can it be stated that transient ischemia is benign with little functional sequelae following resolution of ischemia. We have developed the concepts of the stunned and hibernating myocardium. Critical to these developments was recognition of the phenomenon of prolonged contractile dysfunction, specifically as it related to myocardial ischemia: either a previous ischemic event (stunned myocardium), a chronic ischemic event (hibernating myocardium), or an irreversible ischemic event (infarcted myocardium).

We now recognize that there are a number of clinical conditions that may be associated with stunned myocardium, including reperfusion following thrombolytic therapy, angioplasty or myocardial revascularization, and unstable angina. Similarly, hibernating myocardium may be associated with several clinical conditions, including surgically reversible chronic myocardial asynergy following previous myocardial infarction and reversible asynergy associated with ischemic cardiomyopathy. Considerable gains in the treatment of these clinical conditions may result from our understanding of the phenomena of stunned and hibernating myocardium.

In this brief overview, we focus on myocardial stunning, including a historical perspective of coronary occlusion, and definition, classification, mechanisms, and clinical implications of myocardial stunning. This overview is provided for orientation for the articles that follow. It should be recognized that the information contained here essentially has been abstracted from recent works in the area, including the excellent reviews of Braunwald (3), Bolli (5), Kloner (6), and others.

CORONARY ARTERY OCCLUSION: HISTORICAL PERSPECTIVE

In 1982 Braunwald and Kloner (3) reviewed the history of coronary artery occlusion. Their overview and that of others suggest three periods of development: 1) early history (1698-1935), during which the effects of ligation or occlusion of a coronary artery were first appreciated; 2) middle period (1935-1970), during which the effects of brief occlusions on function, metabolism, and morphological changes in the myocardium were determined; and 3) recent history (1970-present), during which investigators focused on the relationship between myocardial ischemia and contractile dysfunction, introducing the concepts of stunned and hibernating myocardium.

Early History (1698-1935): Coronary Ligation Effects

In 1698 Chirac (7) ligated a coronary artery in a dog and found that the heart ceased to beat following ligation. As reported by Braunwald and Kloner (3), this was the earliest recorded investigation of the effects of coronary artery ligation, demonstrating the importance of this phenomenon. The effects of coronary ligation on intraventricular hemodynamics were first noted approximately 200 years later, in 1895, when Porters ligated the coronary artery and found that the systolic ventricular pressure decreased whereas diastolic ventricular pressure increased. Seventeen years later, the relationship between permanent occlusion of the coronary artery and myocardial infarction was established by Herrick (9).

Middle Period (1935-1970): Brief Occlusion Effects

The early experiments essentially involved complete ligation of a coronary artery and investigation of subsequent phenomena. However, it was not until a classical work of Tennant and Wiggers (10) that the effects of brief periods of coronary artery occlusion were studied. This pivotal work established that within 60 seconds of coronary occlusion, significant decreases in active systolic shortening occur and lead to passive systolic lengthening. Thus, their open chested canine model of acute myocardial ischemia established the important relationship between reversible ischemia and regional mechanical dysfunction. Numerous investigations followed over the next 35 years, leading to our understanding of the effects of brief periods of coronary occlusion on the mechanical (functional), metabolic (biochemical), and morphological (histologic) markers of function. In addition, regional differences across the myocardium were explored, allowing differentiation of subendocardial, intramyocardial, and subepicardial physiology. From these investigations it became clear that total coronary occlusions of 20 minutes or longer usually were associated with irreversibly damaged subendocardial regions serviced by that coronary artery—changes that were documented by morphological evidence of necrosis: release of cardiac enzymes, depletion of biochemical energy stores, and irreversible histologic changes. Even with reperfusion these changes persisted. The second principal finding of investigations during this period was that with briefer periods of coronary occlusion (<20 min), myocardial ischemia was precipitated, but such ischemia was reversible once coronary flow was restored. These investigations suggested that with restoration of flow, abnormalities of function, metabolism, and structure reverse, and the myocardium reverts to its normal (preischemic) physiological state.

Recent History (1970-Present): Ischemic Dysfunction

In contrast to the above thinking, investigations over the last 20 years have demonstrated that even with a single brief occlusion of a coronary artery, lasting as short as 5 minutes, residual myocardial injury persists, despite restoration of flow and resolution of ischemia (2,11,15). It is clear that such "nonlethal ischemia" is associated with prolonged structural, metabolic, and functional changes of the myocardium, which may remain quite abnormal for days to weeks after restoration of flow. Not only had it been established that segment function, wall motion, and thickening remained abnormal after reestablishment of perfusion, but metabolic and morphological changes persist as well. For example, in the central ischemic zone, ATP concentration has been documented to fall to 50% of its preischemic control value after 15 minutes of coronary occlusion, and remains reduced (75% of control) after 3 days of reperfusion (16). Morphological and ultrastructural changes in the myocardium also persist for days after establishment of normal coronary flow and resolution of ischemia (3,5,6,17). Impaired myocardial relaxation, depletion of glycogen granules, modulation of nuclear chromatin, and intermyofibrillar and mitochondrial edema persist for 3 days or longer after a 15-minute occlusion.

These studies, which were performed over the last two decades, have supported the concept of prolonged postischemic contractile dysfunction, and ushered in the era of stunned myocardium. Over these last two decades, experimental investigations in a large number of species have laid the foundation for our understanding of the stunned myocardium and the mechanisms responsible for postischemic contractile dysfunction. Multiple models have been examined and have expanded the scope of myocardial stunning to include single and multiple reversible episodes, partly irreversible episodes, and global ischemia. In addition, there even may be evidence that exercise-induced ischemia may be a model for stunning (5,6). More challenging is the understanding of the mechanisms of myocardial stunning. In this last decade, substantial advances have been made in this area as well, including investigation of a broad spectrum of potential mechanisms such as free radical production, excitation-contraction uncoupling, altered calcium flux, microvascular dysfunction, and impaired energy production and use. Finally, advances have been made in the clinical arena, including development of new technologies that may more sensitively detect dysfunction (transesophageal echocardiography and multiple-lead electrocardiography), and investigation of potentially important therapies such as free radical scavengers, adenosine-regulating agents, and calcium channel blockers (18).

Thus, the concept of postischemic contractile dysfunction has emerged, and its importance is under active investigation.

DEFINITION OF MYOCARDIAL STUNNING

Myocardial stunning has been defined in a number of ways, depending on the experimental model or clinical circumstance under consideration. To enable discussion of the mechanisms and classifications of stunning, it is necessary to develop a definition that is comprehensive yet straightforward.

A DEFINITION OF MYOCARDIAL STUNNING

Certain elements are common to all applicable models of stunning, namely: (1) the presence of contractile dysfunction; (2) the existence of preceding state of ischemia secondary to limitation in coronary flow; (3) the reestablishment of perfusion following ischemia; (4) the absence of residual ischemia; (5) the absence of irreversible damage (viable tissue); and (6) a specific temporal characteristic of dysfunction—prolonged but transient—lasting hours to days.

For our purposes, we propose the following working definition of stunning:

Myocardial Stunning is contractile dysfunction,which:

(1) persists following reperfusion, and

(2) is not accompanied by ischemia or irreversible damage, and

(3) is prolonged, but transient (lasting hours to days).

Relationship of Stunned Myocardium to Hibernating and Necrotic Myocardium

Differentiation of stunned myocardium from hibernating myocardium and infarcted myocardium is confusing at times. The essential features differentiating these conditions are the presence of ischemia, the reversibility of contractile dysfunction, and the time to recovery of contractile function. Table 1 summarizes these comparisons.

Table 1. Ventricular dysfunction and ischemia.

	Ischemic State	*Ventricular Dysfunction*	*Time to Recovery of Ventricular Function*
Myocardial infarction	irreversible ischemia	irreversible	infinite
Hibernating myocardium	chronic ischemia	reversible`	months to years
Stunned myocardium	no ischemia	reversible	days to weeks

Stunned myocardium is not associated with active ischemia, and contractile function is restored over a period of days to weeks following establishment of reperfusion. In contrast, hibernating myocardium is associated with chronic ischemia, but does share the common feature of reversible contractile function, however, the time to recovery of contractile function is usually much longer than with stunned myocardium, taking months to years. Finally, myocardial infarction is associated with "irreversible ischemia" (cell death), and irreversible contractile dysfunction.

Other Characteristics of Stunned Myocardium

In addition to the above characteristics, stunned myocardium may be associated with other functional, biochemical, and histologic abnormalities. Both systolic and diastolic dysfunction may occur with stunning. After 15 minutes of occlusion following 3 hours of reperfusion, not only is systolic contraction compromised, but isovolemic relaxation is impaired as well—manifested by paradoxical diastolic shortening and prolonged diastolic relaxation time (19). Preliminary data supporting diastolic dysfunction also exist in humans (20). The stunned myocardium also is associated with biochemical abnormalities. Multiple studies have demonstrated immediate depression of ATP levels, followed by a slow recovery, similar to the time course of contractile function recovery (11,21). However, surprisingly, the phosphocreatine concentration is normal or even above normal (22), suggesting that mitochondrial phosphorylation is not affected. Additionally, recruitment of myocardium by inotropic stimuli is a common characteristic of stunned myocardium (22,23), suggesting that although ATP energy stores are decreased, production is not markedly impaired and is able to match metabolic needs. Finally, the stunned myocardium routinely exhibits a histologic picture in which the salvaged myocytes are normal. However, electron microscopic abnormalities have been observed, including twisted configuration of the cristae of the mitochondria and the presence of vacuolar structures (17).

Thus, the stunned myocardium is characterized by a complex set of functional, biochemical, and histologic changes dependent on the model chosen.

CLASSIFICATION OF MYOCARDIAL STUNNING

Prolonged postischemic contractile dysfunction, or myocardial stunning, has been demonstrated in multiple experimental and clinical settings. Experimental models have included a number of species subjected to multiple types of ischemic challenges. Therefore, classification of stunning is difficult given the large number of experimental and clinical conditions in which stunning may occur, and the broad spectrum of pathological findings associated with these conditions.

Simplistically, stunning can result from decreases in coronary blood flow (producing regional or global ischemia) or increases in oxygen demand (such as that induced by exercise). In this regard, the classification recently suggested by Bolli (5) is particularly applicable and is summarized below.

Stunning Secondary to Decreases in Coronary Blood Flow Regional Ischemia

Three models have been used to produce stunning by regionally decreasing coronary blood flow. In the first, the classical model, coronary occlusion is applied for less than 20 minutes, and myocardial necrosis does not occur (canine model), but prolonged postischemic dysfunction develops (21,24). In the second model, the multiple occlusion model, multiple shorter (5-10 min) coronary occlusive episodes occur, each of which produce stunning, and all of which result in the cumulative contractile dysfunction (25). Characteristic of this model is progressive dysfunction, with the severity of dysfunction being highest with the first occlusion and becoming smaller with each subsequent occlusion. Dysfunction develops gradually (vs. the single occlusion model), and results in a greater total ischemic burden because of the repeated occlusions. In the third model, the mixed ischemia/infarction model, occlusion lasts more than 20 minutes but less than 3 hours (26-28). As a result, the vulnerable subendocardium suffers irreversible damage; however, the subepicardial region may be salvaged by reperfusion (11,29). Thus, regional dysfunction in the subendocardium is permanent—consistent with infarction; whereas, in the subepicardium, dysfunction is reversible—consistent with stunning. In this model, the myocardial architecture is complex, exhibiting a spectrum of ischemia-dysfunction patterns. The distribution of such patterns depends on the duration of occlusion, the degree of blood flow reduction, and the severity of subsequent injury.

Stunning Secondary to Decreases in Coronary Blood Flow: Global Ischemia

Two models have been suggested (5). In the first, the isolated heart model, isolated hearts, when reperfused after transient ischemia, do not suffer irreversible injury but recover, and intracellular pH and phosphocreatine content return to preischemic levels (22,30). Although several experiments have verified that conditions mimicking stunning can exist, this model is complex, being dependent on species, temperature, duration of ischemia, and perfusate composition. Therefore, demonstration of cell viability and recovery of contractile abnormalities is difficult. In the second model, the cardioplegic arrest model, global ischemia during cardioplegic arrest is followed by prolonged contractile dysfunction. The evidence for this global ischemic model is much more substantial than the isolated heart model, and a number of reports have demonstrated prolonged right and left contractile dysfunction after cardioplegic arrest *in vivo*, lasting for 24 hours or more (18,31,32).

Stunning Secondary to Increased Oxygen Demand

Postexercise contractile dysfunction has been documented in several experimental studies in animals given a flow limiting coronary stenosis (33), and in humans with coronary artery disease (34,35). This is an interesting model for it suggests prolonged contractile dysfunction in association with high coronary flow, the primary problem being an increase in myocardial oxygen demand rather than a decrease in myocardial oxygen supply.

Conclusion

Prolonged contractile dysfunction after restoration of coronary flow has been demonstrated in a number of species, under a variety of experimental circumstances and in a large spectrum of clinical circumstances. The diversity of these models suggests that multiple mechanisms for stunning exist, and that there is no unifying pathological model.

MECHANISMS (POTENTIAL) OF MYOCARDIAL STUNNING

Given the diversity of models and classifications for myocardial stunning, it is not surprising that multiple mechanisms have been postulated. Many of these mechanisms apply only to specific models (such as collagen disruption in the multiple-episode model). Therefore, identification of a fundamental set of mechanisms applicable to all models is difficult, if not impossible. Our understanding of these mechanisms, however, is developing rapidly due to advances in both experimental and clinical research. The following classification of mechanisms is derived from the work of Bolli and Kloner, as well as other investigators in this field.

Potentially Important Mechanisms for Myocardial Stunning

There appear to be five potentially important mechanisms for myocardial stunning: (1) free radical production; (2) altered calcium flux with calcium overload; (3) excitation-contraction uncoupling; (4) abnormalities of the microvasculature secondary to accumulation of white blood cells; and (5) abnormalities in high energy phosphate utilization.

(1) Free radical production. A number of studies have suggested that cytotoxic oxygen derived free radicals may precipitate myocardial stunning. Implicated are reactive oxygen metabolites, including the superoxide anion ($\cdot O_2^-$), hydrogen peroxide (H_2O_2), and the hydroxyl radical ($\cdot OH$). These free radical moieties are generated during coronary occlusion and/or during myocardial reperfusion. Evidence for the free radical hypothesis is based mainly on therapeutic trials using scavenging enzymes, including superoxide dismutase and catalase. This evidence is convincing. Use of both of these agents (but neither alone) results in greater recovery of regional contractile function following 15-minute occlusions of coronary arteries in dogs. A number of authors including Bolli (36,37), Przyklenh (38), Myers (35), and Gross (39) have demonstrated that free radical scavengers, antioxidants, iron chelators, and "quenching" agents mitigate postischemic contractile dysfunction. Thus, it appears that oxygen metabolites may play a critical role in the development of myocardial stunning both *in vitro* and *in vivo.*

More recently, the sources of oxygen radicals in the stunned myocardium have been investigated. Two sources have been suggested. The first source, xanthine oxidase, has been studied indirectly using its inhibitor allopurinol. Reversal of dysfunction of the stunned myocardium has been demonstrated following allopurinol administration (40). The second potential source of oxygen radicals is neutrophils. Depletion of leukocytes in the canine model has been shown to mitigate postischemic contractile dysfunction (41). However, other data are less convincing (42,43), and the role of leukocytes in oxyradical mediated dysfunction remains unresolved.

Oxygen radical generation appears to be an important mechanism for myocardial stunning in models of single or repeated ischemic episodes, as well as global ischemia. However, challenging questions remain regarding the sources of free radicals and the efficacy of specific oxygen scavengers.

(2) Altered calcium flux: Calcium overload. It has been postulated that calcium may play an important role in myocardial stunning. Investigations have focused on three areas: a) the sensitivity of the myofilament to calcium; b) the effect of calcium overload; and c) the effects of calcium channel blockers. Regarding *sensitivity of myofilaments to calcium*, the *in vitro* studies do suggest that stunning may be the result of reduced calcium sensitivity rather than availability. Using a canine model, Krause et al. (44) found that the rate of calcium uptake and calcium ATPase activity was reduced, suggesting calcium transport impairment. Other studies using isolated Langendorff-perfused heart models demonstrated decreased sensitivity to exogenous calcium (45). In contrast, the *in vivo* studies (46,47) suggest that calcium transient is paradoxically increased (calcium paradox), and that the sensitivity of the stunned myocardium to intracoronary calcium is not decreased (48). Therefore, decreased sensitivity of myofilaments to calcium does not appear to be an important mechanism. However, there is evidence that calcium overload, secondary to accelerated calcium entry on reperfusion, may be an important mechanism for myocardial stunning. *In vitro* studies have demonstrated that rises in intracellular calcium occur during ischemia and early reperfusion, and are associated with dysfunction (45), perhaps through damage of intracellular organelles associated with contraction. *In vivo* investigations are necessary to confirm these models.

Regarding the effect of calcium channel blockers, a number of agents including verapamil (49), diltiazem (50), and nifedipine (6,51) have been investigated in intact animals. The data seem favorable, demonstrating a complete recovery of dysfunction in regionally stunned myocardium. Whether the effects are due to their direct (vs. peripheral) actions is unknown. A recent study (52) using nifedipine suggests direct beneficial effects. However, the data are not completely conclusive given time course of administration of nifedipine (30 min after reperfusion), since it is presumed that transient calcium overload occurs immediately. Thus, further investigation of the role of calcium channel blockers is necessary.

(3) Sarcoplasmic reticulum dysfunction. Krause (53), Bolli (5), and others have suggested that sarcoplasmic reticulum dysfunction causing excitation-contraction uncoupling results in decreased ability to transport calcium. As a result, calcium release may be attenuated during systole, which could diminish contractile protein activation. In support of this hypothesis are the findings that administration of exogenous calcium restores ventricular function to the pre-ischemic levels (48). In addition, numerous investigators have reported that inotropic agents that increase intercellular calcium can reverse stunning (23,48,54-57). As stated above, however, there is disparity between the *in vitro* and *in vivo* findings (46,47); thus, this mechanism is attractive but requires verification.

(4) Microvascular dysfunction. Several investigators have suggested that coronary microvascular plugging by white blood cells during reperfusion reduces coronary blood flow—the low reflow phenomenon (58,59). Others have suggested that white blood cells are an extracellular source of oxygen derived free radicals (60,61). It has been demonstrated in support of both these potential mechanisms that depletion of neutrophils can enhance the recovery of post-ischemic function (41). These findings only may be applicable to the repetitive-episode model because of the time course of neutrophil accumulation. Therefore, further investigation is necessary to determine the importance of this mechanism.

(5) Impaired ATP use by myofibrils. Regarding ATP production, initially it had been proposed that stunning may result from insufficient ATP production because of loss of adenine nucleotide precursors. This hypothesis was supported by evidence that in the stunned myocardium the pattern of ATP decrement and recovery paralleled that of contractile dysfunction (11,12). However, newer evidence suggests that energy production does not appear to be impaired (5), and the myocardium in fact can respond to high metabolic demands induced by inotropic stimuli (22,23,48,54-57,62).

Regarding ATP use, Greenfield and Swain (63) reported that 15-minute occlusions in dogs reduced creatine kinase activity and adenosine diphosphate. Thus, normal energy used by the myofibrils may be disrupted and may contribute to dysfunction. Although these arguments have been challenged by the inotropic stimulation findings (demonstrating functional reserve) (22,23,48,54-57,62), controversy still exists regarding this potential mechanism.

Other Potential But Less Important Mechanisms

In addition to the above mechanisms, several other mechanisms have been suggested, including impairment of sympathetic neural responsiveness, impairment of myocardial perfusion, and damage of the extracellular collagen matrix (5). The *in vitro* and *in vivo* evidence for these is not as substantial, and at present these are not considered likely mechanisms for myocardial stunning.

Conclusions

Multiple mechanisms have been proposed and are under active investigation. It is clear that any one or more of these mechanisms may be appropriate for a specific model. However, because of the diversity of models that can cause stunning, no single set of mechanisms will apply. A unified theory, or unified set of mechanisms, for myocardial stunning does not appear to be likely.

Further research is necessary to elucidate the differences between the *in vitro* and *in vivo* experimental findings, and to identify effective therapies for treatment of myocardial stunning, such as antioxidants, adenosine-regulating agents, or calcium channel blockers.

CLINICAL IMPLICATIONS OF MYOCARDIAL STUNNING

Myocardial stunning may be an important factor precipitating left ventricular failure (both systolic and diastolic) and subsequent morbidity and mortality. There are a number of clinical scenarios in which prolonged post-ischemic dysfunction may occur. Among these are: a) unstable angina; b) acute myocardial infarction with early reperfusion (spontaneous or therapeutic); c) cardiac surgery with cardioplegic arrest; d) cardiac transplantation; e) silent ischemia; and f) exercised-induced ischemia.

Unstable Angina

Several clinical studies have demonstrated that prolonged regional wall-motion abnormalities occur in patients with unstable angina, even during pain-free periods. Using echocardiography, Nixon et al. (64) demonstrated that ventricular function remained abnormal several days following resolution of angina.

Acute Myocardial Infarction with Early Reperfusion

Therapeutic trials using streptokinase have demonstrated that regional wall motion is impaired after recanalization, and returns to normal gradually over a 1- to 2-week period following reperfusion. Most streptokinase trials found that if thrombolysis was successful, ventricular function gradually improved only days following recanalization (65-68).

Cardiac Surgery with Cardioplegia Arrest

Following cardiac surgery, both left and right ventricular dysfunction occur in all patients during the first 4 hours following surgery. In high risk patients, dysfunction persists beyond 24 hours, despite apparent resolution of myocardial ischemia (18,31,69). Recent evidence also suggests that ischemia is common following successful coronary revascularization, but resolves over the first 12 hours (70,72), however, dysfunction can persist for several days to 1 week following revascularization (73).

Cardiac Transplantation

Data are sparse, but anecdotal reports cite persistent ventricular dysfunction following transplantation, despite lack of evidence of ongoing ischemia during this period.

Silent Ischemia

The early studies of silent ischemia demonstrated repeated episodes of silent ischemia in ambulatory patients with coronary disease. Ventricular function studies demonstrate persistence of dysfunction following resolution of ischemic episodes (74). Recent evidence also demonstrates a high incidence of postoperative silent ischemia associated with ventricular dysfunction, with persistence of dysfunction after resolution of ischemia (31).

Exercise-induced Angina

Recent evidence (34,35) has suggested that in patients with double or triple vessel disease, regional wall-motion abnormalities persist 30 minutes after termination of exercise and resolution of ECG markers of ischemia.

Conclusion

Because of the complexity of the model for myocardial stunning, and the multiple conditions under which it can be produced, it is not surprising that multiple clinical scenarios exist in which prolonged postischemic contractile dysfunction occurs. It is important to recognize that the phenomenon of stunning exists, for the associated dysfunction may be reversible, and may be amenable to therapeutics such as antioxidants, adenosine-regulating agents, and calcium channel blockers.

SUMMARY

In conclusion, *in vitro, in vivo,* and clinical models have established prolonged postischemic contractile dysfunction, or myocardial stunning, as a real entity. Because of the complexity of stunning, classification includes a number of animal and human models. As a result, mechanisms of stunning are quite varied, and no unified theory of stunning is apparent.

Perhaps the most important challenges are to understand differences between the *in vitro* and *in vivo* models, and to investigate human models using therapeutic probes addressing the potentially most important mechanisms. Principal among these are the antioxidants, adenosine-regulating agents, and calcium channel blockers.

REFERENCES

1. Heyndrickx G, Millar R, McRitchie R, et al: Regional myocardial function and electrophysiological alterations after brief coronary artery occlusion in conscious dogs. J Clin Invest 56:978-985, 1975
2. Hyendrickx G, Baig H, Nellens P, et al: Depression of regional blood flow and wall thickening after brief coronary occlusions. Am J Physiol 234:H653-H659, 1978
3. Braunwald E, Kloner R: The stunned myocardium: Prolonged post-ischemic ventricular dysfunction. Circulation 66:1146-1149, 1982
4. Braunwald E, Rutherford J: Reversible ischemic left ventricular function: Evidence for the "hibernating myocardium." (Editorial) J Am Coll Cardiol 8:1467-1470, 1986
5. Bolli R: Mechanism of myocardial "stunning." Circulation 82:723-738, 1990
6. Kloner R, Przyklenk K, Patel B: Altered myocardial states: The stunned and hibernating myocardium. Am J Med 86(Suppl 1 A):14-22, 1989
7. Chirac P: De Motu Cordis. Adverseria Analytica 121, 1698
8. Porter T: On the results of ligation of the coronary arteries. J Physiol (Lond) 15:121, 1895

9. Herrick J: Clinical features of sudden obstruction of the coronary arteries. J Am Med Assoc 59:2015, 1912
10. Tennant R, Wiggers C: The effect of coronary occlusion on myocardial contraction. Am J Physiol 112:351-361, 1935
11. Ellis S, Henscke C, Sandor T, et al: Time course of functional and biochemical recovery of myocardium salvaged by reperfusion. Am J Cardiol 1:1047-1055, 1983
12. Puri P: Contractile and biochemical effects of coronary reperfusion after extended periods of coronary occlusion. Am J Cardiol 36:244, 1975
13. Weiner J, Apstein C, Arthur J, et al: Persistence of myocardial injury following brief periods of coronary occlusion. Cardiovasc Res 10:678-686, 1976
14. Wood J, Hanley H, Entman M, et al: Biochemical and morphological correlates of acute experimental myocardial ischemia in the dog. (IV. energy mechanisms during very early ischemia.) Circ Res 44:52, 1979
15. Hess M, Barnhart G, Crute S, et al: Mechanical and biochemical effects of transient myocardial ischemia. J Surg Res 26:175, 1979
16. DeBoer F, Ingwal J, Kloner R, et al: Prolonged derangements of canine myocardial purine metabolism after a brief coronary artery occlusion not associated with anatomic evidence of necrosis. Proc Natl Acad Sci USA 77:5471, 1980
17. Kloner R, Ellis S, Carlson M, et al: Coronary reperfusion for the treatment of acute myocardial infarction: Post-ischemic ventricular dysfunction. Cardiology 70:233-246, 1983
18. Mangano D: Perioperative cardiac morbidity. (Review) Anesthesiology 72:153-184, 1990
19. Przyklenk K, Patel B, Kloner R: Diastolic abnormalities of postischemic "stunned" myocardium. Am J Cardiol 60:1211 - 1213, 1987
20. Wijns W, Serruys P, Slager C: Effect of coronary occlusion during percutaneous transluminal angioplasty in humans on left ventricular chamber stiffness and regional diastolic pressure-radius relations. J Am Coll Cardiol 7:455-463, 1986
21. Kloner R, Ellis S, Lange R, et al: Studies of experimental coronary artery reperfusion: Effects of infarct size, myocardial function, biochemistry, ultrastructure, and microvascular damage. Circulation 68(Suppl I):I8-15, 1983
22. Ambrosio G, Jacobus W, Bergman C, et al: Preserved high energy phosphate metabolic reserve in globally "stunned" hearts despite reduction of basal ATP content and contractility. J Mol Cell Cardiol 19:953-964, 1987
23. Arnold J, Braunwald E, Sandor T, et al: Inotropic stimulation of reperfused myocardium with dopamine: Effects on infarct size and myocardial function. J Am Coll Cardiol 6:1026-1034, 1985
24. Jennings R, Reimer K: Factors involved in salvaging ischemic myocardium: Effects of reperfusion of arterial blood. Circulation 68(Suppl l):l25-1-36, 1983

25. Nicklas J, Becker L, Bulkley B: Effects of repeated brief coronary occlusion on regional left ventricular function and dimension in dogs. Am J Cardiol 56:473-478. 1985
26. Theroux P, Ross JJ, Franklin D, et al: Coronary arterial reperfusion: III. Early and late effects on regional myocardial function and dimensions in conscious dogs. Am J Cardiol 38:599-606, 1976
27. Lavallee M, Cox D, Patrick T, et al: Salvage of myocardial function by coronary artery reperfusion 1,2, and 3-hours after occlusion in conscious dogs. Circ Res 1983,53:235-247, 1983
28. Bush L, Buja L, Samowitz W, et al: Recovery of left ventricular segmental function after long-term reperfusion following temporary coronary occlusion in conscious dogs: Comparison of two- and four-hour occlusions. Circ Res 53:248-263, 1983
29. Reimer K, Jennings R: The "wavefront phenomenon" of myocardial ischemic death. II. Transmural progression of necrosis within the framework of ischemic bed size (myocardium at risk) and collateral flow. Lab Invest 40:633-644, 1979
30. Taegemeyer H, Roberts A, Raine A: Energy metabolism in reperfused heart muscle: Metabolic correlates to return of function. J Am Coll Cardiol 6:864-870, 1985
31. Mangano D: Biventricular function after myocardial revascularization in humans: Deterioration and recovery patterns during the first 24 hours. Anesthesiology 62:571-577, 1985
32. Brundage B, Massie B, Botvinick E: Improved regional ventricular function after successful surgical revascularization. J Am Coll Cardiol 3:902-908, 1984
33. Homans D, Sublett E, Dai X, et al: Persistence of regional left ventricular dysfunction after exercise-induced myocardial ischemia. J Clin Invest 77:66-73, 1986
34. Robertson W, Fegenbaum H, Armstrong W, et al: Exercise echocardiography: A clinically practical edition in the evaluation of coronary artery disease. J Am Coll Cardiol 2:1085-1091, 1983
35. Camici P. Araujo L, Spinks T: Increased uptake of ^{18}F-fluorodeoxyglucose in postischemic myocardium of patients with exercise-induced angina. Circulation 74:81-88, 1986
36. Myers M, Bolli R, Lekich R., et al: Enhancement of recovery of myocardial function by oxygen-free radical scavengers after reversible regional ischemia. Circulation 72:915-921, 1985
37. Jeroudi M, Triani F, Patel B, et al: Effect of superoxide dismutase and catalase, given separately, on myocardial "stunning." Am J Physiol 259(3):H889-H901, 1990
38. Przyklenk K, Kloner R: Superoxide dismutase plus catalase improved contractile function in the canine model of the "stunned" myocardium. Circ Res 58:148-156, 1986
39. Gross G, Farber N, Hardman H, et al: Beneficial actions of superoxide dismutase and catalase in "stunned" myocardium of dogs. Am J Physiol 250:H372-H377, 1986

40. Charlat M, O'Neill P, Egan J, et al: Evidence for a pathogenetic role of xanthine oxidase in the "stunned" myocardium. Am J Physiol 252:H566-H577, 1987
41. Engler R, Covell J: Granulocytes cause reperfusion ventricular dysfunction after 15-minute ischemia in the dog. Circ Res 61:20-28, 1987
42. O'Neill P, Charlat M, Hartley C, et al: Neutrophil depletion fails to attenuate post-ischemic myocardial dysfunction. (Abstract) Circulation 74 (Suppl II):II-349, 1986
43. Go L, Murry C, Richard V, et al: Myocardial neutrophil accumulation during reperfusion after reversible or irreversible ischemic injury. Am J Physiol 255:H1188-H1198, 1988
44. Krause S, Jacobus W, Becker L: Alterations in sarcoplasmic reticulum Ca^{2+} transport in the post-ischemic "stunned" myocardium. (Abstract) Circulation 74(Suppl II):II-67, 1986
45. Kusuoka HG, Porterfield J, Weisman H, et al: Pathophysiology and pathogenesis of stunned myocardium. Depressed Ca^{2+} activation of contraction as a consequence of reperfusion-induced cellular calcium overload in ferret hearts. J Clin Invest 79:950-961, 1987
46. Kusuoka H, Koretsune Y, Chacko V, et al: Excitation-contraction coupling in postischemic myocardium: Does failure of activator Ca^{2+} transients underlie stunning? Circ Res 66:1268-1276, 1990
47. Guarnieri T: Direct measurement of (Ca^{2+}) in early and late reperfused myocardium. (Abstract) Circulation 80(Suppl II):II-241, 1989
48. Ito B, Tate H, Kobayashi M, et al: Reversibly injured, postischemic canine myocardium retains normal contractile reserve. Circ Res 61:834-846, 1987
49. Przyklenk K, Kloner R: Effect of verapamil on postischemic "stunned" myocardium: Importance of the timing of the treatment. J Am Coll Cardiol 11:614-623, 1988
50. Taylor A, Golino P, Eckels R, et al: Differential enhancement of postischemic segmental systolic thickening by diltiazem. J Am Coll Cardiol 15:737-747, 1990
51. Lamping K, Gross G: Improved recovery of myocardial segment function following a short coronary occlusion in dogs by nicorandil, a potential new antianginal agent, and nifedipine. J Cardiovasc Pharmacol 7:158-166, 1985
52. Przyklenk K, Ghafari G, Eitzman D, et al: Nifedipine administered after reperfusion oblates systolic contractile dysfunction of postischemic "stunned" myocardium. J Am Coll Cardiol 13:1176-1183, 1989
53. Krause S, Jacobus W, Becker L: Alterations in cardiac sarcoplasmic reticulum calcium transport in the postischemic "stunned" myocardium. Circ Res 65:526-530, 1989
54. Mercier J, Lando U, Kanmatsuse K, et al: Divergent effects of inotropic stimulation on the ischemic and severely depressed reperfused myocardium. Circulation 66:397-400, 1982
55. Ellis S, Wynne J, Braunwald E, et al: Response of reperfusion-salvaged, stunned myocardium to inotropic stimulation. Am Heart J 107:9-13, 1984

56. Bolli R, Zhu W, Myers M, et al: Beta-adrenergic stimulation reverses postischemic myocardial dysfunction without producing subsequent functional deterioration. Am J Cardiol 56:964-968, 1985
57. Heusch G, Schafer S, Kroger K: Recruitment of inotropic reserve in "stunned" myocardium by the cardiotonic agent AR-L 57. Basic Res Cardiol 83:602-610, 1988
58. Kloner R, Alker K: Effect of streptokinase on intramyocardial hemorrhage, infarct size, and the no-reflow phenomenon during coronary reperfusion. Circulation 70:513-521, 1984
59. Engler R, Schmid-Schoenbein G, Pavelec R: Leukocyte capillary plugging in myocardial ischemia and reperfusion in the dog. Am J Physiol 111:98-111, 1983
60. McCord J: Are free radicals a major culprit? In Hearse DJ, Yellen DN (eds): Therapeutic Approaches to Myocardial Infarct Size Limitation. New York, Raven Press, pp. 209-218, 1984
61. Romson J, Hook B, Kunkel S, et al: Reduction of the extent of ischemic myocardial injury by neutrophil depletion in the dog. Circulation 67:1016-1023, 1983
62. Becker L, Levine J, DiPaula A, et al: Reversal of dysfunction in post-ischemic stunned myocardium by epinephrine and postextrasystolic potentiation. J Am Coll Cardiol 7:580-589, 1986
63. Greenfield R, Swain J: Disruption of myofibrillar energy use: Dual mechanisms that may contribute to post-ischemic dysfunction in stunned myocardium. Circ Res 60:283-289, 1987
64. Nixon J, Brown C, Smitherman T: Identification of transient and persistent segmental wall motion abnormalities in patients with unstable angina by two-dimensional echocardiography. Circulation 65:1497-1503, 1982
65. Anderson J, Marshall H, Bray B: A randomized trial of intracoronary streptokinase in the treatment of acute myocardial infarction. N Engl J Med 308:1313-1318, 1983
66. Stack R, Phillips HI, Grierson D: Functional improvement of jeopardized myocardium following intracoronary streptokinase infusion in acute myocardial infarction. J Clin Invest 72:84-95, 1983
67. Reduto L, Freund G, Gaeta J, et al: Coronary artery reperfusion in acute myocardial infarction: Beneficial effects of intracoronary streptokinase on left ventricular salvage and performance. Am Heart J 102:1168-1177, 1981
68. Patel B, Kloner R: Analysis of reported randomized trials of steptokinase therapy for acute myocardial infarction in the 1980's. Am J Cardiol 59:501-504, 1987
69. Mangano D, London M, Tubau J, et al: Dipyridamole thallium-201 scintigraphy as a preoperative screening test. Circulation 84:493-502, 1991
70. Knight A, Hollenberg M, London M, et al: Perioperative myocardial ischemia: Importance of the preoperative ischemic pattern. Anesthesiology 68:681-688, 1988
71. Smith R, Leung J, Mangano D, et al: Postoperative myocardial ischemia in patients undergoing coronary artery bypass graft surgery. Anesthesiology 74:464-473, 1991

72. Siliciano D, Mangano D: Postoperative myocardial ischemia: Mechanisms and therapies. In Estafanous F (ed): Opioids in Anesthesia. Boston, Butterworth Publishers, pp. 164-178, 1990
73. Ballantyne C, Verani M, Short H, et al: Delayed recovery of severely "stunned" myocardium with the support of a left ventricular assist device after coronary artery bypass graft surgery. J Am Coll Cardiol 10:710-712, 1987
74. Mathias P, Kenn N, Blevins R, et al: Coronary vasospasm as a cause of stunned myocardium. Am Heart J 113:383-385

PHOSPHODIESTERASE INHIBITORS

Jerrold.H. Levy, MD

PHOSPHODIESTERASE INHIBITORS

Introduction

Phosphodiesterase, a ubiquitous enzyme in biologic systems, functions to terminate the actions of cyclic 3',5'-nucleotides (i.e., cyclic AMP) by catalyzing its hydrolysis (1,2). Phosphodiesterase enzymes in the cardiovascular system have different substrate specificities, kinetic characteristics, and responses to pharmacologic agents that inhibit phosphodiesterases (1,2). Aminophylline, the phosphodiesterase inhibitor most clinicians are familiar with, has other effects that include interfering with adenosine metabolism. The newer cyclic AMP specific phosphodiesterase (PDE) inhibitors (also called Fraction III or low-Km cyclic AMP) are nonsympathomimetic agents that can produce both positive inotropic effects and vasodilation independent of β_1-adrenergic receptor stimulation (1,2).

Multiple forms of these novel drugs are currently under investigation, however, the bipyridines (milrinone and amrinone) and the imidazolones (enoximone) are the intravenous PDE inhibitors used clinically. (1,2). Milrinone is the most recent PDE fraction III inhibitor approved for use in the United States to treat biventricular failure. The role and application of these pharmacologic agents will be reviewed.

Role of B_1-Adrenergic Stimulation, Adenylyl Cyclase, and Cyclic AMP

Inotropic agents increase contractility by increasing cyclic AMP in the myocardial cell. Catecholamines stimulate β_1 adrenergic receptors that are coupled to adenylyl cyclase by guanine nucleotide-binding (G-regulatory) proteins (3-6). Cyclic AMP is the important "second messenger" in the heart that modulates intracellular calcium through the activation of protein kinases (3-6). Protein kinases phosphorylate proteins at several subcellular sites,

T. H. Stanley and P. L. Bailey (eds.), Anesthesiology and the Cardiovascular Patient, 195–202.

including the sarcolemma, the sarcoplasmic reticulum, and the troponin-tropomyosin regulatory complex on the myofilaments (3-6). Phosphorylation of the voltage-dependent calcium channels of the sarcolemma increases the intracellular influx of calcium during each depolarization and, thereby, the amount of calcium in the cell (3-6). Subsequent binding of intracellular calcium to troponin C leads to actin-myosin crossbridging and myocardial contraction. The extent of intracellular calcium binding, and the subsequent force of myocardial contraction, increase in direct proportion to the amount of intracellular calcium available, which is regulated by availability of adenylyl cyclase and cyclic AMP. As a result, the force of systolic contraction is increased. Cyclic AMP also affects the diastolic relaxation of the heart through phosphorylation of sites on the sarcoplasmic reticulum and contractile apparatus (5).

Patients who present with chronic heart failure and/or ventricular dysfunction have down-regulation of β_1-adrenergic receptors (i.e., a severe reduction in receptor density). In these patients, the β_1-receptor pool typically undergoes severe receptor loss (as much as 60%-70%) while the level of β_2-receptors remains unchanged (7-9). The selective depletion of β_1-receptors in heart failure leads to a shift in the proportion of β_1- versus β_2-receptors from approximately 80:20 (in normal myocardial tissue) to 60:40 in the failing human myocardium (7-9). β-receptor down-regulation and density loss are thought to be caused by chronic stimulation from activation of the renin-angiotensin system in heart failure, changes that increases endogenous norepinephrine release from the sympathetic nervous system to compensate for the low cardiac output states. Because β_1-mediated activation of adenylyl cyclase is the primary mechanism by which intracellular cAMP is produced, the progressive loss of β_1-receptor function can diminish contractility.

In experimental models, acute changes in β-adrenergic receptor function can also occur during cardiac surgery and cardiopulmonary bypass. Schwinn reported only 15% β-adrenergic receptor desensitization upon termination of cardiopulmonary bypass in healthy dogs with normal hearts (11). However, patients undergoing cardiac surgery and cardiopulmonary bypass usually have varying degrees of myocardial dysfunction. A 15% decrease in β-adrenergic receptors in patients with pre-existing low ejection fractions and ventricular dysfunction may contribute to difficulty in weaning from cardiopulmonary bypass. Schwinn also found a decrease in β-adrenergic receptor density in post-cardiopulmonary bypass biopsies suggesting that receptor down-regulation occurs in response to endogenous catecholamines released during the perioperative period.

Implications of β_1-Down Regulation

The clinical implications in patients with congestive heart failure and adrenergic neuroeffector abnormalities are potentially important. Patients with chronic increases in norepinephrine levels associated with heart failure will have neurotransmitter depletion, thus indirect acting pharmacologic agents like dopamine will have less effects than direct-acting β_1-adrenergic agents (12). Bristow has also suggested there is insignificant β-adrenergic receptor reserve available. Catecholamine-induced stimulation of β_1-adrenergic receptors will activate adenylyl cyclase, but at submaximal levels. Although there will be a decreased response in adenylyl cyclase to administration of β_1-specific agents, acute pharmacologic restoration of β_1-adrenergic responsiveness can potentially be obtained by combining catecholamines with phosphodiesterase inhibitors.

Phosphodiesterase Inhibitors

Phosphodiesterase inhibitors are nonglycosidic, nonsympathomimetic agents that can produce both positive inotropic effects and vasodilation (18,19). The bipyridines (amrinone and milrinone), the imidazolones (enoximone), and the methylxanthines (aminophylline) are the ones most widely available. They have a unique mechanism of action, functioning independently of the β_1-adrenergic receptor. Papaverine, a benzylisoquinoline derivative isolated from opium, is a nonspecific phosphodiesterase inhibitor and vasodilator used by cardiac surgeons for its ability to dilate the internal mammary artery.

Phosphodiesterase inhibitors bypass the β_1-adrenergic receptor to increase cyclic AMP and increase ventricular contractility, without significantly increasing the heart rate, by selective inhibition of phosphodiesterase fraction III, a cyclic AMP-specific phosphodiesterase enzyme (19,20). Aminophylline, a nonspecific phosphodiesterase inhibitor, routinely produces tachycardia due in part to its ability to inhibit adenosine. Phosphodiesterase inhibitors increase cyclic AMP in vascular smooth muscle and vasodilate both arterial and capacitance beds (19). Amrinone, milrinone, and enoximone increase cardiac output, while decreasing pulmonary capillary wedge pressure, systemic vascular resistance, and pulmonary vascular resistance, and represent unique agents that effectively manage biventricular dysfunction in cardiac surgical patients (20-24).

Chronic oral administration of milrinone and enoximone have demonstrated no beneficial long-term effect, but rather an increase in mortality. It is not surprising that long-term administration of any positive inotropic agent will have potential adverse effects over time. Whenever we administer inotropic support, it is always accompanied by hemodynamic monitoring, since tachyphylaxis or other adverse hemodynamic effects are likely to occur with prolonged administration of any inotropic agent. There is also an important difference between *acute* and *chronic* therapeutic interventions. Inotropic agents in an intravenous form are used to treat acute biventricular dysfunction, to facilitate separation from cardiopulmonary bypass, to treat acute ventricular dysfunction following cardiac or noncardiac surgery, and to increase cardiac output in patients awaiting cardiac transplantation. In these settings, continuous hemodynamic monitoring is used to help guide our therapeutic interventions. The use of phosphodiesterase inhibitors that bypass down-regulated β_1-adrenergic receptor-mediated pathways is an important therapeutic option. Because studies involving chronic, oral administration of phosphodiesterase inhibitors have shown negative results, this data should not be extrapolated to the use of any inotropic agent to treat *acute* biventricular dysfunction in the perioperative period. By bypassing β_1 adrenergic receptors that are down-regulated, PDE inhibitors offer unique benefits for *acute*, but not *chronic*, therapy.

Effects on Vascular Responses

Phosphodiesterase inhibitors lower calculated systemic vascular resistance by relaxing both arteriolar and venous vascular smooth muscle. They also decrease pulmonary artery occlusion pressure and increase cardiac output in patients with biventricular dysfunction by multiple mechanisms including arterial vasodilation, improving the inotropic state, and increasing venous capacitance, as well as decreasing venous return to the failing heart without increasing heart rate. The net effect is to decrease myocardial wall tension and myocardial oxygen consumption, as has been demonstrated with amrinone in patients with chronic heart failure (25).

Concomitant Administration with Catecholamines

Stimulation of a down-regulated heart with increasing concentrations of β_1-adrenergic agents will produce smaller increases in cyclic AMP formation for given levels of β_1-adrenergic receptor stimulation (10). The newer cyclic-AMP-specific phosphodiesterase inhibitors (drugs like amrinone, milrinone, and enoximone) bypass the β_1-adrenergic receptor and act additively with catecholamines to increase β_1-adrenergic receptor responsiveness (13-18).

Combination therapy with catecholamines and phosphodiesterase inhibitors can have additive effects to restore beta adrenergic responsiveness to the down-regulated β_1-adrenergic receptor (19-24). The concept of combination therapy has been reported using enoximone, a phosphodiesterase inhibitor, with catecholamines to increase cardiac output in severe heart failure (22-24). Patients in cardiogenic shock already receiving adrenergic support, enoximone was administered as a loading dose of 0.5 mg/kg. Pulmonary artery occlusion pressure decreased and cardiac index increased markedly. A second study investigated the effects of the addition of small boluses of enoximone to adrenergic agents in low flow states associated with heart failure or postoperative states after cardiac surgery. Each of the patients was treated with dobutamine; 12 patients were also treated with dopamine and 4 with norepinephrine. Enoximone was administered as small, but increasing intravenous boluses. No significant change in mean arterial pressure was observed, but cardiac index increased markedly after enoximone, 0.25 mg/kg.

For the bipyridine phosphodiesterase inhibitors, Gage reported "additive" effects when a loading dose of amrinone (2 mg/kg) was infused in patients with heart failure receiving dobutamine at 10.9 µg/kg per minute (19). Other reports include beneficial therapeutic use of amrinone and enoximone with the sympathomimetic agents epinephrine, norepinephrine, or dopamine in higher dosage ranges (22-24). Norepinephrine, epinephrine, or dopamine can also be used in combination with the phosphodiesterase inhibitors to support systemic arterial pressures as indicated.

Cyclic-AMP-specific phosphodiesterase inhibitors also provide unique mechanisms of systemic vasodilation, as well as attenuating the constrictive effects of catecholamines (25-27). Although catecholamines are administered as a starting infusion, all phosphodiesterase inhibitors must be administered initially as a loading dose to obtain therapeutic levels, followed by an infusion if levels are to be maintained in a therapeutic range (28-32).

Administration and Therapeutic Levels

With all of the PDE inhibitors, loading and infusion doses are required in order to obtain appropriate therapeutic levels. For amrinone, a loading dose of 1.5 to 2.0 mg/kg is required to achieve a minimum therapeutic concentration of 1.7 µg/ml in cardiac surgical patients when weaning from cardiopulmonary bypass (CPB) (29). Administering a loading dose alone will provide an initial therapeutic concentration for 30 to 60 minutes for most of the phosphodiesterase inhibitors. The half life of amrinone in cardiac surgical patients is approximately 3.5 hours.

We found milrinone has an elimination half-life of approximately 70-90 minutes in patients who receive the drug at the end of CPB (30). This is significantly less than the 210 minutes we reported with amrinone. By loading the patient with a 50 μg/kg dose of milrinone, followed by an infusion of 0.5 μg/kg/min, therapeutic levels of 100-300 ng/ml are obtained (30).

Table 1 lists initial loading doses and continuous infusion rates. All phosphodiesterase inhibitors produce dose-dependent vasodilation. They should be administered over 5 to 10 minutes, however, to attenuate the peak plasma concentration and the associated vasodilation.

Table 1. Loading and infusion doses for the phosphodiesterase inhibitors.

Drug	*Loading Dose*	*Infusion*
Amrinone	1.5-2.0 mg/kg	5-20 μg/kg/min
Enoximone	0.5-1.0 mg/kg	5-10 μg/kg/min
Milrinone	50-75 μg/kg	0.375-0.75 μg/kg/min
Aminophylline	5-6 mg/kg	0.25-0.9 mg/kg/min

REFERENCES

1. Beavo JA, Reifsnyder DH. Primary sequence of cyclic nucleotide phosphodiesterase enzymes and the design of selective inhibitors. TIPS 11:150-155, 1990
2. Evans DB. Overview of cardiovascular physiologic and pharmacologic aspects of selective phosphodiesterase peak III inhibitors. Am J Cardiol. 63:9A-11A, 1989
3. Rasmussen H. The calcium messenger system. N Engl J Med 314:1094-1101, 1164-70, 1986
4. Royster RL. Intraoperative administration of inotropes in cardiac surgery patients. J Cardiothorac Anesth 4(55):17-28, 1990
5. Katz AM. Cyclic adenosine monophosphate effects on the myocardium: a man who blows hot and cold with one breath. J Am Coll Cardiol 2:143-9, 1983
6. Trautwein W, Hescheler J. Regulation of cardiac L-type calcium current by phosphorylation and G proteins. Annu Rev Physiol 52:257-74, 1990
7. Bristow MR, Ginsburg R, Minobe W, et al. Decreased catecholamine sensitivity and β-adrenergic receptor density in failing human hearts. N Engl J Med 307:205-211, 1982
8. Bristow MR, Port JD, Hershberger RE, et al. The β-adrenergic receptor-adenylate cyclase complex as a target for therapeutic intervention in heart failure. Eur Heart J 10(suppl B):45-54, 1989

9. Bristow MR, Hershberger RE, Port JD, et al. β-adrenergic pathways in nonfailing and failing human ventricular myocardium. Circulation 82(suppl):I12-I25, 1990
10. Bristow MR, Sandoval AB, Gilbert EM, et al. Myocardial a- and β-adrenergic receptor in heart failure: is cardiac-derived norepinephrine the regulatory signal? Eur Heart J 9:35-40, 1988
11. Schwinn DA, Leone BJ, Spahn DR, Chesnut LC, Page SO, McRae RL, Liggett SB. Desensitization of myocardial β-adrenergic receptors during cardiopulmonary bypass. Evidence for early uncoupling and late downregulation. Circulation 84:2559-2567, 1991
12. Port JD, Gilbert EM, Larrabee P, et al. Neurotransmitter depletion compromises the ability of indirect acting amines to provide inotropic support in the failing human heart. Circulation 81:929-938, 1990
13. Benotti JR, Grossman W, Braunwald E, et al. Hemodynamic assessment of amrinone. N Engl J Med 299:1373-1377, 1987
14. Levy JH, Ramsay J, Bailey JM: Pharmacokinetics and pharmacodynamics of phosphodiesterase-III inhibitors. J Cardiothorac Anesth 6(Suppl 5):7-11, 1990
15. Baim DS, McDowell AV, Cherniles J, Monrad ES, Parker JA, Edelson J, Braunwald E, Grossman W. Evaluation of a new bipyridine inotropic agent - milrinone - in patients with severe congestive heart failure. N Engl J Med 309:748-756, 1983
16. Fitzpatrick PG, Cinquegrani MP, Vakiener AR, et al. Hemodynamic and regional blood flow response to milrinone in patients with severe congestive heart failure: a dose-ranging study. Am Heart J 114:97-105, 1987
17. Gonzalez M, Desager J-P, Jacquemart J-L, Chenu P, Muller T, Installe E. Efficacy of enoximone in the management of refractory low output states following cardiac surgery. J Cardiothorac Anesth 2:409-418, 1988
18. Benotti, JR, Grossman W, Braunwald E, et al. Effects of amrinone on myocardial energy metabolism and hemodynamics in patients with severe congestive heart failure due to coronary artery disease. Circulation 62:28-36, 1980
19. Gage J, Rutman H, Lucido D, et al. Additive effects of dobutamine and amrinone on myocardial contractility and ventricular performance in patients with severe heart failure. Circulation 74:367-373, 1986
20. Robinson RJS, Tchervenkov C. Treatment of low cardiac output after aortocoronary artery bypass surgery using a combination of norepinephrine and amrinone. J Cardiothorac Anesth 3:229-233, 1987
21. Olsen KH, Kluger J, Fieldman A. Combination high dose amrinone and dopamine in the management of moribund cardiogenic shock after open heart surgery. Chest 94:503-506, 1988
22. Boldt J, Kling D, Moosdorf R, Hempelmann G. Enoximone treatment of impaired myocardial function during cardiac surgery: combined effects with epinephrine. J Cardiothorac Anesth 4:462-468, 1990
23. Vincent JL, Leon J, Melot BC, Kahn RJ. Addition of phosphodiesterase inhibitors to adrenergic agents in acutely ill patients. Intl J Cardiology 28:S7-S11, 1990

24. Uretsky BF, Hua J. Combined intravenous pharmacotherapy in the treatment of patients with decompensated congestive heart failure. Amer Heart J, June, 1991
25. Levy JH, Salmenpera MT, Meyer K, Harrison D. Phosphodiesterase inhibitors dilate human internal mammary artery in vitro. Anesthesiology A1118(S), 1991
26. Levy JH, Bailey JM. Effects of amrinone on vascular resistance and capacitance in humans. Chest 105: 62-64, 1994
27. Silver PJ, Lepore RE, O'Connor B, et al. Inhibition of the low Km cyclic AMP phosphodiesterase and activation of the cyclic AMP systsem in vascular smooth muscle by milrinone. J Pharmacol Exp Ther 247:34-42, 1988
28. Edelson J, Stroshane R, Benziger DP, et al. Pharmacokinetics of the bipyridines amrinone and milrinone. Circulation. 73(suppl III):145-152, 1986
29. Bailey JM, Levy JH, Rogers G, Szlam F, Hug CC. Pharmacokinetics of amrinone during cardiac surgery. Anesthesiology 75:961-968, 1991
30. Bailey JM, Levy JH, Kikura M, Szlam F, Hug CC. Pharmacokinetics of milrinone: during cardiac surgery. Anesthesiology 81: 616-622, 1994
31. Borow KM, Come PC, Neumann A, Baim DS, Braunwald E, Grossman W. Physiologic assessment of the inotropic, vasodilator and afterload reducing effects of milrinone in subjects without cardiac disease. Am J Cardiol. 55:1204-1209, 1985
32. Jaski BE, Fifer MA, Wright RF, Braunwald E, Colucci WS. Positive inotropic and vasodilator actions of milrinone in patients with severe congestive heart failure: dose-response relationships and comparison to nitroprusside. J Clin Invest. 75:643-649, 1985

ISCHEMIC MITRAL VALVE REGURGITATION, MITRAL VALVE REPAIR AND TEE

Norbert P. de Bruijn, MD, FACC

Over the last decade, mitral valve repair has developed from an interesting fad to a widely accepted technique of preserving a patient's native valve resulting in better preserved left ventricular function, better exercise tolerance and fewer postoperative complications. Transesophageal echocardiography (TEE) has been instrumental in stimulating this development because of its unique potential to aid in the evaluation of the mitral valve. From an anatomical and (patho)physiological point of view, both before surgery is undertaken and immediately after, TEE helps ensure that patients leave the operating room with a satisfactory result.

ISCHEMIC MITRAL REGURGITATION

At a time when hospital mortality for adult cardiac operations is continuing to fall, risk in patients undergoing combined coronary bypass-mitral valve surgery remains relatively high. Efforts to improve results have been directed toward a more general application of mitral valve reconstruction in this population, tailoring the type of repair to the pathological anatomy underlying the valve dysfunction.

The explanation for suboptimal surgical results after mitral valve replacement is not entirely clear. Reduced long-term survival has been associated with several risk factors, such as isolated mitral regurgitation, NYHA Class IV congestive heart failure and the ischemic etiology of valvular incompetence. Even in the mid-to-late 1980s, acute valve replacement for ischemic incompetence in the Duke series was associated with a hospital mortality in excess of 50%, when mortality for other elective isolated valve replacement operations was 5.6% (1).

Although the exact pathophysiology of mitral valve incompetence is not always obvious preoperatively, categorization of patients according to the etiology of valve regurgitation is important from a prognostic and technical

T. H. Stanley and P. L. Bailey (eds.), Anesthesiology and the Cardiovascular Patient, 203–206.

viewpoint. Primary mitral valve dysfunction is usually related to myxomatous degeneration or rheumatic involvement of valve tissue. Myxomatous degeneration of the mitral valve is characterized by leaflet prolapse, chordal rupture, or both, and is almost always accompanied by chronic annular dilatation and central incompetence of one or both leaflets. Rheumatic valvular involvement typically produces leaflet retraction, fibrotic thickening and calcification.

In ischemic mitral regurgitation, valve incompetence directly follows an acute myocardial infarction and can be divided into three types:

1. Posterior papillary muscle dysfunction in which regurgitation and congestive failure are coincident with the onset of a large posterior wall infarction. Combinations of localized posterior annular dilatation, loss of papillary muscle shortening, and anatomical leaflet defects produce localized lateral valve prolapse and incompetence at the posterior commissural region. The clinical picture in some of these patients can fluctuate considerably over time.
2. Papillary muscle rupture is the second type of ischemic mitral incompetence and is the least common type (0.1% of CAD patients undergoing cardiac catheterization).
3. The third type consists of patients with diffuse left ventricular dysfunction from multiple infarctions, and the accompanying regurgitation is associated with generalized ventricular and annular dilatation. In our experience this group is probably the most common.

Operative mortality associated with mitral valve surgery in patients with severe mitral regurgitation and cardiogenic shock due to myocardial infarction is extremely high. Currently, our preference is to insert an intraaortic balloon pump in order to reverse organ failure. Although the mortality of this conservative treatment is high, many appropriately managed critically ill patients subsequently become satisfactory surgical candidates. Other patients in whom prompt surgical treatment may be ill advised are elderly patients with multiorgan failure. It is advisable to follow patients with posterior papillary muscle dysfunction for a period of time in order to properly assess the ultimate magnitude of regurgitation and need surgery.

Whenever possible, patients with papillary muscle dysfunction who present within several hours of infarct onset should undergo reperfusion therapy. Successful early reperfusion with thrombolytics or PTCA frequently produces rapid and dramatic recovery of mitral valve competence and hemodynamic stabilization.

INTRAOPERATIVE TEE AND OPERATIVE PROCEDURE

After placement of the TEE probe (preferably a biplane or multiplane probe) it is important to adjust patients' afterload to a level where they will be expected to function postoperatively. Appropriate afterload is necessary to form an accurate impression concerning the severity of mitral regurgitation. The mitral valve is examined in multiple planes, if at all possible, and the anatomy described in terms of leaflet motion (restriction or prolapse), leaflet thickness and integrity, annular size and shape, presence of calcification/fibrosis, presence of elongated or ruptured chordae, and regional wall motion (especially of the inferior LV wall). Subsequently Doppler color flow imaging is used to describe the amount of mitral regurgitation as well as the direction of the regurgitant jet, which can impart additional information about the valve's pathology. It is probably optimal to first perform coronary artery surgery and reexamine the mitral valve after revascularization. Frequently bypass grafting of the right coronary artery will restore mitral valve competence. However, this approach is time consuming and in practice we often decide the surgical course to be taken prior to aortic crossclamping. In the vast majority of patients with pure ischemic mitral valve regurgitation, annuloplasty is all that is usually required. Most of these patients have little or no residual mitral regurgitation and their long-term survival has been satisfactory (2).

In patients in whom there is mitral regurgitation secondary to myxomatous degeneration, often there is central leaflet incompetence. Frequently the insufficiency is caused by dilatation of the posterior part of the annulus in combination with elongation or actual rupture of one or more chordae. The first step in the valve repair is resection of the middle scallop of the posterior leaflet, with or without undermining of the lateral scallops. The effect of this procedure is to move the posterior annulus anteriorly, more so by undermining the lateral scallops (sliding annuloplasty), and to remove any redundant posterior leaflet tissue.

In practice this repair converts the posterior leaflet from a mobile, flexible structure into a stiff shelf, which acts as a "door jamb" to anterior leaflet "door." Elongated chordae are shortened into troughs in the papillary muscles, in order to move the apposition point of the leaflets well into the ventricle. In our institution, we exclusively employ Carpentier annuloplasty rings, which are semi-rigid, to reinforce the mitral annulus. The ring is sized so that the anterior leaflet completely covers the ring. This ensures adequate coaptation with the posterior leaflet. It is important that the leaflets are not moved too far into the ventricle or systolic anterior motion of the anterior leaflet, generally with LV outflow tract obstruction, will result.

In primary mitral valve disease the chordae tendineae can be too short or broken. Appropriate surgical interventions include lengthening or replacement of the chordae or transplantation of chordae from one leaflet to the other. Perforations in the leaflets can be carefully closed and vegetations can be shaved of.

In the case of mitral stenosis, the results are not nearly as favorable as in mitral regurgitation. It is critical that the mitral commissures, which are not just the two leaflets meeting but which form a skirt, are left intact or mitral regurgitation will result. The presence of retracted chords, thickened leaflets, and annular calcification make repair more difficult and less rewarding.

After valve repair it is crucial that valve function be evaluated under appropriate hemodynamic loading conditions, so that an accurate evaluation of post-repair valve function can be obtained. There is ample evidence (3) that residual mitral regurgitation after surgery for either primary valve disease or ischemic mitral regurgitation is an important predictor of patient survival, even more so than patient age or left ventricular ejection fraction.

The application of TEE plays crucial role in the assessment of patients with mitral valve disease and dysfunction and has contributed significantly to the successful application of valvular repair surgery.

REFERENCES

1. Rankin JS, Hickey MS, Smith LR, et al. Current management of mitral valve incompetence associated with coronary artery disease. J Card Surg 4:25-42, 1989
2. David TE. Techniques and results of mitral valve repair for ischemic mitral regurgitation. J Card Surg 9(suppl):274-277, 1994
3. Sheikh KH, Rankin JS, de Bruijn NP et al. Intraoperative transesophageal Doppler color flow imaging used to guide patient selection and operative treatment of ischemic mitral regurgitation. Circulation 84:594-604, 1991

CARDIOVASCULAR ACTIONS OF DESFLURANE

David C. Warltier, MD, PhD

Desflurane (difluoromethyl-1-fluoro-2,2,2-trifluoroethyl ether; I-653), a structural analog of isoflurane, possesses remarkable metabolic stability. It has very low blood- and tissue-gas partition coefficients which facilitates rapid anesthetic induction, alterations in anesthetic depth, and emergence in a variety of clinical settings. The hemodynamic actions of desflurane have been explored in detail in experimental animals and humans.

CARDIOVASCULAR ACTIONS OF DESFLURANE IN EXPERIMENTAL ANIMALS

Weiskopf et al. (1) examined the cardiovascular effects of desflurane (end-tidal concentrations of 0.8, 1.2, and 1.6 MAC) and directly compared these effects to those produced by nearly equianesthetic concentrations of isoflurane in chronically instrumented swine. Desflurane caused an increase in heart rate which was greatest at 0.8 MAC and dose-related decreases in mean arterial pressure. Cardiac output was maintained at 0.8 MAC, but decreased at 1.2 and 1.6 MAC. A decrease in systemic vascular resistance was observed at the lowest concentration but was not further depressed at the higher concentrations. Depression of systemic hemodynamics and myocardial function were evident, but desflurane did not affect overall tissue perfusion as oxygen transport and consumption and mixed venous oxyhemoglobin saturation were unchanged from the conscious state. The cardiovascular effects of desflurane were not distinguishable from those produced by isoflurane.

The cardiovascular safety of high concentrations of desflurane and isoflurane were also explored in swine (2). Using the ratio of lethal-to-anesthetic concentration as an index of margin of safety, it was found that had an index of (2.5) and isoflurane (3:0) an index of 2.5 for desflurane relatively greater than the ratio reported for other volatile anesthetics (e.g., halothane approximately 2.0). The concentration of desflurane producing cardiovascular collapse was greater than that resulting in apnea. Thus, cardiovascular compromise during spontaneous ventilation is unlikely. This study (2) also suggested that desflurane

T. H. Stanley and P. L. Bailey (eds.), Anesthesiology and the Cardiovascular Patient, 207–217.

may produce more profound cardiovascular depression than isoflurane when administered in concentrations greater than 1.5 MAC.

Weiskopf et al. (3) investigated the arrhythmogenic potential of desflurane in response to administration of epinephrine in swine. The rate of infusion of epinephrine needed to cause premature ventricular contractions during anesthesia with desflurane was similar to the rate required during equianesthetic concentrations of isoflurane. In addition, epinephrine infusions resulted in similar increases in mean arterial pressure and heart rate in both desflurane and isoflurane groups. In contrast, ventricular ectopy occurred at lower infusion rates of epinephrine when swine were anesthetized with halothane. Other investigations have shown that anesthetic adjuvants such as atracurium, succinylcholine, atropine, fentanyl, and thiopental administered during desflurane or isoflurane anesthesia do not produce unexpected or potentially disadvantageous cardiovascular effects.

Desflurane was found to produce significant decreases in cerebral vascular resistance and increases in cerebral blood flow (4). Desflurane also caused dose-related decreases in mean arterial pressure and systemic vascular resistance with relative maintenance of cardiac index, supporting the findings of Weiskopf et al. (1) in swine. Desflurane provided adequate cerebral perfusion to meet the demands of cerebral oxygen consumption during profound desflurane-induced hypotension (5). These parallel decreases in both cerebral blood flow and oxygen consumption and maintenance of adequate cerebral perfusion are similar to those previously described for halothane and isoflurane.

The systemic and coronary hemodynamic actions of desflurane were studied in the presence and absence of autonomic nervous system blockade and directly compared to the effects produced by isoflurane, halothane, and enflurane in chronically instrumented dogs in an investigation by Pagel et al. (6). While many similarities between the hemodynamic effects of desflurane and isoflurane were identified, some differences between these anesthetics were noted as well. Desflurane maintained mean arterial pressure to a greater degree than did isoflurane (up to 1.75 MAC; Figure 1). In addition, while isoflurane produced a decrease in calculated systemic vascular resistance, no changes in resistance were observed during administration of desflurane. Desflurane appeared to maintain myocardial contractility as assessed by left ventricular peak positive dP/dt and dP/dt_{50} to a greater degree than did isoflurane in dogs with intact autonomic nervous system function. These differences between isoflurane and desflurane were abolished in the presence of pharmacological blockade of the autonomic nervous system, suggesting that desflurane may produce less depression of sympathetic tone and autonomic reflexes than

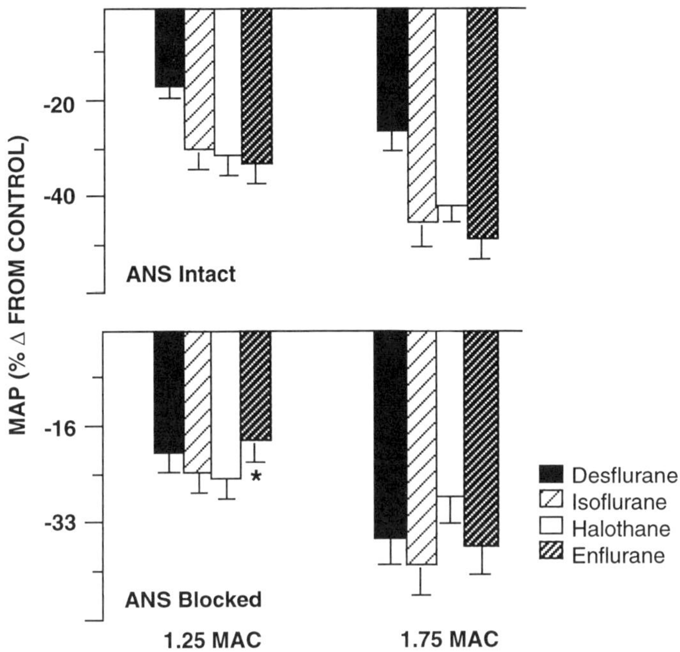

Figure 1. Histograms depicting the effects of volatile anesthetics (1.25 and 1.75 MAC) on mean arterial pressure (MAP) in autonomically (ANS) intact and blocked chronically instrumented dogs. All values are significantly ($p < 0.05$) different from the baseline conscious control. Desflurane reduced MAP to a lesser ($p < 0.05$) degree than isoflurane, enflurane, or halothane in ANS intact dogs (upper panel), an effect which was abolished with ANS blockade (lower panel). *Significantly ($p < 0.05$) different from the same anesthetic at the same concentration in ANS dogs.

isoflurane and, therefore, result in greater maintenance of mean arterial pressure and contractile function at any given level of anesthetic depth. Desflurane also caused less cardiovascular depression than did equianesthetic concentrations of halothane or enflurane. Both desflurane and isoflurane increased diastolic coronary blood flow and decreased diastolic coronary vascular resistance, indicating that desflurane, like isoflurane but not halothane or enflurane, may produce coronary vasodilation. In contrast to isoflurane, however, when heart rate was prevented from increasing during autonomic nervous system blockade, desflurane caused no change in coronary flow.

Merin et al. (7), in a concurrent investigation, also examined the effects of desflurane and isoflurane on cardiovascular dynamics and regional blood flow in the chronically instrumented dog. These investigators (7) demonstrated that desflurane and isoflurane produced nearly identical hemodynamic effects at several equianesthetic concentrations, including similar decreases in mean arterial pressure and myocardial contractility as assessed by left ventricular peak positive dP/dt. Desflurane maintained hepatic arterial blood flow and hepatic vascular resistance. In contrast, isoflurane produced an increase and decrease, respectively, in these variables. The combined total hepatic blood flow (portal plus hepatic arterial) was reduced by high concentrations of desflurane reflecting a decrease in the portal flow component. In contrast, total hepatic blood flow was unchanged by isoflurane. Neither desflurane nor isoflurane significantly effected renal blood flow.

Because desflurane may produce mild coronary vasodilation similar to isoflurane, the theoretical potential exists for this new anesthetic to produce a redistribution of coronary collateral blood flow away from ischemic myocardium ("coronary steal") during an increase in blood flow to normal zones. Hartman et al. (8) studied the effects of desflurane on the regional distribution of myocardial blood flow in a chronically-instrumented canine model of multivessel coronary artery disease. The results of this investigation indicated that desflurane did not redistribute blood flow away from collateral-dependent myocardium to normal regions *via* a "coronary steal" mechanism when heart rate and mean arterial pressure were restored to postocclusion control levels (Figure 2). Similar results were obtained in analogous investigations with isoflurane, in direct contrast to the findings obtained with adenosine, a potent coronary vasodilator which produced pronounced "coronary steal" despite correction of heart rate and mean arterial pressure to control values. Although isoflurane and desflurane may produce small decreases in coronary vascular resistance, the agents are simply not strong enough vasodilators to cause coronary steal.

The effects of desflurane on left ventricular mechanics during systole and diastole have been examined in chronically instrumented dogs with pharmacologic blockade of the autonomic nervous system (9,10). Contractility was evaluated using the preload recruitable stroke work (PRSW) versus end diastolic segment length (EDL) relationship, a linear and relatively afterload-insensitive extension of the Frank-Starling concept which has been shown to be a reliable index of inotropic state. The PRSW versus EDL relationship was calculated from left ventricular pressure-segment length diagrams generated by sequential constriction of the inferior vena cava with a hydraulic vascular occluder. PRSW versus EDL slope was decreased to equal degrees by desflurane and

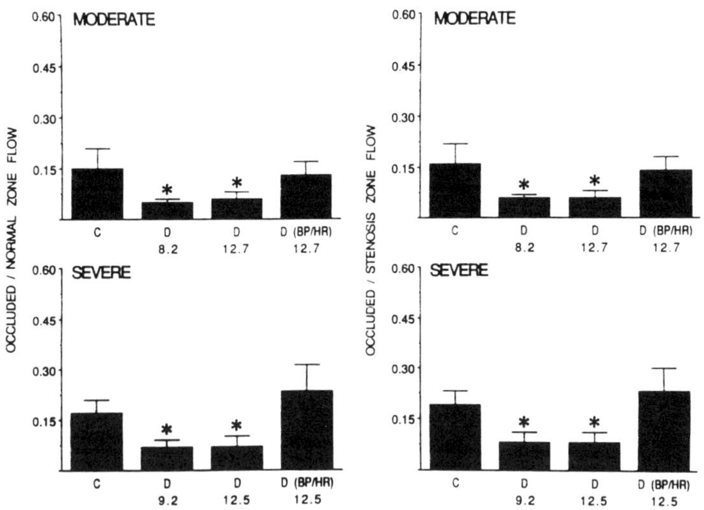

Figure 2. Ratio of occluded to normal zone (left panels) or occluded to stenosis zone (right panels) myocardial blood flows in chronically instrumented dogs with moderate (top panels) or severe (bottom panels) left circumflex coronary artery stenosis. Data obtained during the conscious state (C), during two concentrations of desflurane (D), and with blood pressure and heart rate returned to levels present in the conscious state (BP/HR) during the high concentration of desflurane. *Significantly ($p < 0.05$) different from the conscious state.

isoflurane, indicating that these agents produced equivalent direct decreases in myocardial contractility (Figure 3).

Left ventricular diastolic function has been shown to significantly influence systolic performance in several pathologic states including ischemic heart disease, left ventricular hypertrophy, and cardiomyopathy. Desflurane, isoflurane, and halothane prolong isovolumic relaxation to a similar degree as evaluated by an invasively-derived time constant of relaxation (10). In addition, while halothane impaired passive ventricular filling, desflurane and isoflurane had no effect on ventricular compliance. Thus, desflurane and isoflurane also appeared to produce equivalent depression of ventricular function during diastole.

In summary, although desflurane and isoflurane produce similar cardiovascular effects, some subtle differences between these agents have been noted

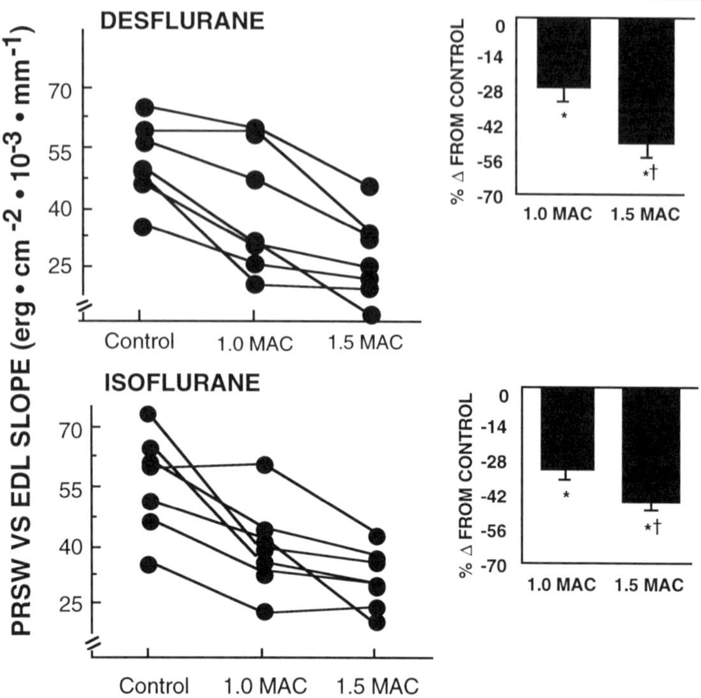

Figure 3. Preload recruitable stroke work (PRSW) versus end diastolic segment length (EDL) slope for each chronically instrumented dog (N=7) during conscious control and 1.0 and 1.5 MAC desflurane (top panel) or isoflurane (bottom panel). Figure insets depict data represented as percent change from control. *Significantly ($p < 0.05$) different from control. †Significantly ($p < 0.05$) different from 1.0 MAC. No differences were observed between desflurane and isoflurane groups at either anesthetic concentration.

in experimental animals. In general, however, the similarities in the cardiovascular effects produced by these agents are quite striking.

CARDIOVASCULAR ACTIONS OF DESFLURANE IN HUMANS

Weiskopf et al. (11) studied the steady state cardiovascular actions of desflurane in volunteers mechanically ventilated to maintain normocarbia. Desflurane caused dose-dependent decreases in mean arterial pressure and systemic vascular resistance and increases in right heart filling pressures and heart rate. These findings were similar to the effects produced by isoflurane. In addition, desflurane did not change cardiac index, left ventricular ejection fraction, or the velocity of left ventricular circumferential fiber shortening (V_{cfs}) as assessed by echocardiography. These findings suggest that desflurane may produce less depression of myocardial contractility than other halogenated agents in man. Mixed venous oxyhemoglobin saturation, oxygen consumption, and the ratio of oxygen transport to oxygen consumption remained constant in this study, indicating that desflurane maintains adequate tissue perfusion despite producing significant declines in perfusion pressure.

It has been established that the duration of halothane and enflurane anesthesia effect the hemodynamic profiles produced by these volatile agents. Therefore, Weiskopf et al. (11) also studied the cardiovascular actions of desflurane after a prolonged period of anesthesia (7 hours). Prolonged anesthesia with desflurane resulted in less cardiovascular depression than during the first 90 minutes of anesthesia. Indices of cardiac filling including central venous pressure and left ventricular cross- sectional area (as assessed by echocardiography) did not differ between the early and late periods at either 0.83 or 1.66 MAC desflurane. In contrast, heart rate and cardiac index were higher after prolonged anesthetic exposure at both concentrations than during the first 90 minutes. Other variables including left ventricular ejection fraction, V_{cfs}, and skeletal muscle blood flow did not change during prolonged anesthesia.

The hemodynamic effects of combined desflurane and nitrous oxide anesthesia were studied in male volunteers by Cahalan et al. (12). Desflurane-nitrous oxide anesthesia caused dose-dependent decreases in mean arterial pressure, cardiac index, systemic vascular resistance and left ventricular stroke work index and increases in pulmonary arterial and central venous pressures. No significant changes in heart rate were observed when desflurane was combined with nitrous oxide. The combination of these two agents also modestly increased left ventricular end diastolic cross-sectional area and decreased V_{cfs}, systolic wall stress and left ventricular ejection fraction indicating myocardial depression. The cardiovascular responses to tetanic electrical stimulation of the ulnar nerve were investigated in male volunteers during desflurane anesthesia (13). Stimulation of the ulnar nerve increased in heart rate, mean arterial pressure, cardiac output, and pulmonary arterial pressure at 0.8 and 1.2 MAC desflurane. In contrast, these hemodynamic responses were attenuated at 1.66 MAC.

Several investigations have been undertaken to determine the efficacy and safety of desflurane in patients with coronary artery disease. Thomson et al. (14) directly compared desflurane to isoflurane in patients undergoing coronary artery bypass graft surgery. After anesthetic induction with thiopental and fentanyl, desflurane or isoflurane was administered maintaining systolic blood pressure and heart rate at near preanesthetic levels. Vasoactive drugs or additional fentanyl were used to control hemodynamics if end-tidal anesthetic concentrations between zero and 2 MAC could not maintain hemodynamics within predefined limits. The cardiovascular actions of desflurane and isoflurane prior to cardiopulmonary bypass were very similar. In addition, the anesthetic requirements needed to maintain stable hemodynamics were indistinguishable between desflurane and isoflurane groups. During stressful stimuli, e.g., intubation or sternotomy, systolic pressure increased significantly more during isoflurane than during desflurane anesthesia. No differences in the incidence of electrocardiographic changes indicative of myocardial ischemia prior to cardiopulmonary bypass, perioperative myocardial infarction, or perioperative mortality were identified between desflurane and isoflurane groups.

Helman et al. (15) also examined the impact of desflurane in patients with coronary artery disease by comparing the risk of myocardial ischemia during desflurane versus sufentanil anesthesia. Myocardial ischemia was detected by continuous Holter electrocardiography (prior to, during, and 48 hours following surgery) and echocardiography in patients undergoing elective coronary artery bypass graft surgery. The authors reported that increases in heart rate and systemic and pulmonary artery pressures were more common and required a greater use of esmolol during induction with desflurane (in the absence of any opioid) than with sufentanil. An increased incidence of ischemia as detected by electrocardiographic changes and regional wall motion abnormalities occurred in the desflurane group in the induction period concomitant with increases in heart rate and arterial pressure. During maintenance of anesthesia, hemodynamics were well controlled by desflurane and the risk of ischemic events not significantly increased. No differences in adverse cardiac outcome (ventricular failure requiring intra-aortic balloon pump placement, myocardial infarction, or cardiac death) between desflurane and sufentanil were identified. This was the first investigation that reported the "sympathomimetic type" actions of desflurane.

SYMPATHOMIMETIC ACTIONS OF VOLATILE ANESTHETIC AGENTS

Some of the older inhaled anesthetics such as cyclopropane, nitrous oxide and diethylether are known to produce cardiovascular stimulation. The newer volatile anesthetics depress sympathetic nervous system activity during steady-state conditions, but it has recently been discovered that several volatile anesthetics may also cause sympathetic stimulation during induction of anesthesia or following a rapid change in anesthetic depth. For example, isoflurane (16,17) and desflurane (17,18) transiently increase heart rate and arterial pressure when the end-tidal concentrations of these agents are rapidly changed to those exceeding 1 MAC. Interestingly, this has only recently been described for isoflurane despite its introduction into clinical practice many years ago. The mechanism of the hyperdynamic circulatory response is unknown but is clearly mediated through the sympathetic nervous system as concentrations of norepinephrine, epinephrine and vasopressin are increased and sympathetic nerve activity can be clearly demonstrated. It may also have a component of parasympathetic withdrawal. These findings have led to the hypothesis that activation of receptors in airways or the lungs by high inspired concentrations of pungent anesthetics may be the initiating factor, however, other mechanisms such as direct activation of afferent pathways (e.g., direct baroreceptor stimulation) or a direct central nervous system response cannot be ruled out.

The increase in heart rate and arterial pressure observed following isoflurane or desflurane is transient in nature (lasts less than 6 minutes) and is greatly diminished with subsequent changes in anesthetic depth (tachyphylaxis) possibly due to adaptation of afferent receptors or depletion of neurotransmitters from sympathetic nerves and adrenal medulla. Studies by Ebert and Muzi and Weiskopf and Eger have convincingly demonstrated that the hypertension and tachycardia observed during administration of volatile anesthetics can be markedly attenuated by slowly increasing anesthetic depth or by a host of pharmacological agents including opioids, $alpha_2$ agonists, and beta blocking agents. It is important for the clinician to recognize that during administration of the volatile anesthetic agents, an increase in heart rate and arterial pressure may not be solely due to "light anesthesia" but may in fact be directly related to the volatile anesthetic.

CONCLUSIONS

In summary, the investigations completed to date have shown that desflurane produces a systemic hemodynamic profile in humans which is almost indistinguishable from other volatile anesthetics such as isoflurane. Furthermore, significant differences between the cardiovascular actions of desflurane and isoflurane have been identified in volunteers during spontaneous and controlled ventilation in the presence and absence of nitrous oxide. Finally, there is no evidence of desflurane-induced cardiovascular morbidity in patients with coronary artery disease.

REFERENCES

1. Weiskopf RB, Holmes MA, Eger II EI, et al: Cardiovascular effects of I653 in swine. Anesthesiology 69:303-309, 1988
2. Weiskopf RB, Holmes MA, Rampil IJ, et al: Cardiovascular safety and actions of high concentrations of I-653 and isoflurane in swine. Anesthesiology 70:793-798, 1989
3. Weiskopf RB, Eger E2, Holmes MA, et al: Epinephrine-induced premature ventricular contractions and changes in arterial blood pressure and heart rate during I-653, isoflurane, and halothane anesthesia in swine. Anesthesiology 70:293-8, 1989
4. Lutz LJ, Milde JH, Milde LN: The cerebral functional, metabolic, and hemodynamic effects of desflurane in dogs. Anesthesiology 73:125-131, 1991
5. Milde LN, Milde JH: The cerebral and systemic hemodynamic and metabolic effects of desflurane-induced hypotension in dogs. Anesthesiology 74:513-518, 1991
6. Pagel PS, Kampine JP, Schmeling WT, Warltier DC: Comparison of the systemic and coronary hemodynamic actions of desflurane, isoflurane, halothane, and enflurane in the chronically instrumented dog. Anesthesiology 74:539-51, 1991
7. Merin RG, Bernard J-M, Doursout M-F, et al: Comparison of the effects of isoflurane and desflurane on cardiovascular dynamics and regional blood flow in the chronically instrumented dog. Anesthesiology 74:568-574, 1991
8. Hartman JC, Pagel PS, Kampine JP, et al: Influence of desflurane on regional distribution of coronary blood flow in a chronically instrumented canine model of multivessel coronary artery obstruction. Anesth Analg 72:289-99, 1991
9. Pagel PS, Kampine JP, Schmeling WT, Warltier DC: Influence of volatile anesthetics on myocardial contractility in vivo: desflurane versus isoflurane. Anesthesiology 74:900-907, 1991
10. Pagel PS, Kampine JP, Schmeling WT, Warltier DC: Alteration of left ventricular diastolic function by desflurane, isoflurane, and halothane in the chronically instrumented dog with autonomic nervous system blockade. Anesthesiology 74:1103-14, 1991
11. Weiskopf RB, Cahalan MK, Eger II EI, et al: Cardiovascular actions of desflurane in normocarbic volunteers. Anesth Analg 73:143-156, 1991
12. Cahalan MK, Weiskopf RB, Eger II EI, et al: Hemodynamic effects of desflurane/nitrous oxide anesthesia in volunteers. Anesth Analg 73:157-164, 1991
13. Yasuda N, Weiskopf RB, Cahalan MK, et al: Does desflurane modify circulatory responses to stimulation in humans? Anesth Analg 73:175-179, 1991
14. Thomson IR, Bowering JB, Hudson RJ, et al: A comparison of desflurane and isoflurane in patients undergoing coronary artery surgery. Anesthesiology 75:776-781, 1991
15. Helman J, Leung J, Bellows W, et al: Desflurane anesthesia and myocardial ischemia: Comparative risk vs. sufentanil anesthesia in patients undergoing coronary artery bypass graft surgery. Anesthesiology 75:A1124, 1991

16. Yli-Hankala A, Randell T, Seppala T, Lindren L: Increases in hemodynamic variables and catecholamine levels after rapid increase in isoflurane concentration. Anesthesiology 78:266-271, 1993
17. Weiskopf RB, Moore MA, Eger II EI, et al: Rapid increase in desflurane concentration is associated with greater transient cardiovascular stimulation than with rapid increase in isoflurane concentration in humans. Anesthesiology 80:1035-1045, 1994
18. Ebert TJ, Muzi M: Sympathetic hyperactivity during desflurane anesthesia in healthy volunteers. A comparison with isoflurane [see comments]. Anesthesiology 79:444-453, 1993

OBJECTIVE ASSESSMENT OF CARDIAC FUNCTION IN VASCULAR SURGERY

Pierre Foëx, MD

INTRODUCTION

It is well recognized that patients undergoing peripheral vascular surgery are at risk for postoperative cardiac complications of anesthesia and surgery (1,2). This relates directly to the prevalence of coronary artery disease and/or hypertensive heart disease in such patients. However, as coronary artery disease may be asymptomatic, the preoperative assessment may fail to elicit symptoms or signs of coronary disease. Thus, postoperative complications may occur in patients in whom the absence of symptoms or signs of heart disease may have been falsely reassuring.

CLINICAL RISK INDICES

Medical history and clinical examination are of considerable importance. In many patients, risk factors will be identified and some risk stratification will be possible. The cardiac risk index developed by Goldman and colleagues (3) has been used and in subsequent studies of this index the proportion of cardiac complications has been shown to be much higher in vascular than in nonvascular patients. Other indices of cardiac risks, such as those developed by Detsky and colleagues (4) or Larsen and colleagues (5) can be used. Recent papers focusing on the cardiac risks in vascular surgical patients have emphasized the value of available clinical indices as predictors of adverse cardiac outcome (6-9). However, our own experience with such indices in vascular surgical patients has proved disappointing as only few patients fulfilled the criteria for high risk. Thus, the majority of cardiac complications occurred in patients regarded as relatively low risk. This is not surprising as these indices were developed on data collected from patients presenting for general rather than vascular surgery.

T. H. Stanley and P. L. Bailey (eds.), Anesthesiology and the Cardiovascular Patient, 219–228.

CHEST RADIOGRAPH

The cost-effectiveness of the routine chest radiograph has been questioned (10), yet this test continues to be used extensively as a preoperative screening test. In patients with coronary heart disease, cardiomegaly (heart shadow greater than 50% of the diameter of the thorax) is usually associated with poor left ventricular function (ejection fraction less than 50%). In patients with valvular heart disease, the heart shadow may be pathognomonic of the disorder. However, cardiac dimensions do not closely correlate with the ejection fraction. In patients with hypertensive heart disease, a prominent left ventricle is often associated with poor diastolic function even though systolic function may be normal. Inspection of the thoracic aortic shadow is essential, especially in patients presenting for surgery of the abdominal aorta because of the therapeutic implications of the association of thoracic and abdominal aortic aneurysms. Signs of pulmonary emphysema, presence of pleural effusions, presence of hitherto undiagnosed intrathoracic neoplasms also must be taken into consideration in deciding on the operability of the patient.

ELECTROCARDIOGRAM

The resting electrocardiogram is normal in 25 to 50% of patients with coronary heart disease. Yet a recent electrocardiogram is essential to identify dysrhythmias and conduction disorders, signs of previous myocardial infarction, myocardial ischemia, and signs of atrial or ventricular hypertrophy (and/or strain). The implications of ECG abnormalities can be summarized as follows:

1. Signs of right atrial and/or ventricular hypertrophy suggest the presence of pulmonary outflow tract obstruction, pulmonary valve stenosis or, more frequently, pulmonary hypertension. In patients with these features, preoperative measurement of pulmonary artery pressure, if not previously available, may be indicated as well as its monitoring during the perioperative period. In such patients episodes of hypoxemia, be it at induction of anesthesia or during the recovery period, may cause right ventricular failure associated with acute circulatory failure because of dramatic hypoxia-induced increases in pulmonary artery pressure. Postoperative artificial ventilation may be indicated as the increase in oxygen consumption during recovery may exceed the

patient's ability to increase oxygen delivery. Though evaluation for ease of intubation is carried out routinely in all patients, it has to be particularly thorough in patients presumed to have pulmonary hypertension as unforeseen difficulties at intubation may cause life-threatening hypoxemia associated with cardiovascular collapse.

2. Signs of left ventricular hypertrophy, especially associated with strain patterns, are likely to indicate the presence of reduced left ventricular compliance. This may justify the insertion of a pulmonary artery catheter for the measurement of the pulmonary capillary wedge pressure (PCWP) as right and left ventricular filling pressures may differ substantially. Fluid replacement is likely to be more appropriate if based on PCWP rather than CVP measurements.

3. Signs of previous myocardial infarction must be noted as extensive Q waves in the precordial leads are likely to be associated with reduced left ventricular function.

4. Signs of myocardial ischemia must be considered in the context of the past medical history of the patient. Persistence of myocardial ischemia long after myocardial infarction may indicate the presence of a ventricular aneurysm. If it has appeared *de novo* after previous infarction it may suggest a recent extension or the development of a new area of ischemia. Patients with such features should be considered for further investigations of wall motion (suspected ventricular aneurysms) or coronary angiography.

5. Any rhythm other than sinus rhythm must be regarded as a marker of increased risk as it often indicates the presence of myocardial damage. Conduction disorders must be carefully evaluated as anesthesia may precipitate the development of complete heart block. The indication for the preoperative implantation of a temporary (or permanent) pace-maker must be based on the ECG and on the presence or absence of symptoms suggestive of acute cerebral hypo-perfusion (see Table 1).

Table 1. Indications for temporary pacemakers.

Symptomatic first degree heart block
Symptomatic second degree Mobitz I heart block
Second degree Mobitz II heart block
Third degree heart block
Symptomatic bifascicular block
Left bundle branch block and first degree heart block
Sick sinus syndrome
Slow rates unresponsive to drugs

EXERCISE ECG

Several of the major determinants of myocardial oxygen consumption are affected by exercise, namely increases in heart rate, wall tension, and contractility. As oxygen extraction does not usually increase with exercise, the increases in demand have to be met by increases in coronary blood flow. These are achieved by marked, locally regulated, reductions in coronary vascular resistance. When the coronary arteries are moderately or severely obstructed, such reductions in coronary vascular resistance cannot occur and exercise causes angina or silent ischemia. Exercise ECG has a high specificity in predicting the presence of coronary artery disease. It gives a clear indication of coronary reserve. Unfortunately, in many patients with peripheral vascular disease, claudication limits its usefulness and physical stress may have to be replaced by pharmacological stress such as the infusion of dobutamine (11). In vascular surgical patients who are able to exercise, the maximum achievable heart rate is a predictor of cardiovascular complications of anesthesia and surgery as an inverse relationship exists between incidence of complications and maximum heart rate (12). In the presence of a severe limitation of exercise capacity, coronary angiography may be required as coronary angioplasty or coronary bypass graft may be indicated, particularly prior to major intra-abdominal vascular surgery.

AMBULATORY ECG MONITORING

Continuous ambulatory ECG monitoring is of considerable value in the diagnosis of dysrhythmias and conduction disorders as the frequency of dysrhythmias and the presence or absence of more severe conduction disorders may facilitate decisions regarding the need for drug therapy of dysrhythmias or pacemaker insertion. In addition the detection of episodes of silent myocardial ischemia may identify patients in whom the risk of cardiovascular complications of anesthesia and surgery may be increased (13-18). Silent myocardial ischemia is most likely to occur in patients with known coronary heart disease (19) and in those with untreated or poorly controlled hypertension (20,21). In these patients ambulatory ECG monitoring may help to identify those with a particularly high risk.

ECHOCARDIOGRAPHY

Echocardiography is an important means of noninvasively assessing regional wall motion, global ventricular function and valvular anatomy. M-mode echocardiography represents a one-dimensional view of the heart plotted against time—whereas two-dimensional (2D) echo-cardiography allows evaluation of an entire sector of single-dimension beams. Observations can be made regarding wall thickness, end-diastolic and end-systolic dimensions; ejection fraction; segmental wall motion abnormalities; and presence of valvular heart disease. Advances in Doppler flow technology make it possible to measure flow across heart valves and to calculate pressure gradients. In addition, the patterns of mitral flow are an indicator of left ventricular stiffness that complements the observation of the speed of ventricular thinning.

In patients with ischemic heart disease the extent of previous myocardial infarction can be estimated as well as the presence of a ventricular aneurysm. Segmental hypokinesia is also easily detected. The ejection fraction can be computed from different views of the heart (22). In hypertensive heart disease, the extent of left ventricular hypertrophy can be evaluated as well as the dynamics of relaxation.

NUCLEAR CARDIAC IMAGING

Over the past 25 years, nuclear imaging has made significant advances. It is now a safe, accurate, and reproducible method for assessment of myocardial perfusion and infarction, and ventricular function. Scintillation cameras detect gamma rays emitted by radio labeled drugs. Two main techniques are used: myocardial imaging and blood pool scanning (radionuclide ventriculography).

Myocardial Scintigraphy

Myocardial imaging is used extensively to determine the presence and size of myocardial infarction and of areas of reversible hypoperfusion. Hot-spot imaging relies on the avidity of infarcted segments for technetium-99m pyrophosphate. Exaggerated uptake may be detected as early as 12 to 16 hours after myocardial infarction and maximum abnormality is observed after 48 to 72 hours. This technique is of particular value when the standard ECG is uninterpretable (left bundle branch block) or cardiac enzymatic changes may be masked by other tissue effects.

Cold-spot imaging is much more relevant to the preoperative assessment of vascular surgical patients as the uptake of thallium-201 identifies the normally perfused myocardium. Areas of ischemia appear as cold spots. As thallium is distributed within the myocardium in proportion to blood flow, areas of relative hypoperfusion are also detected. Myocardial scintigraphy may be obtained at rest or during either exercise or the administration of drugs such as dipyridamole (coronary vasodilator) or dobutamine. If scans are obtained during exercise (or during the infusion of dipyridamole or dobutamine) and 3 to 4 hours later, regional improvements in uptake denote the presence of areas of reversible ischemia (poor uptake during stress, better uptake at rest). Several studies have shown a clear correlation between reversible ischemia detected by myocardial scintigraphy and adverse outcome (23-25). In sharp contrast, the more recent study of Baron and colleagues (26) has shown, in a group of vascular surgical patients, that myocardial scintigraphy was not a particularly useful predictor of adverse cardiovascular outcome as presence of reversible ischemia was not a significant predictor when the data was subjected to multivariate analysis. By contrast, these authors found clinical criteria to be significant multivariate predictors of adverse cardiovascular outcome. However, as the study included only a small number of patients with reversible ischemia detected by myocardial scintigraphy, the lack of predictive value may simply reflect the low prevalence of reversible ischemia.

RADIONUCLIDE VENTRICULOGRAPHY

Gated blood-pool imaging (MUGA scan, radionuclide ventriculography) relies on technetium-99m to label serum albumin or red cells. Following equilibration of the radiolabelled albumin or red cells in the intravascular space, including the blood passing through the heart, images of the heart cavities can be obtained. Radioactivity is counted over 300 to 500 cardiac cycles and is gated to the ECG so that changes in counts throughout the cardiac cycles may be obtained. Multiple methods of analysis are applied to the images so that global ejection fraction, regional ejection fractions, and synchrony of contraction are determined. A major advantage of radionuclide ventriculography over echocardiography is that it is not observer dependent and measurements are highly reproducible. The same dose of labeled albumin or red cell may be utilized to obtain images at rest and during stress. The latter may be physical exercise or pharmacological challenge using dipyridamole or dobutamine. Exercise or pharmacological challenges should cause an increase in global ejection fraction and regional wall motion. A reduction of the global ejection fraction or marked reductions in regional ejection fraction, indicate the presence of reversible ischemia. Thus, radionuclide ventriculography provides a direct measure of ventricular function and an indirect assessment of myocardial perfusion. A number of studies of vascular and nonvascular surgical patients have shown that low ejection fraction is associated with a substantial increase in the risk of post-operative adverse events (3,7,27-32). In contrast with these studies, Baron and colleagues found that a low ejection fraction was only a significant predictor of acute left ventricular failure in the postoperative period (26). They concluded that radionuclide ventriculography was of little value for risk prediction. However, the prevalence of patients with a low ejection fraction was very low, and it may not be legitimate to generalize their conclusion as in other groups of patients low ejection fraction may be much more prevalent. Our own experience of radionuclide ventriculography based on over 200 patients is that approximately 55% have an ejection fraction greater than 50%; 45% have either an ejection fraction of greater than 50% associated with wall motion abnormalities (16%), or an ejection fraction lower than 50% (28% of all patients). Of all patients with an abnormal radionuclide ventriculogram, 8% had an ejection fraction less than 30%. This is in sharp contrast with the data of Baron and colleagues. In their study, almost 85% of patients had an ejection fraction greater than 50%, and only 15% had an ejection fraction smaller than 50%. Only 2% had an ejection fraction less than 35%, while the remaining 13% had an ejection fraction comprised between 35 and 50%. Clearly, when a high proportion of patients are found to have a low ejection fraction, radionuclide ventriculography becomes a useful test as it is difficult to predict the ejection fraction on pure clinical data. However, preliminary analysis of our series suggests that in patients presenting for major vascular surgery, absence of history of coronary disease, absence of Q waves on the ECG, and absence of a nonspecific ST segment or T wave abnormalities is almost always associated with an ejection fraction greater than 50% which increases with exercise. Thus, simple clinical criteria and the ECG make it possible to substantially reduce the number of tests done and to concentrate efforts on patients in whom the ejection fraction is more likely to be abnormal.

On a purely empirical basis, we tend to use the results of radionuclide ventriculograms as follows: 1) Large reductions in ejection fraction (>10%) with exercise or pharmacological challenge indicate the need for coronary angiography. 2) Ejection fractions of less than 20% justify a complete re-appraisal of the management strategy for intra-abdominal vascular surgery as crossclamping of the aorta may cause acute, irreversible, cardiac dilatation and failure; if surgery can be carried out with side-clamping of the aorta, the risks are probably less. 3) Ejection fractions between 20 and 30% indicate a very high risk for complications and there must be compelling reasons for surgery. If such compelling reasons do exist, the management strategy may include the pre-operative insertion of a pulmonary artery catheter and optimization of left ventricular function on the ICU prior to anesthesia and surgery. 4) Ejection fractions between 30 and 40% indicate an increased risk, and justify the perioperative insertion of a pulmonary artery catheter. When the ejection fraction is above 40%, this type of monitoring may not be necessary. Our approach is at variance with the approach often used in the USA where most patients undergoing major vascular surgery would be monitored with a pulmonary artery catheter in addition to the routine monitoring of arterial and central venous pressure. Though interesting, the measurement of the pulmonary capillary wedge pressure is unlikely to contribute to improved management in patients with normal or only moderately compromised left ventricular function unless there are other risk factors, such as compromised pulmonary function. In addition, the small risks and the costs of pulmonary artery catheterization must be taken into consideration.

REFERENCES

1. Diehl JT, Cali RF, Hertzer NR, Beven EG. Complications of abdominal aortic reconstruction. An analysis of perioperative risk factors in 557 patients. Ann Surg 197:49-56, 1983
2. Mackey WC, O'Donnell TF, Callow AD. Cardiac risk in patients undergoing carotid endarterectomy: impact on perioperative and long-term mortality. J Vasc Surg 11:226-234, 1990
3. Goldman L, Caldera DL, Nussbaum SR, et al. Multifactorial index of cardiac risk in noncardiac surgical procedures. N Engl Med 297:845-850, 1977
4. Detsky AS, Abrams HB, Forbath N, Scott JG, Hilliard JR. Cardiac assessment for patients undergoing non-cardiac surgery: a multifactorial clinical risk index. Arch Intern Med 146:2131-2134, 1986
5. Larsen SF, Olesen E, Jacobsen H, et al. Prediction of cardiac risk in non-cardiac surgery. Eur Heart J 8:179-185, 1987
6. Jeffrey CC, Lunsman J, Cullen DJ, Brewster DC. A prospective evaluation of cardiac risk index. Anesthesiology 1983:58: 462-464. 1983

7. Goldman L. Multifactorial Index of cardiac risk in non-cardiac surgery. 10-year status report. J Cardiothor Anesth 1:237-244, 1987
8. Wong T, Detsky AJ. Preoperative risk assessment for patients having peripheral vascular surgery. Ann Intern Med 116:743-753, 1992
9. Jivegard L, Frid I, Haljamae H, Hallenberg B, Holm J, Johansson SR. Cardiac risk and peripheral vascular surgery: new approach based on a multifactorial risk index. Br J Surg 80:354-358, 1993
10. Sagel SS, Evens RG, Forrest JV, Bramson RT. Efficacy of routine screening and lateral chest radiographs in a hospital-based population. New Engl J Med 1974: 291:1001-1004, 1974
11. Hoffmann R, Lethen H, Kleinhans E, Weiss M, Flachskampf FA, Hanrath P. Comparative evaluation of bicycle and dobutamine stress echocardiography with perfusion scintigraphy and bicycle electrocardiogram for identification of coronary artery disease. Am J Cardiol 72:555-559, 1993
12. McPhail N, Calvin JE, Shariatmadar A, Barber GG, Scobie TK. The use of preoperative exercise testing to predict cardiac complications after arterial reconstruction. J Vasc Surg 7:60-68, 1988
13. Raby KE, Barry J, Creager MA, Crook F, Weisberg MC, Goldman L. Detection and significance of intraoperative and postoperative myocardial ischemia in peripheral vascular surgery. JAMA 268: 222-227, 1992
14. Raby KE, Goldman L, Creager MA, et al. Correlation between preoperative ischemia and major cardiac events after peripheral vascular surgery. N Engl J Med 321:1296-1300, 1989
15. Ouyang P, Gerstenblith G, Furman WR, Golueke PJ, Gottlieb SO. Coronary artery disease: frequency and significance of early postoperative silent myocardial ischemia in patients having peripheral vascular surgery. Am J Cardiol 64:1113-1116, 1989
16. Pasternack PF, Grossi EA, Baumann FG, et al. The value of silent ischemia monitoring in the prediction of perioperative myocardial infarction in patients undergoing peripheral vascular surgery. J Vasc Surg 10:617-625, 1989
17. Mangano D, Browner W, Hollenberg M, London M, Tubau J, Tateo I. Association of perioperative myocardial ischaemia with cardiac morbidity and mortality in men undergoing noncardiac surgery. N Engl J Med 323:1781-1788, 1990
18. Mangano DT, Browner WS, Hollenberg M, Tateo IM. Long-term cardiac prognosis following noncardiac surgery. JAMA 268:233-239, 1992
19. Muir AD, Reeder MK, Foëx P, Ormerod OJM, Sear JW, Johnston C. Preoperative silent myocardial ischaemia: Incidence and predictors in a general surgical population. Br J Anaesth 67:373-377, 1991
20. Hemming AE, Howell S, Sear JW, Foëx P. Admission blood pressure is predictive of silent myocardial ischaemia in treated hypertension. Br J Anaesth 1993, 71:760P, 1993
21. Allman KG, Muir A, Howell SJ, Hemming AE, Sear JW, Foëx P. Resistant hypertension and preoperative silent myocardial ischaemia in surgical patients. Br J Anaesth 73:574-578, 1994

22. Folland ED, Parisi AF, Moynihan PF. Assessment of left ventricular ejection fraction and volumes by real-time, two-dimensional echocardiography. Circulation 60:760-766, 1979
23. Boucher CA, Brewster DC, Darling RC, Okada RD, Strauss HW, Pohost GM. Determination of cardiac risk by dipyridamole-thallium imaging before peripheral vascular surgery. N Engl J Med 312:389-394, 1985
24. Leppo J, Plaja J, Gionet M, Tumolo J, Paraskos JA, Cutler BS. Noninvasive evaluation of cardiac risk before elective vascular surgery. J Am Coll Cardiol 9:269-276, 1987
25. Lette J, Waters D, Lassonde J, et al. Multivariate clinical models and quantitative dipyridamole-thallium imaging to predict cardiac morbidity and death after vascular reconstruction. J Vasc Surg 14:160-169, 1991
26. Baron JF, Mundler O, Bertrand M, et al. Dipyridamole-thallium scintigraphy and gated radionuclide angiography to assess cardiac risk before abdominal aortic surgery. N Engl J Med 330:663-669, 1994
27. Dirksen JT, Kjoller E. Cardiac predictors of death after non-cardiac surgery evaluated by intention to treat. Lancet 297:1011-1013, 1988
28. Fiser WP, Thompson BW, Thompson AR, Eason C, Read RC. Nuclear cardiac ejection fraction and cardiac index in abdominal aortic surgery. Surgery 94:736-739, 1983
29. Fletcher JP, Antico VF, Grunwald S, Kershaw LZ. Prediction of cardiac risk in aortic surgery by gated heart pool scan. Br J Surg 76: 26-2, 1989
30. Pasternack PF, Imparato AM, Bear G, et al. The value of radionuclide angiography as a predictor of perioperative myocardial infarction in patients undergoing abdominal aortic aneurysm resection. J Vasc Surg 1:320-325, 1984
31. Mc Cann RL, de Wolfe WG. Resection of abdominal aortic aneurysm in patients with low ejection fraction. J Vasc Surg 10:240-244, 1989
32. Mantha S, Roizen MF, Barnard J, Thisted RA, Ellis JE, Foss J. Relative effectiveness of four preoperative tests for predicting adverse cardiac outcome after vascular surgery: a meta-analysis. Anesth Analg 79:422-433, 1994

CARDIOPULMONARY BYPASS AND THE BRAIN

John C. Drummond, MD, FRCPC

The impact of cardiopulmonary bypass (CPB) on the brain deserves discussion; the available literature suggests that stroke occurs with an incidence of 2 to 10% (1). In addition, the rate of neuropsychologic dysfunction shortly after cardiopulmonary bypass (CPB) can exceed 50%. With respect to the latter, the incidence is clearly related to the duration of testing after CPB. The metanalysis by Robinson et al. of CABG patients revealed reported rates of neuropsychologic dysfunction for the immediate post-CPB period (5-8 days) of 11-75%; of 11-40% after 6-12 weeks; and of 5% at 6 months or longer (2).

This review will examine first the causes of neurologic damage occurring during CPB and then the physician-controllable factors that may be relevant to the prevention of these events. Thereafter, the modalities available for monitoring the well-being of the brain during CPB will be reviewed, as will pharmacologic protection of the brain. Finally, management of the patient with combined carotid/coronary disease will be reviewed.

THE CAUSES OF NEUROLOGIC DAMAGE

Causes of neurologic damage invariably fall into one of two categories: embolization and hypoperfusion.

Embolization

1. Embolization is probably the most common cause. Macroembolization of debris from either the aortic root or valve is the most common cause of focal stroke. The importance of the aortic root as a source of embolic debris has been emphasized recently (3-5). Neuropsychologic dysfunction is probably largely the result of microembolization of air, platelet aggregates and other debris from either the surgical field or the oxygenator. The occurrence of microembolization has been well-confirmed by both intraoperative transcranial Doppler (TCD) recordings (6) and by pathologic study (7). Specific histologic lesions known as

T. H. Stanley and P. L. Bailey (eds.), Anesthesiology and the Cardiovascular Patient, 229–246.

SCADs (small capillary arteriolar dilations) have been identified in the brains of both humans and experimental animals (7). TCD data confirm the high incidence of embolic events during cardiopulmonary bypass and identify the periods of aortic manipulation (cross-clamp application and cross-clamp release) as being the periods with the highest frequency of embolic events (8,9). However, embolic events are recognized to occur throughout the period of cardiopulmonary bypass, though the precise etiology of these events is not often apparent. These additional events are relevant because the extent of neuropsychologic dysfunction is proportional to the duration of cardiopulmonary bypass (10).

Hypoperfusion

2. Hypoperfusion can occur in association with primary cardiac events either pre- or postbypass or, potentially, as a consequence of elective use of low mean arterial pressures during cardiopulmonary bypass. Either circumstance maybe compounded by a low hematocrit. Hypoperfusion may also occur as a consequence of cannulation misadventures, including aortic dissection.

Reducing the incidence of neurologic damage associated with CPB has been a focus of interest for over 30 years (11). A multitude of variables have been identified as associated with postoperative deficits. Some, such as age, years of education and genetic makeup (12), are beyond the control of the operating team, while others can be influenced. Table 1 lists the various factors that can be manipulated by the operating team and that have potential relevance to the incidence of damage. The list omits duration of bypass,[a] which appears to be a correlate of postoperative dysfunction (10,14), but which is largely a function of the required surgical procedure.

ACID-BASE MANAGEMENT: ALPHA-STAT VS. PH-STAT

The issue of whether blood gases are best managed by an alpha-stat (normal $PaCO_2$ in patient, blood warmed to 37°C) or a pH-stat (normal $PaCO_2$ at patient temperature) protocol has undergone much discussion and investigation. Largely, on the basis of the observation that pressure autoregulation of cerebral blood flow (CBF) appears to be preserved during alpha-stat but not pH-

[a]Age and duration of CBP are frequently listed as correlating with post-operative neurologic injury. However, one investigation that analyzed 50 possible contributing factors found, while both age and duration of CBP were significantly associated with injury on univariate analysis, that multivariate analysis did not confirm the relationship (13). This suggests that it may, in fact, be another factor or factors such as extent and severity of vascular disease, that is the primary correlate.

Table 1. Factors with potential relevance to neurologic injury during CPB.

Perfusion pressure/Pump flow
Temperature management
Flow pattern: pulsatile vs. non-pulsatile
Filters
Oxygenators
Glucose management

stat management (15), the argument can be made that the brain's physiologic behavior is more "normal" with the former. There are other physiologic differences between the two approaches. $CMRO_2$ is lower using a pH-stat approach. However, while the difference may be substantial in profoundly hypothermic subjects (i.e., CMR 35-40% lower with pH-stat management at 17°C), available information suggests that the threshold for the appearance of this difference may only just be reached at temperatures commonly employed during CPB (16,17). Furthermore, the mechanism and significance of the difference in CMR is unclear. Because $PaCO_2$ is maintained at a higher level with a pH-stat approach in a hypothermic patient, CBF is greater and a state of luxury perfusion exists. This has been used as an argument against pH-stat protocols because of the concern that higher flows might deliver additional embolic material to the brain and thereby contribute to microembolization-related neuropsychologic dysfunction. Because of these two arguments, alpha-stat management is by far the most commonly used approach today and at least two investigations have demonstrated better neurologic or neuropsychologic performance after hypothermic CPB for CABG in patients managed by an alpha-stat protocol (17,18). The possible exception to the general adoption of alpha-stat management may be procedures in which circulatory arrest is intended. In those circumstances, higher CBF levels pre-arrest might contribute to more rapid and homogeneous cooling of the brain.

PERFUSION PRESSURE/PUMP FLOW

The use of relatively low perfusion pressures has been popular among cardiac surgeons for several reasons. These include: a decreased likelihood of vascular injuries (i.e., dissection); decreased damage to blood elements; and decreased collateral bleeding into the surgical field. There are reasonable data to support the concept that CBF will be adequately maintained to mean arterial pressures as low as 30 mm Hg during CPB with moderate hypothermia (19).

[Note that this may not be the case with profound hypothermia (17-22°C) which has been shown to impair autoregulation (20)].

However, most centers prefer to use higher average mean arterial pressures (MAPs) (e.g., 50 mm Hg) to allow some margin for error. Furthermore, recent data appear to indicate that the subset of patients with severe atherosclerosis of the proximal aorta have a reduced incidence of stroke when managed with high MAPs (80-100 mm Hg) on CPB (1).

A MAP of 30 mm Hg seems remarkably low at first glance. But it is worth remembering that cerebral perfusion pressure rather than MAP is the important determinant of CBF at these low pressures. Cerebral perfusion pressure (CPP = MAP – ICP) is substantially influenced by ICP, especially at low MAPs. Drainage of the right heart by siphon to the venous reservoir results in right heart pressures during CPB that are zero and perhaps sometimes even negative. While ICP has not been measured systematically in humans on cardiopulmonary bypass, it is this reviewer's suspicion that these very low right heart (and therefore jugular venous) pressures result in an ICP lower during bypass than in a normal recumbent patient. Unrecognized compression of the neck, e.g., by twill tape ties used to secure endotracheal tubes, has the potential to raise intracranial pressure and reduce the cerebral perfusion associated with mean arterial pressures of 30 mm Hg from marginal to frankly inadequate.

Within the range of intact pressure autoregulation CBF does not appear to vary with pump flow during moderate hypothermic bypass using either alpha or pH-stat ABG management (21).

TEMPERATURE MANAGEMENT—HYPOTHERMIA

There is little doubt of the protective benefit of hypothermia in the context of hypothermic circulatory arrest. These procedures could not be accomplished safely without hypothermia. The protective effect is probably largely a consequence of reduction in the rate of oxygen utilization for both electrophysiologic activity and membrane/organelle homeostasis. Hypothermia has additional and apparently specific effects on cerebral biochemistry that may also play a role. These include: inhibition of neurotransmitter release; inhibition of protein kinase C translocation; and preservation of the enzymes, calcium-calmodulin kinase II and ubiquitin (22). It also appears probable that mild to moderate hypothermia contributes to cerebral protection in the context of CABG or valvular surgery. However, this action cannot be as emphatically confirmed. While there is an enormous body of experimental (animal) literature to confirm the efficacy of moderate hypothermia (temperature reduction of 2-6°C) in the setting of standardized focal ischemic insults, until very recently, there has been no confirmation of its efficacy in the setting of CPB (23). Intuitively, granted that the macro and microembolic events that are recognized to occur during CPB are decidedly focal in nature, one would anticipate a beneficial effect. In particular, in the circumstances of embolization of air or platelet/white cell aggregates, which could be expected to dissipate with the passage of time, a protective strategy to "see the brain through" until such emboli were dissipated could be effective. However, at least one investigation has failed to confirm the benefits of hypothermia. McLean et al. studied 201 patients randomized to either normothermic or hypothermic CPB (<28°C) and observed no difference in neuropsychologic outcome (24). Interpretation of these data should take into account the observation that there was no evidence of residual dysfunction at three-month follow-up in *either* group. This could mean either that their methods were not sufficiently sensitive or, that in the context of well managed CPB, temperature reduction may have little to add to the benefits achieved by expedient surgery using a membrane oxygenator with appropriate filtration and appropriate maintenance of perfusion pressure.

Other studies of hypothermia have been performed. The recent development of the concept that normothermic cardioplegia with blood may be preferable to hypothermic cardioplegic techniques for myocardial protection has resulted in an increased number of institutions performing normothermic CPB. This has made the need for clarification of any potential benefit of hypothermia more pressing since hypothermia is now less likely to be used as a matter of routine. The surgical group at Emory University sought to determine whether this practice had any influence on neurologic outcome. They compared neurologic outcome in two cohorts of patients, including one (n=493) that underwent near normothermic bypass and normothermic blood cardioplegia and a second (n= 379) managed with a hypothermic technique (29-30°C) with hypothermic blood cardioplegia. The incidence of neurologic events was significantly higher in the normothermic group (4.7 vs 1.8%) (23). This study provides some support for the potential advantages of a hypothermic CPB technique. However, the study was not ideal in that the experimental groups in the study of Craver et al. were non-concurrent. Additional support for the potential benefits of hypothermia are provided by an investigation by Cook et al. who examined the frequency of cerebral venous desaturation ($SjvO_2 \leq 50\%$) and found that the incidence differed significantly between normothermic (37°C) and hypothermic (27°C) patients (54% vs. 12%, respectively) (25).

From these data, one might construct an argument that moderate hypothermia might be most appropriate in patients at greater risk for focal stroke including those with substantial atheromatous disease of the aortic root, those scheduled to undergo open chamber procedures, and, perhaps those patients in whom a lengthy period of CPB is anticipated. Not all would accept this view as adequately substantiated. In all probability, the discussion of the merits of hypothermic CPB will continue.

TEMPERATURE MANAGEMENT—HYPERTHERMIA

There is also a credible body of experimental information to confirm the adverse effects of hyperthermia in the setting of acute cerebral ischemia. A logical extrapolation of this literature is that overheating of the brain should be avoided in contexts in which focal ischemic events have occurred or may occur. Nonetheless, the practice of expediting rewarming by delivery of blood as warm as 40°C during CPB is not uncommon. There has been only one attempt to examine the neurologic implications of this phenomenon systematically (26). That report, available only in abstract form, describes the results of memory function testing three months post CPB in 150 patients who were grouped retrospectively according to the maximum nasopharyngeal temperature observed during rewarming. Patients with maximum recorded temperatures >38°C had poorer scores than those ≤38°C. It appears, to this reviewer, prudent to avoid overwarming the brain, especially in the period following removal of the aortic cross-clamp. The delivery of blood above physiologic temperatures, e.g., 37.5 to 38°C, appears ill advised.

FLOW PATTERN: PULSATILE VS. NON-PULSATILE

Existing literature suggests that microcirculatory function in many vascular beds is improved by pulsatile flow (PF), as opposed to non-pulsatile flow (NPF). A reviewer, new to the area, might be surprised by the limited extend to which pulsatile techniques are employed; the only large trial comparing the two methods appears to confirm substantial benefits of PF. In that prospective, randomized trial in 350 CPB patients, total mortality, the incidence of low cardiac output states and the necessity of intra-aortic balloon pump support were all lower in the PF group (27). Some of the specific physiologic advantages of PF that have been identified are listed in Table 2. [Relevant references published prior to 1983 are provided in the very comprehensive review by Hickey et al. (28).] Yet, in spite of a significant body of data appearing to justify the use of PF, it is not widely employed. The reason may be in part that there are substantial discrepancies among the many studies comparing these flow modalities such

Table 2. Potentially beneficial physiologic effects of pulsatile perfusion (28).*

Lower peripheral vascular resistance
Less capillary red cell sludging
Less edema formation/better preservation of lymph flow
Better preservation of renal blood flow and function
Better preservation of myocardial blood flow (during fibrillation), metabolism and function
Lower levels of catecholamines
Lower levels of renin, angiotensin II, and antidiuretic hormone
Better preservation of pituitary response to TRH
Lesser elevation of thromboxane (vasoconstrictor, platelet proaggregant)
Greater elevation of prostacyclin (vasodilator, platelet antiaggregant)
More rapid core cooling and rewarming (29)

*For each entry, there is a least one published investigation in support, although in many instances additional investigations may have revealed no difference between pulsatile and non-pulsatile perfusion. However, no item was included in this table if there was a published investigation indicating an advantage of non-pulsatile over pulsatile perfusion.

that the advantages of PF have not been consistently apparent. By way of explanation of these discrepancies, Hickey et al. point out emphatically that "pulsatile" flow has been loosely defined and even less well quantitated by the majority of investigators (28) and that the precise characteristics of the pulsatile waveform may be important in determining the physiologic effects achieved.

While not all investigations confirm differences, the vast majority indicate either a benefit to pulsatile perfusion or no difference between the two modalities. Exceptions include two reports demonstrating increased levels of free hemoglobin (though no differences in hematocrit) with PF (30,31). These observations serve to highlight the potential physiologic disadvantage of PF. It might be speculated that the variations in dP/dt that occur at both the pump heads and in the great vessels and could be associated with an increased risk of damage to blood elements and to the vascular tree. These considerations, in addition to the added expense of PF devices may have contributed to the limited use of this mode of perfusion. More important may be the absence of data supporting any beneficial effect of PF on the brain.

Investigations of the effect of perfusion technique on cerebral physiology in the context of typical CPB routines have identified some differences in cerebral physiology, though once again there are discrepancies. An investigation performed in rabbits revealed no differences in CBF or CMR at either normothermia or 27°C (32,33), whereas two investigations in normothermic dogs found CBF to be greater during PF than NPF (34,35). In a third investigation in dogs, there were no differences in CBF over a broad range of MAPs at either 37°C or 25°C, but CBF was marginally greater during PF when MAP fell below the apparent lower limit of autoregulation (36). This latter difference was much less apparent at 25°C than at normothermia. A single human investigation has compared CBF and CMR during PF and NPF (37). It identified no differences between PF and NPF, however the group sizes are too small (NPF=14; PF=8) for the study to be viewed as definitive. That same study also compared neurologic outcome 7 days after CPB. There were no differences but group size and the use of only a neurologic examination, without neuropsychologic testing, renders this aspect of the study inconclusive. A second larger and more appropriately designed trial also examined the impact of perfusion technique as part of a prospective investigation in 312 CPB patients on 50 perioperative variables. Fifty-seven percent of the patients underwent NPF, the remainder PF. Multivariate analysis identified no influence of perfusion modality. Accordingly, it is difficult to argue forcefully for an advantage of PF.

If there is a cerebral benefit to PF it probably occurs in the setting of deep hypothermic circulatory arrest (DHCA) or low flow bypass in association with profound hypothermia. Several investigations performed in dogs have demonstrated that, after a period of DHCA, the cerebral physiologic state recovers more rapidly with PF than with NPF (38-42) and one of those investigations also demonstrated improved neurologic outcome (40). As an aside, PF has also been shown to result in higher levels of CBF than NPF within the ischemic territory produced by middle cerebral artery occlusion in the dog (34). There are also data to suggest that, with the use of low flow perfusion (25 ml/kg/min) and profound hypothermia, the cerebral microenvironment (lactate, pH) is better maintained by PF than NPF (38). Consistent with the implication of more efficient cerebral perfusion with PF is the observation, in the setting of DHCA, that both cooling and rewarming are accomplished more rapidly with a concomitant reduction in total bypass time (29).

In summary, the available information does not provide substantial impetus for the routine use of PF in the majority of CPB procedures. However, PF may deserve wider application in the context of DHCA, and perhaps other situations, in which periods of low cerebral perfusion, either focally or globally, are anticipated.

FILTERS

The concept that filters, in particular on the arterial line, can reduce embolization is well established (6,43). One study has confirmed that filtration can have a beneficial effect on the incidence of neuropsychologic dysfunction (6). Typically, filters with mesh pore of 25-40 microns are used on both the cardiotomy return and the arterial perfusion line.

OXYGENATORS

The concept that membrane oxygenators generate fewer particulate emboli than either bubble of disk oxygenators is well established. This difference has been shown to correlate with a better postoperative status in several endpoints including cognitive function, CT scan evidence of cerebral damage, and frequency of retinal vessel occlusion (44-46).

GLUCOSE MANAGEMENT

In spite of an overwhelming body of laboratory information that provides firm support for the notion that elevation of serum glucose occurring prior to a standardized ischemic episode results in a worsened neurologic outcome, the limited attempts to examine this phenomenon in the context of cardiopulmonary bypass have failed to demonstrate any variation in outcome related to plasma glucose level (47,48). In a study of 107 CPB patients, Metz and Keats saw no increase in neurologic deficit among patients given glucose during the procedure as compared with those from whom it was withheld (47). That study, however, was subjected to sharp criticism in an accompanying editorial because of an apparent lack of sensitivity of the neurologic assessment methods used (49). A second investigation involving fewer (60) patients and apparently more sensitive methods also observed no difference in neurologic outcome (48). That investigation, reported in abstract form in 1991, has yet to appear in peer-reviewed form. In spite of these negative investigations, because there is little benefit of an elevated glucose level, it seems reasonable to recommend that hyperglycemia be avoided. However, in this reviewer's opinion, "tight" management of plasma glucose during cardiopulmonary bypass has a significant potential to result in postbypass hypoglycemia. This concern is based on the observation that plasma glucose levels frequently rise substantially during bypass and then decreases spontaneously at the conclusion of bypass. This phenomenon has been attributed to poor splanchnic (including pancreatic) perfusion during bypass with re-establishment of pancreatic perfusion with the renewal of pulsatile flow. Managing a theoretic risk (neurologic damage associated with increased plasma glucose) with a therapy that carries the risk of an event (profound hypoglycemia) that also can be neurologically injurious is difficult to justify.

MONITORING THE BRAIN DURING CPB

EEG Monitoring During Cardiopulmonary Bypass

The only systematic attempt to determine whether the commonly available two-channel EEG processors can serve to identify ischemic conditions during CPB or prevent adverse outcome failed to confirm the efficacy of these devices (50). Nonetheless, there are anecdotal reports suggesting that gross cerebral ischemic events related to cannulation or cross-clamp misadventures can be identified by simple EEG processors. These events include aortic dissection (51) or cross-clamp misplacement resulting in occlusion of the right innominate artery. While two-channel EEG has not been predictive of neuropsychologic dysfunction, there have been two investigations suggesting that the use of processors that examine eight or more channels can be used to identify and guide corrective maneuvers in the event of ischemia due to hypoperfusion. These reports suggest that the results obtained with these devices can be used to predict postoperative neuropsychologic dysfunction (52-55).

Cerebral Venous Oxygen Saturation Monitoring

$SjvO_2$ is another potential index of the adequacy of cerebral perfusion. It suffers from some technical limitations. Chief among these is the fact that mixing of cerebral venous blood at the confluence of sinuses is incomplete and, as a result, an individual jugular bulb may not represent average global perfusion (56). In addition, and probably as a consequence of the variable degree of mixing of blood from cortical and subcortical compartments, the threshold values that constitute "abnormal" are not well defined. In general, a saturation below 50% for a period of five minutes is viewed as being abnormal. Exploration of the use of this technique has revealed the relatively common occurrence of reduced jugular venous saturation during normothermic CPB (25) and during rewarming after hypothermic CPB (57-59), especially when rewarming is rapid (58). It has been speculated that this is a function of increased demand (due to rising brain parenchyma temperature) in the face of incomplete recovery of the normal flow-metabolism coupling. There is no proof to support this speculation and the concept that very vulnerable neurons would recover function more rapidly than the less metabolically fastidious vascular smooth muscle cells seems counterintuitive. Nonetheless, the phenomenon appears to be a real one in terms of the reduction of $SjvO_2$ that occurs, and there are data that indicate that patients in whom jugular desaturation following rewarming occurs, have a greater incidence of postoperative neuropsychologic dysfunction (59). The management implications of these observations are not yet agreed upon, although it has been reported that rewarming desaturation is less likely to occur when higher carbon dioxide tensions are employed during the rewarming period (i.e., more in keeping with a pH-stat style of management).

Near Infrared Spectroscopy (NIRS)

NIRS has the potential to provide a measure of mean cerebral hemoglobin saturation. Various investigators have attempted to examine the correlation between transcranial NIRS values and jugular bulb saturation. Correlations have been reported as both poor (60) and reasonable (61). It is conceivable that after further methodologic development and further evaluation to define critical thresholds, this technology could be used to identify circumstances of inadequate cerebral perfusion (caused by either inadequate perfusion pressures or vascular occlusive events) and to define the safe duration of periods of circulatory arrest. However, further refinement appears necessary. The only commercial device available was the Somanetics INVOS 3100 cerebral oximeter which became available in May of 1993. However, in November of 1993, the United States Food and Drug Administration rescinded Somanetics' approval to market the device because of perceived inadequacies in the data previously submitted. Somanetics has subsequently identified deficiencies in the initial device and a revised version, the 3100A is currently undergoing clinical trials.

PHARMACOLOGIC PROTECTION DURING CPB

The administration of pharmacologic agents as specific cerebral protectants in the setting of CPB is not routine. This is in spite of the apparent demonstration by Nussmeier et al. of protection by thiopental in the setting of open heart procedures (62). That study entailed approximately 90 patients in each of the control and thiopental groups. EEG silence was maintained by the continuous infusion of thiopental starting prior to atrial cannulation and continued until the discontinuation of CPB. Ten days following the procedure, neurologic or psychologic deficits were present in seven of the control patients and none of those who received thiopental ($P < 0.25$). The use of thiopental has nonetheless not become widespread. Why? First, a subsequent study by Zaidan et al. failed to demonstrate a similar protective benefit in the setting of coronary artery bypass grafting (63). Accordingly, the Nussmeier result, if applicable at all, may be relevant only to the setting of open heart procedures. Secondly, several of the circumstances of the Nussmeier study have lead to the suspicion that the favorable result may be specific to the circumstances of CPB used in that investigation, namely near normothermic bypass (34°C), bubble oxygenators and no arterial line filtration. Thirdly, thiopental resulted in a greater requirement for pressor utilization in the period immediately following CPB and was associated with a somewhat longer time to extubation. Fourthly, it was pointed out that one fewer neurologic deficit in the control group or one additional deficit in the thiopental group would have rendered the result nonsignificant.

Other anesthetic agents that are capable of producing considerable suppression of the EEG have been considered as potential cerebral protectants. However, the experimental literature regarding the protective effects of these various anesthetics in the setting of focal ischemia have failed to confirm any protective efficacy for etomidate, propofol or isoflurane beyond that achieved by any control state consisting of adequate anesthesia with other agents.

There was some interest in the evaluation of either dextrophan or dextromethorphan, both glutamate receptor antagonists, for cerebral protection in the setting of CPB. This reviewer is not familiar with any publication that evolved from the preliminary investigations of those agents.

Calcium channel blockers (CCBs) have been shown to have some efficacy in the setting of other focal cerebral insults including stroke and subarachnoid hemorrhage. There has also been preliminary indication of efficacy in the setting of CPB. In a small study group, Forsman et al. found better neuropsychologic function ("verbal fluency and visual retention") 6 months after CPB in patients who received nimodipine during CPB (n=13) than in control subjects (n=15) (64). Subsequently, Tuman et al. reported in abstract form that patients undergoing CPB who were on CCBs for other reasons had a lower incidence of postoperative neurologic deficit (65). This latter report has not subsequently appeared in peer-reviewed form. Subsequent to these promising preliminary suggestions of a benefit of CCBs, however, a prospective, randomized trial of the impact of perioperative nimodipine on neurologic/neuropsychologic outcome after valve replacement surgery was recently discontinued because of excess mortality in the nimodipine group as a consequence of "major surgical bleeding" (66). This is likely to discourage further evaluation of CCBs, at least those of the dihydropyridine group, as neuroprotectants in the setting of CPB.

COMBINED CAROTID/CABG SURGERY

When the patient has carotid and coronary artery disease, should the procedures be combined or staged? If staged, should the coronary surgery precede or follow the carotid surgery?

This topic is addressed by a relatively large body of literature, but within that literature, there is no appropriately designed prospective and randomized trial. The literature certainly allows one to choose his/her favorite approach and find a paper to support it. To this reviewer, that literature appears to be driven more by author conviction and influenced by local skills, procedures, habits and patient selection than by careful science. However, a very thorough review of this topic was provided by Moore et al. in their "Multidisciplinary consensus statement from the Ad Hoc Committee, American Heart Association" which provided "Guidelines for carotid endarterectomy" (67). They performed a review of the 56 English language papers addressing this topic. Their analysis reveals that the perioperative stroke rate was not significantly different if the carotid/CABG procedures were combined or if the carotid endarterectomy was performed before CABG. However, the incidence of stroke was greater when CABG preceded CEA. These data build a reasonable argument against performing the CABG first in the presence of surgical carotid artery disease. Does this mean that CEA should precede CABG? Their analysis revealed that the frequency of myocardial infarction and death were significantly greater when the CEA was performed as a staged procedure before the CABG. This latter observation is not surprising given that, even among patients who are not candidates for CABG surgery who undergo a CEA, myocardial infarction is the leading cause of death. Their data appear to argue that carotid endarterectomy should rarely be performed as preparation of a patient who is scheduled to undergo a subsequent CABG procedure.

Readers interested in a thorough review of the changes in cerebral physiology associated with cardiopulmonary bypass should refer to the extensive review by Schell et al. (68). Those interested in a further discussion of the etiology and identification of neurologic events associated with cardiopulmonary bypass should review the proceedings of the "Conference on Cardiopulmonary Bypass: CNS Dysfunction After Cardiac Surgery" (December 10-11, 1994), published in the *Annals of Thoracic Surgery*, 59: 1287-1362, 1995.

REFERENCES

1. Hartman GS, Yao FS, Bruefach M, et al. Cardiopulmonary bypass at high pressure reduces stroke incidence in patients with TEE diagnosed severe aortic atheromatous disease [abstract]. Anesth Analg 80:SCA52, 1995
2. Robinson M, Blumenthal JA, Burker EJ, et al. Coronary artery bypass grafting and cognitive function: A review. J Cardiopulmonary Rehabil 10:180-9, 1990
3. Wareing TH, Davila-Roman VG, Daily BB, et al. Strategy for the reduction of stroke incidence in cardiac surgical patients. Ann Thorac Surg 55:1400-8, 1993
4. Blauth CI, Cosgrove DM, Webb BW, et al. Atheroembolism from the ascending aorta; an emerging problem in cardiac surgery. J Thorac Cardiovasc Surg 103:1104-12, 1992
5. Wolman RL, Aggarwal A, Kanchuger M, et al. Risk factors for adverse neurologic outcome following intracardiac surgery [abstract]. Anesth Analg 80:SCA58, 1995
6. Pugsley W, Klinger L, Paschalis C, Treasure T. The impact of microemboli during cardiopulmonary bypass on neuropsychological functioning. Stroke 25:1393-1399, 1994
7. Challa VR, Moody DM, Troost BT. Brain embolic phenomena associated with cardiopulmonary bypass. J Neurol Sci 117:224-231, 1993
8. Barbut D, Hinton RB, Szatrowski TP. Cerebral emboli detected during bypass surgery are associated with clamp removal. Stroke 25:2398-2402, 1994
9. Stump DA, Rogers AT, Kon ND, et al. When emboli occur during coronary artery bypass graft surgery. Anesthesiology 79:A49, 1993
10. Murkin JM. Neurologic dysfunction after CAB or valvular surgery: Is the medium the miscreant? [editorial]. Anesth Analg 76:213-4, 1993
11. Gilman S. Cerebral disorders after open-heart operations. N Engl J Med 272:489-98, 1965
12. Newman MF, Croughwell ND, Blumenthal JA, et al. Predictors of cognitive decline after cardiac operation. Ann Thorac Surg 59:1329-30, 1995
13. Shaw PJ, Bates D, Cartlidge NE, et al. An analysis of factors predisposing to neurological injury in patients undergoing coronary bypass operations. Q J Med 72:633-46, 1989
14. Kuroda Y, Uchimoto R, Kaieda R, et al. Central nervous system complications after cardiac surgery: A comparison between coronary artery bypass grafting and valve surgery. Anesth Analg 76:222-7, 1993
15. Rogers AT, Stump DA, Gravlee GP, et al. Response of cerebral blood flow to phenylephrine infusion during hypothermic cardiopulmonary bypass: Influence of Pa_{CO_2} management. Anesthesiology 69:547-551, 1988
16. Prough DS, Rogers AT, Stump DA, et al. Hypercarbia depresses cerebral oxygen consumption during cardiopulmonary bypass. Stroke 21:1162-6, 1990
17. Stephan H, Weyland A, Kazmaier S, Henze T, Menck S, Sonntag H. Acid-base management during hypothermic cardiopulmonary bypass does not

affect cerebral metabolism but does affect blood flow and neurological outcome. Br J Anaesth 69:51-57, 1992
18. Venn GE, Patel RL, Chambers DJ. Cardiopulmonary bypass: perioperative cerebral blood flow and postoperative cognitive deficit. Ann Thorac Surg 59:1331-5, 1995
19. Govier AV, Reves JG, McKay RD, et al. Factors and their influence on regional cerebral blood flow during nonpulsatile cardiopulmonary bypass. Ann Thor Surg 38:592-600, 1984
20. Greeley WJ, Ungerleider RM, Smith LR, Reves JG. The effects of deep hypothermic cardiopulmonary bypass and total circulatory arrest on cerebral blood flow in infants and children. J Thorac Cardiovasc Surg 97:737-45, 1989
21. Rogers AT, Prough DS, Roy RC, et al. Cerebrovascular and cerebral metabolic effects of alterations in perfusion flow rate during hypothermic cardiopulmonary bypass in man. J Thorac Cardiovasc Surg 103:363-368, 1992
22. Maher J, Hachinski V. Hypothermia as a potential treatment for cerebral ischemia. Cerebrovasc Brain Metab Rev 5:277-300, 1993
23. Craver JM, Bufkin BL, Weintraub WS, Guyton RA. Neurologic events after coronary bypass grafting: further observations with warm cardioplegia. Ann Thorac Surg 59:1429-34, 1995
24. McLean RF, Wong BI, Naylor CD, Snow WG. Cardiopulmonary bypass, temperature, and central nervous system dysfunction. Circulation 90:II-250-255, 1995
25. Cook DJ, Oliver WC, Orszulak TA, Daly RC. A prospective, randomized comparison of cerebral venous oxygen saturation during normothermic and hypothermic cardiopulmonary bypass. J Thorac Cardiovas Surg 107:1020-9, 1994
26. Buss MI, McLean RF, Wong BI, et al. Rewarming after cardiopulmonary bypass and neurological function. Anesth Analg 80:SCA50, 1995
27. Taylor KM, Bain WH, Davidson KG, Turner MA. Comparative clinical study of pulsatile and non-pulsatile perfusion in 350 consecutive patients. Thorax 37:324-30, 1982
28. Hickey PE, Buckley MJ, Philbin DM. Pulsatile and nonpulsatile cardiopulmonary bypass: review of a counterproductive controversy. Ann Thorac Surg 36:720-37, 1983
29. Williams GD, Seifen AB, Lawson NW, et al. Pulsatile perfusion versus conventional high-flow nonpulsatile perfusion for rapid core cooling and rewarming of infants for circulatory arrest in cardiac operation. J Thorac Cardiovasc Surg 78:667-77, 1979
30. Goto M, Kudoh K, Minami S, et al. The renin-angiotensin-aldosterone system and hematologic changes during pulsatile and nonpulsatile cardiopulmonary bypass. Artifical Organs 1993;17:318-22, 1993
31. Dapper F, Neppl H, Wozniak G, et al. Effects of pulsatile and nonpulsatile perfusion mode during extracorporeal circulation—a comparative clinical study. Thorac Cardiovasc Surg 40:345-51, 1992

32. Hindman BJ, Dexter F, Ryu KH, Smith T, Cutkomp J. Pulsatile versus nonpulsatile cardiopulmonary bypass: No difference in brain blood flow or metabolism at 27°C. Anesthesiology 80:1137-47, 1994
33. Hindman BJ, Dexter F, Smith T, Cutkomp J. Pulsatile versus nonpulsatile flow: No difference in cerebral blood flow or metabolism during normothermic cardiopulmonary bypass in rabbits. Anesthesiology 82:241-50, 1995
34. Tranmer BI, Gross CE, Kindt GW, Adley GR. Pulsatile versus nonpulsatile blood flow in the treatment of acute cerebral ischemia. Neurosurg 731:724-31, 1986
35. Dernevik L, Arvidsson S, William-Olsson G. Cerebral perfusion in dogs during pulsatile and nonpulsatile extracorporeal circulation. J Cardiovasc Surg 26:32-5, 1985
36. Sadahiro M, Haneda K, Mohri H. Experimental study of cerebral autoregulation during cardiopulmonary bypass with or without pulsaile perfusion. J Thorac Cardiovasc Surg 108:446-54, 1994
37. Henze T, Stephan H, Sonntag H. Cerebral dysfunction following extracorporeal circulation for aortocoronary bypass surgery: no differences in neuropsychological outcome after pulsatile versus nonpulsatile flow. Thorac Cardiovasc Surg 38:65-8, 1990
38. Watanabe T, Washio M. Pulsatile low-flow perfusion for enhanced cerebral protection. Ann Thorac Surg 56:1478-81, 1993
39. Watanabe T, Washio M. Cerebral cellular response to profound hypothermia. Cardiol Young 3:383-93, 1993
40. Anstadt MP, Stonnington MJ, Tedder M, et al. Pulsatile reperfusion after cardiac arrest improves neurologic outcome. Ann Surg 214:478-88, 1991
41. Onoe M, Mori A, Watarida S, et al. The effect of pulsatile perfusion on cerebral blood flow during profound hypothermia with total circulatory arrest. J Thorac Cardiovasc Surg 108:119-25, 1994
42. Anstadt MP, Tedder m, Hegde SS, et al. Pulsatile versus nonpulsatile reperfusion improves cerebral blood flow after cardiac arrest. Ann Thorac Surg 56:453-61, 1993
43. Padayachee TS, Parsons S, Theobold R, et al. The effect of arterial filtration on reduction of gaseous microemboli in the middle cerebral artery during cardiopulmonary bypass. Ann Thorac Surg 45:647-9, 1988
44. Carlson RG, Lande AJ, Ivey LA, et al. The Lande-Edwards membrane oxygenator for total cardiopulmonary support in 110 patients during heart surgery. Surgery 72:913-9, 1972
45. Muraoka R, Yokota M, Aoshima M, et al. Subclinical changes in brain morphology following cardiac operations as reflected by computed tomographic scans of the brain. J Thorac Cardiovasc Surg 81:364-9, 1981
46. Blauth CI, Smith PL, Arnold JV, et al. Influence of oxygenator type on the prevalence and extent of microembolic retinal ischemia during cardiopulmonary bypass. Assessment of digital image analysis. J Thorac Cardiovasc Surg 99:61-9, 1990
47. Metz S, Keats AS. Benefits of a glucose-containing priming solution for cardiopulmonary bypass. Anesth Analg 72:423-34, 1991

48. Frasco P, Croughwell N, Blumenthal J, et al. Association between blood glucose level during cardiopulmonary bypass and neuropsychiatric outcome (abstract). Anesthesiology 75:A55, 1991
49. Lanier WL. Glucose management during cardiopulmonary bypass: cardiovascular and neurologic implications. Anesth Analg 72:423-7, 1991
50. Bashein G, Nessly ML, Bledsoe SW, Townes BD. Electroencephalography during surgery with cardiopulmonary bypass and hypothermia. Anesthesiology 76:878-91, 1992
51. Michaels I, Sheehan J. EEG changes due to unsuspected aortic dissection during cardiopulmonary bypass. Anesth Analg 63:946-8, 1984
52. Edmonds HL, Griffiths LK, van der Laken J. Quantitative electroencephalographic monitoring during myocardial revascularization predicts postoperative disorientation and improves outcome. J Thorac Cardiovasc Surg 103:555-63, 1992
53. Arom KV, Cohen DE, Strobl FT. Effect of intraoperative intervention on neurological outcome based on electroencephalographic monitoring during cardiopulmonary bypass. Ann Thorac Surg 48:476-83, 1989
54. Edmonds HL, Slater AD, Shields CB. Electroencephalographic monitoring during cardiac surgery [Letter]. Anesthesiology 78:208, 1993
55. Chabot RJ, Gugino VE. Quantitative electroencephalographic monitoring during cardiopulmonary bypass [Letter]. Anesth 78:209-10, 1993
56. Murkin JM. Monitoring cerebral oxygenation (Editorial). Can J Anaesth 41:1027-32, 1994
57. Croughwell ND, Frasco PB, Blumenthal JA, et al. Warming during cardiopulmonary bypass is associated with jugular bulb desaturation. Ann Thorac Surg 52:827-32, 1992
58. Nakajima T, Kuro M, Hayashi Y, Kitaguchi K, Uchida O, Takaki O. Clinical evaluation of cerebral oxygen balance during cardiopulmonary bypass: online continuous monitoring of jugular venous oxyhemoglobin saturation. Anesth Analg 74:630-5, 1992
59. Croughwell ND, Newman MF, Blumenthal JA, et al. Jugular bulb saturation and cognitive dysfunction after cardiopulmonary bypass. Ann Thorac Surg 58:1702-8, 1994
60. Bryce R, Proper J, Cook D, W Oliver J, Orszulak T, Daly R. Comparison of oxyhemoglobin saturations determined by transcranial infrared spectroscopy and co-oximetry during hypothermic cardiopulmonary bypass [abstract]. Anesth Analg 80:S61, 1995
61. Amory D, Pan L, Asinas R, Li JK-J, Kalatzis-Manolakis E. Relationship between continuous jugular venous oxygen saturation and regional cerebral oxygen saturation during cardiac surgery [abstract]. The Annual Meeting of the Society for Cardiovascular Anesthesia 288, 1993
62. Nussmeier NA, Arlund C, Slogoff S. Neuropsychiatric complications after cardiopulmonary bypass: Cerebral protection by a barbiturate. Anesthesiology 64:165-170, 1986
63. Zaidan JR, Klochany A, Martin WM, Ziegler JS, Harless DM, Andrews RB. Effect of thiopental on neurologic outcome following coronary artery bypass grafting. Anesthesiology 74:406-411, 1991

64. Forsman M, Olsnes BT, Semb G, Steen PA. Effects of nimodipine on cerebral blood flow and neuropsychological outcome after cardiac surgery. Br J Anaesth 65:514-520, 1990
65. Tuman KJ, McCarthy RJ, Spiess BD, Ivankovich AD. Do calcium channel blockers decrease neurologic deficits after intracardiac operations? Anesth Analg 70:S413, 1990
66. Wagenknecht LE, Furberg CD, Hammon JW,et al. Surgical bleeding: unexpected effect of a calcium antagonist. Brit Med J 310:776-7, 1995
67. Moore WS, Barnett HJ, Beebe HG, Bernstein EF, Brener BJ, Brott T. Guidelines for carotid endarterectomy—a multidisciplinary consensus statement from the ad hoc committee. Circulation 91:566-579, 1995
68. Schell RM, Kern FH, Greeley WJ, Schulman SR. Cerebral blood flow and metabolism during cardiopulmonary bypass. Anesth Analg 76:849-65, 1993

CLINICAL NEUROLOGIC AND DEVELOPMENTAL STUDIES AFTER CARDIAC SURGERY UTILIZING HYPOTHERMIC CIRCULATORY ARREST AND CARDIOPULMONARY BYPASS *

Gil Wernovsky, MD, Richard A. Jonas, MD, Paul R. Hickey, MD, Adre J. du Plessis, MD, Jane W. Newburger, MD, MPH

INTRODUCTION

The dramatic reduction in surgical mortality associated with repair of congenital heart anomalies in recent decades has been accompanied by a growing recognition of adverse neurologic sequelae in some survivors. Central nervous system (CNS) abnormalities may be a function of coexisting brain abnormalities (1,2) or acquired events unrelated to surgical management (e.g., paradoxical embolus, brain infection, effects of chronic cyanosis) (3), but CNS insults appear to occur most frequently during or immediately after surgery. In particular, support techniques used during neonatal and infant cardiac surgery—cardiopulmonary bypass (CPB), profound hypothermia and circulatory arrest—have been implicated as important causes of brain injury. This paper will review the effects of CPB and deep hypothermic circulatory arrest (DHCA) on neurodevelopmental outcome.

CARDIOPULMONARY BYPASS

During hypothermic CPB, there are multiple perfusion variables which might influence the risk of brain injury (Table 1). These include (but are probably not limited to) the total duration of CPB (4), duration and rate of core cooling (5), pH management during core cooling (6-10), duration of circulatory arrest (11-16), type of oxygenator (17-20), presence of arterial filtration (19-21), depth of hypothermia (22-25), hematocrit and precirculatory arrest glucose

*Reproduced with permission from CARDIOLOGY IN THE YOUNG. Vol. 3, pp. 308-316, 1993.

T. H. Stanley and P. L. Bailey (eds.), Anesthesiology and the Cardiovascular Patient, 247–264.

Table 1. Factors potentially influencing brain injury during cardiopulmonary bypass .

pH Management During Core Cooling
Duration of Circulatory Arrest
Anticoagulation
Type of Oxygenator
Arterial Filtration
Depth of Hypothermia
Hematocrit
Pre-Circulatory Arrest [Glucose]

concentration (26-27). Undoubtedly, there is interaction between these various elements, and CNS injury following CPB is most likely multifactorial.

An extensive literature exists on the CNS effects of CPB, primarily in adult populations (28-31). Extrapolation of the adult experience to infants with congenital heart disease must be made cautiously, as the degree of hypothermia used in adults is usually only mild to moderate, and circulatory arrest is only rarely used. Longer bypass times have been associated with higher frequencies of neurologic injury (4,14). Suggested mechanisms include activation of complement (32), various metabolic perturbations (33) and embolism (particulate, air) (18,21). Both microembolic and macroembolic phenomena have been implicated in the pathogenesis of cerebral damage following CPB (14,18-21,34-36). Filtration of arterial blood during CPB has been demonstrated to reduce the number of circulating emboli. A serial neuroimaging study by McConnell et. al (35) using magnetic resonance imaging reported measurable increases in ventricular volumes and subarachnoid spaces in 14 of 15 children studied undergoing repair on CPB.

PERFUSION VARIABLES

A. Deep Hypothermic Circulatory Arrest

DHCA has been increasingly used in centers with expertise in neonatal and infant cardiac surgery. The major surgical advantage of this technique is the absence of perfusion cannulae and blood from the operative field. The use of DHCA assumes that there is a "safe" duration that is inversely related to body temperature; the organ with the shortest "safe" period is the brain. Evidence for transient cerebral injury during DHCA comes from numerous laboratory and clinical investigations. While laboratory studies have focused primarily on cerebral blood flow/metabolism abnormalities (37-45) and histologic changes

(15), clinically based studies have primarily emphasized the incidence of seizures, choreoathetosis and long-term developmental abnormalities.

Experimental studies in animals on brain structure and function after use of DHCA have suggested that, at a core temperature of 15°C to 2°C, a 30-minute total arrest time is "safe" with respect to CNS damage (15,46-50). Conflicting results have been reported with DHCA times between 45 and 60 minutes (15,19,48-50). Electrophysiologic studies using electroencephalography (EEG) and somatosensory cortical evoked potentials have shown that at least transient cerebral dysfunction does occur after these prolonged periods of DHCA (51-52). The reappearance latency and latency to continuous EEG activity have been related to duration of circulatory arrest. Cerebral blood flow and metabolism studies suggest altered autoregulation during profound hypothermia (40-42) and during reperfusion following DHCA (39). Finally, the serum level of creatinine kinase, brain isoenzyme (CK-BB), has been reported by Rossi et al. (53) to be significantly higher among children who had surgery using DHCA than among those with closed procedures (i.e., without CPB or DHCA). The duration of DHCA had a marked influence on peak concentration of CK-BB, presumably reflecting the severity of cerebral ischemic insult. However, extrapolation of these laboratory abnormalities to clinically relevant findings, especially long-term cognitive and developmental issues, has only rarely been performed.

Early Postoperative Sequelae of DHCA

Seizures are the most frequently observed neurologic consequence of cardiac surgery using DHCA, with a reported incidence of 4 to 25% (16,52,54,55). Both focal and generalized seizures have been described, usually occurring on the first through fourth postoperative day. The immature brain has a lower seizure threshold and the frequency of seizures in the neonatal and infantile period is higher than at any other stage of life (56). The trend toward early neonatal repair of complex congenital cardiac lesions thus potentially shifts this population towards higher risk for seizures.

However, there is no universally accepted definition of "seizure activity" in the neonate and young infant, the age group in which DHCA is most often used. The differences between normal behavior patterns, abnormal but non-ictal behavior and true seizure activity are less distinct in the newborn than at any other age (56), and often present a bedside diagnostic challenge in the intensive care unit setting. Of the different clinical seizure patterns described, (i.e., clonic, tonic, myoclonic and "subtle" seizures) (57), it is the motor automatism and autonomic paroxysms of subtle seizures that are most difficult to distinguish from the normal movements of the young infant or the abnormal nonictal behavior patterns of the encephalopathic or sedated infant (58-59). Long term video-EEG has been increasingly utilized in the detection of seizures in children. This technology allows simultaneous (15-16) channel EEG recordings to be compared with visual examination of the patient and/or various physiologic monitoring tracings in patients after cardiac surgery. Studies utilizing long term video-EEG recording in newborns (not following cardiac surgery) have shown a high incidence of "silent" electrocortical ictal activity not manifest clinically (16,60). These"EEG seizures" occur most often in the setting of stupor/coma, after the onset of anticonvulsant therapy and in pharmacologically paralysed infants.

Thus, defining the "true" incidence of postoperative seizures is complex. The incidence of clinical seizures may be overestimated, due to the difficulties in distinguishing between normal and abnormal movements in neonates and young infants. Conversely, the incidence of EEG-seizures may be underestimated, in part because the frequent use of paralytic or sedative agents (e.g., benzodiazepines) in the early postoperative period obscures the clinical manifestations of seizure activity.

Although the long-term prognosis after hypoxic-ischemic seizures in the (normothermic) neonate may be guarded, the long-term significance of seizures occurring after hypothermic CPB with DHCA is unknown. The most powerful criteria for predicting outcome in non-cardiac patients suffering neonatal and early infantile seizures are 1) the underlying etiology of the seizure and 2) the background features of the interictal EEG. These criteria are not easily applied to the neonate or infant with seizures following cardiac surgery, as the exact etiologic mechanism(s) are not always clear. Although any of the usual metabolic, vascular and infectious etiologies may underlie these seizures, there appears to be a group (possibly the majority) of transient ictal events peculiar to this population. These seizures appear to have several distinguishing features. They tend to present in the second 24 hours after surgery, may be either generalized or focal clinical events and are easily controlled with anticonvulsants. Follow-up studies on this group of patients is limited, with no well controlled prospective studies in print at present. A largely anecdotal study (61) suggested no long-term neurologic morbidity, increased risk for late seizures or need for chronic anticonvulsant therapy in a small group of patients who had clinically "unexplained" seizures following infant cardiac surgery. Finally, the lack of prospectively gathered EEG data and a "normative" EEG database in this population of infants also compromises, at this point, the use of intraoperative or postoperative EEG in long term prognostication.

We recently compared the incidence of perioperative brain injury after hypothermic CPB with DHCA in a group of 171 patients undergoing the arterial switch operation for transposition of the great arteries (16). Patients were randomized to receive predominantly DHCA or predominantly low-flow (50 cc/kg/min) CPB. Anesthetic, other perfusion variables, surgical and postoperative care methods were standardized and identical in the two groups. The groups were comparable with respect to preoperative factors (e.g., hypoxemia, acidosis, apgar scores, socioeconomic status, etc.), cross-clamp time, total support time (i.e., the sum of DHCA and CPB times) and postoperative hemodynamics and hospital course. (62) The period of DHCA ranged from 6 to 59 minutes; this wide range in the duration of DHCA allowed for analysis both by "intention to treat" (DHCA versus low-flow bypass) as well as considering total duration of DHCA as a continuous variable.

Video EEG was performed preoperatively, continuously during the first 48 hours postoperatively and again prior to discharge. Reappearance latencies were defined as the time in minutes from the onset of rewarming to (a) "first EEG activity," (b) "close bursts," (c) "relative continuous" and (d) "continuous". Rhythmic paroxysmal activity on continuous video EEG during the first 48 hours postoperatively was classified as ictal (i.e., EEG seizures) if the duration of the discharge was longer than 5 seconds. Clinical seizures were diagnosed by the medical and nursing staffs of the cardiac intensive care unit, and characteristics of seizures were recorded on a form designed for this purpose. Serial neurologic examinations were performed by a neurologist blinded to treatment assignment before surgery and again 7 to 10 days postoperatively.

Both clinical and EEG seizures occurred significantly more frequently among infants randomized to receive predominantly DHCA. All infants with definite clinical seizures had at least 35 minutes of DHCA; in a logistic regression model using total duration of DHCA, EEG seizures were highly associated with longer duration of DHCA ($p=0.0103$, Figure 1). Infants randomized to DHCA also had longer recovery times to first EEG activity, close bursts and relative continuous activity, with similar relationships identified using duration of DHCA as a continuous variable. However, the frequency of possible or definite abnormalities on the EEG and neurologic examination at the time of discharge (7-10 days postoperative) was comparable between the two groups.

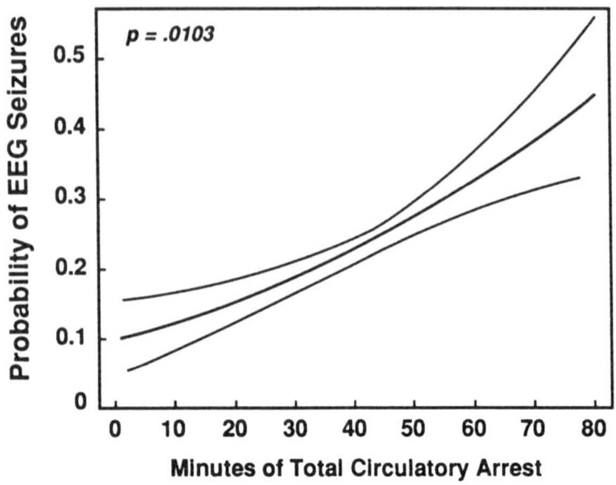

Figure 1. Probability of seizures on continuous video-EEG monitoring as a function of the duration of deep hypothermic circulatory arrest.

The results from this early phase of our clinical trial must be interpreted cautiously. Although the immediate neurologic perturbations were more common in the group assigned to predominantly DHCA, the groups were comparable at hospital discharge. The anatomic, neurologic and developmental correlates of these perioperative abnormalities await ongoing follow-up of this cohort of patients. Cranial MRI, neurologic and developmental testing will take place at one year of age, and serial long-term developmental and intelligence follow-up is currently underway.

Choreoathetosis is an enigmatic and sometimes devastating complication which has been described following cardiac surgery using CPB both with and without DHCA. Factors that have been implicated in the development of choreoathetosis include age beyond infancy (63-67), chronic preoperative hypoxemia (68), depth of hypothermia (69) and the use of DHCA (63,70). The duration and rapidity of core cooling on CPB may result in uneven brain cooling, especially in the deep areas of the basal ganglia and midbrain (71). As choreoathetosis appears to occur sporadically and even epidemically, one might speculate on an infectious agent as a contributing cause in selected patients. Finally, the presence of systemic to pulmonary collaterals may potentially result in a "cerebral steal" from the head and neck vessels into the low-resistance pulmonary vascular bed), contributing to uneven or inadequate brain cooling during core cooling on CPB (71).

The difficulty in implicating various patient-related or perfusion-related parameters to the development of severe choreoathetosis is that thousands of infants and children with similar preoperative characteristics and/or intraoperative CPB management are repaired each year without the development of this unfortunate complication. As choreoathetosis is an exceedingly rare complication of CPB with many potential causes, prospective cohort studies are unlikely to provide sufficient delineation of risk factors. Further case-control studies, ideally multi-institutional, are needed.

Late Postoperative Sequelae of DHCA

Psychological and intellectual development after cardiac surgery in children utilizing DHCA has been addressed in a number of studies, often with conflicting results. Several studies have suggested that the duration of DHCA has little or no important influence on later development (5,10,63,72-76), while others caution against its use (11-13). Many studies contend that patient related variables (e.g., Iow birth weight, preoperative illness, pre-existing neurologic abnormalities, age at operation, duration of cyanosis, socioeconomic status, etc.) play a more significant role in later development than the intraoperative effects of DHCA and CPB. Thus, the identification of an adequate control group is crucial in determining the effects of DHCA on later development.

Blackwood et al. (76) tested 36 children with both cyanotic and acyanotic congenital heart disease before and 4-29 months after surgery, using the patients as their own controls. DHCA was used in 26/36 patients. This study suggested no relationship of either the duration of DHCA or age at operation on developmental quotient (DQ). Higher socioeconomic status was significantly positively correlated with later outcome.

Clarkson and colleagues (75) studied 72 children with heterogeneous forms of congenital heart disease repaired at 0.2-26 months of age using DHCA. Follow-up testing was performed 29-84 months after surgery; results were compared to a matched group of pre-schoolers randomly selected from a sequential group of children born at one hospital. The results suggested no relationship of intelligence quotient (IQ) to either duration of DHCA, age at operation or race; however, low birth weight, pre-operative neurologic abnormalities and low socioeconomic status negatively impacted on later outcome.

Wells et al. (13) studied 31 patients undergoing repair of both cyanotic and acyanotic lesions using DHCA. Three control groups were used; I, 19 children undergoing repair using moderate hypothermic CPB without DHCA; II, 16 siblings of the study patients; and III, 14 siblings of the patients undergoing repair without DHCA. The mean IQ of the DHCA patients was 91 + 4 (SE), lower than each comparison group (group I-102 + 5.2, group II-106 + 4.1, group III-96 + 5.9). The difference between the IQ of the study patients (repaired with DHCA) and their siblings, particularly in the verbal subtests, was linearly related to the duration of DHCA. Patients repaired without DHCA had an IQ which was comparable to their siblings. Age at operation and age at testing were not related to later outcome.

In addition to generalized developmental delay and focal neurologic findings, many authors have commented on more specific long-term sequelae after DHCA and CPB. Expressive language and verbal delays are reported with a fairly high frequency (5,12,13,73,76), as is inattentiveness and "hyperactivity" (12-73). Gross and fine motor delays are common findings (12,76).

Methodologic Limitations. The literature concerning neurodevelopmental effects of cardiovascular support techniques in general and DHCA in particular must be interpreted cautiously; many studies are complicated by numerous (but sometimes unavoidable) methodologic flaws. These include 1) small sample sizes with limited statistical power; 2) heterogeneous (e.g., cyanotic and acyanotic) congenital lesions; 3) different methods of achieving hypothermic conditions, i.e., surface versus core cooling; 4) different ages at operation, testing and follow-up; 5) different testing modalities; 6) failure to identify an adequate "control" population with appropriate identification of social class, birth order and perinatal events; and 7) inadequate adjustment for and/or investigation of preexisting CNS lesions.

Prospective evaluations by neurologists have consistently found a higher incidence of neurologic morbidity compared with findings of cardiologists or cardiac surgeons (77-78). Additionally, most long-term studies focus on IQ or DQ, with a broad definition of normalcy and with only limited attempts to differentiate the potential impact of the independent variables on important component skills (e.g., attention, visual-motor integration, expressive and receptive language). Extrapolation of laboratory-based investigations (e.g., cerebral blood flow) to clinically relevant outcome measures has rarely been performed. Finally, there are inherent difficulties in the developmental assessment of young children, which may limit the inferences one may make vis-a-vis long term functioning. Nonetheless, these preliminary clinical and laboratory studies form the basis of our understanding of the pathophysiology of CNS injury during cardiac surgery and provide the impetus for further investigations.

B. Rate and Duration of Core Cooling

Cerebral protection by hypothermia is based on the premise that there is a significant fall in cerebral metabolic rate and oxygen consumption that is exponentially related to brain temperature (39). Cerebral protection afforded by core cooling on CPB presumes that all areas of the brain are cooled homogeneously on CPB. However, in a recent study by Kern and colleagues (23), variable oxygen saturations were measured in the jugular vein implying continued cerebral metabolism and oxygen extraction prior to DHCA in some patients. Standard monitoring of the tympanic and rectal temperatures did not identify those patients with continued cerebral metabolism. We speculated that inhomogeneous cooling in some patients may be related to aortic cannula position, age or biologic variability. Institutional variability in the rate of core cooling, such as rapid (heat exchanger on CPB maintained at 4-5°C) or more gradual cooling (heat exchanger maintained at 18°C) may also result in different degrees of deep cerebral protection (79). Adjunctive techniques of cerebral cooling, such as topical cooling of the head with ice (45) may further aid in CNS protection.

In a retrospective study (5), we recently reported an association between long-term cognitive development and the duration of core cooling on CPB prior to the institution of DHCA. We studied a group of 28 children between 7 and 53 months of age who underwent surgery between 1983 and 1988. All patients underwent the arterial switch operation for transposition of the great arteries as neonates or young infants. The surgical procedure was performed using a long period of DHCA, with a mean of 64.5 + 9.8 (SD) minutes. The younger (7-30 months) children were tested with the Bayley Scales of Infant Development while the older (30-53 months) children were administered the McCarthy Scales of Children's Abilities. Both tests were age-normed to have a mean score of 100 + 16.

In general, most children scored in the normal range; the mean (SD, range) score on the Mental Development Index of the Bayley scales was 98.6 (10.5, 78-120) and on the General Cognitive Index of the McCarthy scales, 106.3 (11.0, 93-129). The mean scores were not significantly associated with sociodemographic characteristics, preoperative acidosis, hypoxemia or "sickness," age at testing or any other patient-related variable. The duration of DHCA among the patients ranged from 49 to 101 minutes and was not significantly correlated with development ($p=0.41$).

The intraoperative variable most strongly associated with cognitive development was the duration of core cooling prior to DHCA. The relationship appeared to be curvilinear, with the strongest association in the group with shorter cooling times (11-18 min). Within this range of core cooling periods, an increase of 5 minutes of core cooling was associated with a 26-point increase in development score (Figure 2). We speculated that a shorter duration of cooling on CPB prior to an extended period of DHCA might result in watershed areas of inhomogeneous cooling within the brain in which metabolism had not slowed adequately, leaving these areas vulnerable to damage during DHCA.

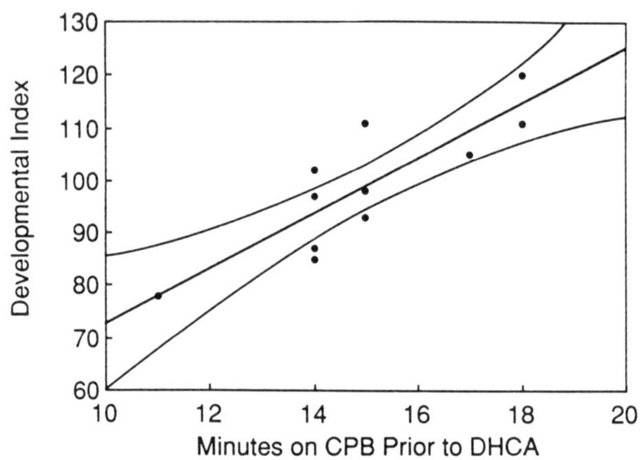

Figure 2. The developmental index (see text) of 11 patients undergoing an arterial switch operation who were cooled rapidly on cardiopulmonary bypass (CPB) prior to deep hypothermic circulatory arrest (DHCA). Modified from Bellinger et. al. (5)

Patients cooled for more prolonged (20-39 min) periods on CPB showed a trend toward worse developmental outcome with longer cooling times, though this association did not reach statistical significance. We speculated that the potential benefits of prolonged core cooling may be offset by the known sources of brain injury related to the length of CPB, such as microembolic events.

The results of this study must be interpreted cautiously, due to the relatively small sample size, retrospective design, different ages at testing and relatively long circulatory arrest times utilized. It is also important to note that all patients were cooled uniformly rapidly, achieving a rectal temperature of less than 20°C in less than 10 minutes. The remainder of the cooling period entailed maintaining hypothermic temperatures while continuing full flow bypass at 150 cc/kg/min.

C. Management of PH During Core Cooling

In a separate, concurrent retrospective study (10), the influence of alpha-stat versus pH-stat management during core cooling was investigated. A group of 16 children were studied between 11 and 79 months of age. All patients had a Senning procedure performed for transposition of the great arteries during the neonatal period or early infancy. The surgical procedure was performed using predominantly deep hypothermic circulatory arrest, with a mean duration of 43.4 + 6.2 (SD) minutes. As with the retrospective arterial switch study (see section B), the younger children were tested with the Bayley Scales, while the older children were tested with the McCarthy Scales. During the period of the study (1983-1988), the pH strategy employed during bypass was changed from pH stat to alpha stat, resulting in a wide range of pH and pCO_2.

Most children scored in the normal range; the median developmental IQ score was 109.0 (range 74-129). The mean scores were not significantly associated with any patient-related variables. The duration of DHCA among the patients ranged from 35-60 minutes and was not significantly correlated with later cognitive development. The mean (+SD, range) core cooling time was 14.5 (6.2, 8-32) minutes in this study group. In contrast to our study of arterial switch patients (who had longer periods of circulatory arrest) (5), core cooling duration was not associated with later outcome.

There was a strong positive correlation between arterial PCO_2 and developmental score (Figure 3). A more acidotic strategy (pH stat) resulted in better

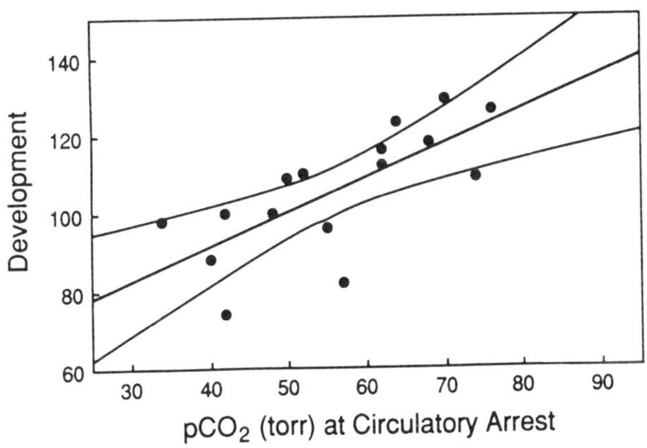

Figure 3. The developmental index (see text) of 16 patients undergoing a Senning procedure related to the PCO_2 at the onset of circulatory arrest. Modified from Jonas et. al. (10)

cognitive function in this group of patients, all of whom had relatively rapid core cooling prior to DHCA. Over the range of approximately 30-80 torr, developmental score increased 8.8 points for every 10 torr increase in PCO_2 ($p=0.002$). We have speculated that the improved cognitive result obtained with the pH stat strategy may be related to the increased cerebral blood flow which might result in more homogeneous brain cooling. In addition, the relative acidosis of the pH stat strategy counteracts the leftward shift in the oxyhemoglobin dissociation curve which results from hypothermia. This effect may be important when rapid core cooling is used, particularly in the early phases of cooling when relatively cool blood may be unable to deliver sufficient oxygen to as yet warm areas of the brain.

The interpretation and generalizability of this study are limited by its small sample size and retrospective nature. These data conflict with recent studies (many of them in adults subjected to only moderately hypothermic continuous cardiopulmonary bypass) demonstrating 1) no important differences between pH stat and alpha stat (80-81) or 2) studies favoring the alpha stat strategy (9,82,83) or even more alkaline strategies (7). To help clarify this issue, a prospective, partially-blinded study is underway at Children's Hospital, Boston, in which neonates and infants undergoing corrective surgery are randomized to either a pH or alpha stat strategy during core cooling.

SUMMARY AND FUTURE DIRECTIONS

DHCA affords the optimal operating environment; a cannulae-free, bloodless field in a still heart. Undoubtedly, DHCA will continue to be beneficial in the repair of complex malformations in neonates and infants. Conflicting data exists regarding its long-term neurologic and developmental effects. Cardiovascular surgeons will need to balance for each individual patient the neurodevelopmental risks with the technical advantages of DHCA.

Potential future adjuncts to brain protection during CPB with DHCA include cerebroplegia, Nmethyl-D-aspartate (NMDA) receptor blockade, oxygen free-radical scavengers and limiting the post-CPB inflammatory response. Perfusion strategies during core cooling (rate, duration, pH management, depth of hypothermia) need to be studied in a controlled fashion, both in the laboratory and clinical environments. Future research should be aimed at optimizing brain protection when DHCA is necessary or desirable.

REFERENCES

1. Berthrong M, Sabiston DC: Cerebral lesions in congenital heart disease: A review of autopsies on one hundred and sixty-two cases. Bull John Hopkins Hospital 89:384-401, 1951
2. Glauser TA, Rorke LB, Weinberg PM, Clancy RR: Congenital brain anomalies associated with the hypoplastic left heart syndrome. Pediatrics 85:984-990, 1990
3. Terplan KL: Patterns of brain damage in infants and children with congenital heart disease. AJDC 125:175, 1973
4. Slogoff ST, Girgis KZ, Keats AS: Etiologic factors in neuro-psychiatric complications associated with cardiopulmonary bypass. Anesth Analg 61:903-911, 1982
5. Bellinger DC, Wernovsky G, Rappaport LA, et al: Cognitive development of children following early repair of transposition of the great arteries using deep hypothermic circulatory arrest. Pediatrics 87:701- 707, 1991
6. Watanabe T, Masamichi M, Orito H, Kobayasi M, Washio M: Brain tissue pH, oxygen tension, and carbon dioxide tension in profoundly hypothermic cardiopulmonary bypass. J Thorac Cardiovasc Surg 100:274-280, 1990
7. Watanabe T, Miura M, Inui K, et al: Blood and brain tissue gaseous strategy for profoundly hypothermic total circulatory arrest. J Thorac Cardiovasc Surg 102:497-504, 1991
8. Johnston WE, Vinten-Johansen J, DeWitt DS, O'Steen WK, Stump DA, Prough DS: Cerebral perfusion during canine hypothermic cardiopulmonary bypass: effect of arterial carbon dioxide tension. Ann Thorac Surg 52:479-489, 1991
9. Willford DC, Moores WY, Ji S, Zhung TC, Palencia A, Daily PO: Importance of acid-base strategy in reducing myocardial and whole body oxygen consumption during perfusion hypothermia. J Thorac Cardiovasc Surg 100:699-707, 1990
10. Jonas RA, Newburger JW, Wernovsky G, Farrell DM, Rappaport LA, Bellinger DC: Alkaline pH strategy during core cooling worsens developmental outcome after circulatory arrest. Circulation 84 (suppl 11):121A, 1991
11. Settergren G, Ohqvist G, Lundberg S, et al: Cerebral blood flow and cerebral metabolism in children following cardiac surgery with deep hypothermia and circulatory arrest. Clinical course and follow-up of psychomotor development. Scan J Thor CV Surg 16:209-215, 1982
12. Wright JS, Hicks RG, Newman DC: Deep hypothermic arrest: observations on later development in children. J Thorac Cardiovasc Surg 77:466-468, 1979
13. Wells FC, Coghill S, Caplan HL, Lincoln C: Duration of circulatory arrest does influence the psychological development of children after cardiac operation in early life. J Thorac Cardiovasc Surg 86:823-831, 1983
14. Muraoka R, Yokota M, Aoshima M, et al: Subclinical changes in brain morphology following cardiac operations as reflected by computed tomographic scans of the brain. J Thorac Cardiovasc Surg 81 :364-369, 1981

15. Fisk GC, Wright JS, Hicks RG, et al: The influence of duration of circulatory arrest at 20OC on cerebral changes. Anaesth Intens Care 4:126-134, 1976
16. Jonas RA, Wernovsky G, Ware J, et al: The Boston circulatory arrest study: perioperative neurologic outcome after the arterial switch operation. Circulation 86 (suppl 1):360A, 1992
17. Barry YA, Labow RS, Keon WJ, Tocchi M, Rock G: Perioperative exposure to plasticizers in patients undergoing cardiopulmonary bypass. J Thorac Cardiovasc Surg 97:900-905, 1989
18. Blauth Cl, Smith PL, Arnold JV, Jagoe JR, Wootton R, Taylor KM: Influence of oxygenator type on the prevalence and extent of mircroembolic retinal ischemia during cardiopulmonary bypass. J Thorac Cardiovasc Surg 99:61-69, 1990
19. Fish KJ: Microembolization: etiology and prevention. In: Hilberman M, ed. Brain injury and protection during heart surgery. Boston: Martinus Nijhoff Publishing, 1988, pp 67-84
20. Nussmeier MA, McDermott JP: Macroembolization: prevention and outcome modification. In: Hilberman M, ed. Brain injury and protection during heart surgery. Boston: Martinus Nijhoff Publishing, 1988, pp 85-108
21. Padayachee TS, Parsons S, Theobold R, Gosling RG, Deverall PB: The effect of arterial filtration on reduction of gaseous microemboli in the middle cerebral artery during cardiopulmonary bypass. Ann Thorac Surg 45:647-649, 1988
22. Wilson GJ, Rebeyka IM, Coles JG, et al: Loss of the somatosensory evoked response as an indicator of reversible cerebral ischemia during hypothermic, low-flow cardiopulmonary bypass. Ann Thorac Surg 45:206-209, 1988
23. Kern FH, Jonas RA, Mayer JE, et al: Temperature monitoring during CPB in infants: does it predict efficient brain cooling? Ann Thorac Surg 54:749-754, 1992
24. Coselli JS, Crawford ES, Beall AC, Mizrahi EM, Hess KR, Patel VM: Determination of brain temperatures for safe circulatory arrest during cardiovascular operation. Ann Thorac Surg 45:638-642, 1988
25. Busto R, Dietrich WD, Globus MYT, et al: Small differences in intraischemic brain temperature critically determine the extent of ischemic neuronal injury. J Cerbrl Blood Flow and Met 7:729-738, 1987
26. Pulsinelli WA, Waldman S, Rawlinson D, Plum F: Moderate hyperglycemia augments ischemic brain damage: a neuropathologic study in the rat. Neur 32:1239, 1982
27. Steward DJ, DaSilva CA, Flegel T: Elevated blood glucose levels may increase the danger of neurological deficit following profoundly hypothermic cardiac arrest. Anesth 68:653, 1988
28. Whitman V, Drotar D, Lambert S, et al: Effects of cardiac surgery with extracorporeal circulation on intellectual function in children. Circulation 160-163, 1973
29. Hammeke TA, Hastings JE: Neuropsychologic alterations after cardiac operation. J Thorac Cardiovasc Surg 96:326-331, 1989

30. Grote CL, Shanahan PT, Salmon P, et al: Cognitive outcome after cardiac operations. J Thorac Cardiovasc Surg 104:1405-1409, 1992
31. Aberg T: Cerebral injury during open heart surgery: studies using functional, biochemical, and morphological methods. In: Hilberman M, ed. Brain injury and protection during heart surgery. Boston: Martinus Nijhoff Publishing, 1988, pp 1-12
32. Kirklin JK, Westaby S, Blackstone EH, et al: Complement and the damaging effects of cardiopulmonary bypass. J Thorac Cardiovasc Surg 86:845-857, 1983
33. Jonas RA: Pathophysiology of cardiopulmonary bypass and its relation to age: metabolic response. In: Jonas RA, Elliott ME, eds. Cardiopulmonary Bypass for Neonates, Infants and Small Children. London: Butterworth-Heinemann, 1993
34. Mathews K, Bale JF, Clark EB, et al: Cerebral infarction complicating Fontan surgery for cyanotic congenital heart disease. Petitur Cartel 7:161-166, 1986
35. McConnell JR, Fleming W, Chi W-K, et al: Magnetic resonance imaging of the brain in infants and children before and after cardiac surgery. A prospective study. AJDC 144:374-378, 1990
36. Moody DM, Belal MA, Calla VR, Johnston WE, Prough DS: Brain microemboli during cardiac surgery or aortography. Ann Neurol 28:477-486, 1990
37. Ekroth R, Thompson RJ, Lincoln C, Scallan M, Rossi R, Tsang V: Elective deep hypothermia with total circulatory arrest: changes in plasma creatine kinase BB, blood glucose, and clinical variables. J Thorac Cardiovasc Surg 97:30-35, 1989
38. Mezrow CK, Sadeghi AM, Gandsas A, et al: Cerebral blood flow and metabolism in hypothermic circulatory arrest. Ann Thorac Surg 54:609-616, 1992
39. Greeley WJ, Kern FH, Ungerleider RM, et al: The effect of hypothermic cardiopulmonary bypass and total circulatory arrest on cerebral metabolism in neonates, infants and children. J Thorac Cardiovasc Surg 101:783-794, 1991
40. Lundar T, Lindberg H, Lindegaard KF, et al: Cerebral Perfusion during Major Cardiac Surgery in Children. Pediatric Cardiology 8:161-65, 1987
41. Greely W, Ungerleider RM, Smith LR, Reves JG: The effects of deep hypothermic cardiopulmonary bypass and total circulatory arrest on cerebral blood flow in infants and children. J Thorac Cardiovasc Surg 97:737-745, 1989
42. Greeley WJ, Ungerleider RM, Kern FH, et al: Effects of cardiopulmonary bypass on cerebral blood flow in neonates, infants, and children. Circulation 80:209-215, 1989
43. Soma Y, Hirotani T, Yozu R, et al: A clinical study of cerebral circulation during extracorporeal circulation. J Thorac Cardiovasc Surg 97:187-193, 1989
44. Kern FH, Ungerleider RM, Quill TJ, et al: Cerebral blood flow response to changes in arterial carbon dioxide tension during hypothermic cardiopulmonary bypass in children. J Thorac Cardiovasc Surg 101:618-622, 1991

45. Mault JR, Ohtake S, Klingensmith ME, et al: Cerebral metabolism and circulatory arrest: effects of duration and strategies for protection. Ann Thorac Surg 55:57-64, 1993
46. Folkerth TL, Angell WW, Fosburg RG, Oury JH: Effect of deep hypothermia, limited cardiopulmonary bypass, and total arrest on growing puppies. In: Recent advances in studies on cardiac structure, Vol. 10. Baltimore: University Park, 1975, pp 411-421
47. Kramer RS, Sanders AP, Lesage AM, Woodhall B, Sealy WC: The effect of profound hypothermia on preservation of cerebral ATP content during circulatory arrest. J Thorac Cardiovasc Surg 56:699, 1968
48. Fisk GC, Wright JS, Turner BB: Cerebral effects of circulatory arrest at 200 C in the infant pig. Anaesth Intens Care 2:33, 1974
49. Wolin LR, Massopust LC Jr, White RJ: Behavioral effects of autocerebral perfusion, hypothermia and arrest of cerebral blood flow in the rhesus monkey. Exp Neurol 39:336, 1973
50. Treasure T, Naftel DC, Conger KA, Garcia JH, Kirklin JW, Blackstone EH: The effect of hypothermic circulatory arrest time on cerebral function, morphology, and biochemistry. J Thorac Cardiovasc Surg 86:761, 1983
51. Coles JG, Taylor MJ, Pearce JM, et al: Cerebral monitoring of somatosensory evoked potentials durinq profoundly hypothermic circulatory arrest. Circulation 70 (suppl): 1-96-1-102, 1984
52. Weiss M, Weiss J, Cotton J, Nicolas F, Binet JP: A study of the electroencephalogram during surgery with deep hypothermia and circulatory arrest in infants. J Thorac Cardiovasc Surg 70:316-329, 1975
53. Rossi R, Ekroth R, Lincoln C, et al: Detection of cerebral injury after total circulatory arrest and profound hypothermia by estimation of specific creatinine kinase isoenzyme levels using monoclonal antibody techniques. Am J Cartel 58:1236-1241, 1986
54. Hicks RG, Poole JL: Electroencephalographic changes with hypothermia and cardiopulmonary bypass in children. J Thorac Cardiovasc Surg 81:781-786, 1992
55. Nussmeier NA, Arlund C, Slogoff ST: Neuropsychiatric complications after cardiopulmonary bypass: cerebral protection by a barbiturate. Anesth 64:165-170, 1986
56. Shewmon DA: What is a neonatal seizure? Problems in definition and quantification for investigative and clinical purposes. J Clin Neurophysiol 7:315-368, 1993
57. Volpe JJ: Neonatal seizures: current concepts and revised classification. Pediatrics 84:422-428, 1989
58. Scher MS, Painter MJ: Controversies concerning neonatal seizures. Ped Clncs of NA 36:281-310, 1989
59. Zelnik N, Nir A, Amit S, lancu TC: Autonomic seizures in an infant: unusual cutaneous and cardiac manifestations. Dev Med Child Neurol 32:74-78, 1990
60. Clancy RR, Legido A, Lewis D: Occult neonatal seizures. Epilepsia 29:256-261, 1988

61. Ehyai A, Fenichel GM, Bender HWJr: Incidence and prognosis of seizures in infants after cardiac surgery with profound hypothermia and circulatory arrest. JAMA 252:3165-3167, 1984
62. Wernovsky G, Jonas RA, Newburger JW, et al: The Boston circulatory arrest study: hemodynamics and hospital course after the arterial switch operation. Circulation 86 (suppl 1) :237A, 1992
63. Brunberg JA, Really EL, Doty DB: Central nervous system consequences in infants of cardiac surgery using deep hypothermia and circulatory arrest. Circulation 50 (suppl 11):60-68, 1974
64. Barratt-Bodes BG: Choreoathetosis as a complication of cardiopulmonary bypass. Ann Thorac Surg 50:693-694, 1990
65. Robinson RO, Samuels M, Pohl KRE: Choreic syndrome after cardiac surgery. Arch Dis Child 63: 1466-1469, 1988
66. Smith-Wical B, Tomasi LG: A distinctive neurologic syndrome after induced profound hypothermia. Pediatric Neurol 6:202-205, 1990
67. Brunberg JA, Doty DB, Really EL: Choreoathetosis in infants following cardiac surgery with deep hypothermia and circulatory arrest. J Petitur 84:232-235, 1974
68. Chaves E, Scaltsas-Persson l: Severe choreoathetosis following congenital heart disease surgery. Neur 38 (suppl):284, 1988
69. DeLeon S, llbawi M, Archiia R, et al: Choreoathetosis after deep hypothermia without circulatory arrest. Ann Thorac Surg 50:714-719, 1990
70. Treasure T: The safe duration of total circulatory arrest with profound hypothermia. Am Heart J 1991
71. Wong PC, Barlow CF, Hickey PR, et al: Factors associated with choreoathetosis after cardiopulmonary bypass in children with congenital heart disease. Circulation 86 (suppl 11):118-126, 1992
72. Messmer BJ, Schallberger U, Gattiker R, Senning A: Psychomotor and intellectual development after deep hypothermia and circulatory arret in early infancy. J Thorac Cardiovasc Surg 72:495-502, 1976
73. Haka-lkse K, Blackwood MJA, Steward DJ: Psychomotor development of infants and children after profound hypothermia during surgery for congenital heart disease. Develop Med Child Neurol 20:62-70,1978
74. Dickinson DF, Sambrooks JE: Intellectual performance in children after circulatory arrest with profound hypothermia in infancy. Arch Dis Child 54:1-6, 1979
75. Clarkson PM, MacArthur BA, Bard-Bodes BG, Whitlock RM, Neutze JM: Developmental progress after cardiac surgery in infancy using hypothermia and circulatory arrest. Circulation 62:855-861, 1980
76. Blackwood MJA, Haka-lkse K, Steward DJ: Developmental outcome in children undergoing surgery with profound hypothermia. Anesth 65:437-440, 1986
77. Ferry PC: Neurologic sequelae of open-heart surgery in children: an "irritating question". AJDC 144:369-373, 1990
78. Sotaniemi KA: Cerebral outcome after extracorporeal circulation. Comparison between prospective and retrospective evaluations. Arch Neurol 40:75-77, 1989

79. Kern FH, Ungerleider RM, Schulman S, et al: Comparison of two strategies of CPB cooling on jugular venous oxygen saturation. Anesth 77:1136A, 1992
80. Baraka AS, Baroody MA, Haroun ST, et al: Effect of alpha stat versus pH stat strategy on oxyhemoglobin dissociation and whole-body oxygen consumption during hypothermic cardiopulmonary bypass. Anesth Analg 74:32-37, 1992
81. Rogers AT, Prough DS, Roy RC, et al: Cerebrovascular and cerebral metabolic effects of alterations in perfusion flow rate during hypothermic cardiopulmonary bypass in man. J Thorac Cardiovasc Surg 103:363-368, 1992
82. Tuppurainen T, Settergren G, Stensved P: The effect of arterial pH on whole body oxygen uptake during hypothermic cardiopulmonary bypass in man. J Thorac Cardiovasc Surg 98:769-773, 1989
83. Murkin JM: Cerebral hyperperfusion during cardiopulmonary bypass: the influence of $PaCO_2$. In: Hilberman M, ed. Brain injury and protection during heart surgery. Boston: Martinus Nijhoff Publishing, 1988, pp 47-66

ACKNOWLEDGMENT

Supported in part by grant HL41786 from the National Heart, Lung and Blood Institute, National Institutes of Health, Bethesda, Maryland, U.S.A..

MAJOR VASCULAR SURGERY OF THE ABDOMINAL AORTA: PROTECTION OF TARGET ORGANS (HEART AND KIDNEY)

Robert N. Sladen, MB, MRCP(UK), FRCP(C)

FUNDAMENTAL PROBLEM

Stress	*vs.*	*Reserve*

Stress:	Aortic Crossclamp
Reserve:	Diffuse Atherosclerosis

Patients have a high incidence of coronary, renovascular and cerebrovascular disease. The typical patient is an elderly, hypertensive, diabetic, obese, heavy smoker with attendant complications.

Response to aortic cross-clamp (AXC) depends on organ system reserve. Potential complications: myocardial infarction, arrhythmias, acute renal failure, stroke.

There is also an increased risk of drug interactions because many patients are on antihypertensive and/or antidiabetic agents. Many patients have significant obstructive lung disease.

Ruptured abdominal aortic aneurysm is a catastrophic event. Even with successful resuscitation and primary repair there is a high incidence of postoperative sequential organ dysfunction (multisystem organ failure) with a forbidding mortality approaching 100%.

Morbidity and Mortality

Cardiac

Although the perioperative mortality of elective aortic aneurysm resection is only 3-5%, the delayed mortality at 3 years is 30-40%, mostly from acute myocardial infarction (1,2). Since 15-20% of patients with ischemic heart disease who present for surgery are asymptomatic, proper work-up is essential. There is a subgroup of patients who might benefit from primary CABG before aortic vascular surgery.

T. H. Stanley and P. L. Bailey (eds.), Anesthesiology and the Cardiovascular Patient, 265–276.

In summary, there is a 60% incidence of coronary artery disease; 25% of patients give a history of angina; 15% have no cardiac history. Myocardial infarction causes 55% of all postop deaths; the mortality from postoperative MI is 70%.

Renal

Of patients who survive surgery for ruptured aortic aneurysm, one-third develop acute renal failure. The mortality in this group is 90%.

The incidence of acute renal failure following elective aortic vascular surgery is now less than 5%, which makes a very cogent case for early operation. However, even in this group the mortality is 50-60% once acute renal failure occurs.

Hemodynamic Stress Factors During Aortic Aneurysm Surgery

Hypertensive Stress

1. Preinduction period (fear, anxiety), especially if line placement is not done with adequate premedication, local anesthetic and care.
2. Laryngoscopy and intubation.
3. Skin incision.
4. Aortic cross-clamping.
5. Emergence (inadequate basal narcosis on awakening in ICU)—exacerbated by hypothermia and vasoconstriction.
6. Post-sequestration period—after capillary leak settles down and intravascular volume expands in the ICU, blood pressure control can become a difficult problem (responds to diuresis).

Hypotensive Stress

1. Anesthetic induction—especially if volume depleted (treated congestive heart failure, excessive diuretics, untreated hypertension)
2. Mesenteric manipulation—vagal effect or kinin activation?
3. Aortic unclamping ("unclamping shock")—sudden reduction in SVR, lactate release, myocardial ischemia induced by AXC.
4. Bleeding—often unrecognized in OR and ICU (hematocrit affected by fluid shifts, abdominal distention can be due to sequestration); exacerbated by coagulopathy.
5. Sequestration ("third spacing")—induced by splanchnic ischemia, degree profound with ruptured aneurysm, suprarenal AXC, preexist-

ing mesenteric insufficiency. Difficult to assess by intake/output, clinical signs (edema, rales), hematocrit.

6. Rewarming in ICU—vasodilatation.

Aortic Cross-clamp: Cardiac Responses

The primary response to AXC is an abrupt increase in *systemic vascular resistance* (SVR)—however, the extent appears to be greater with isolated aortic aneurysm than with aortoocclusive disease and extensive collaterals (3,4).

Normal cardiac function: The typical response is a decrease in venous return from the viscera, with decreased filling pressures (pulmonary artery diastolic, wedge, CVP) and mild to moderate decrease in cardiac output.

Myocardial ischemia: Increased filling pressures, acute ischemia, arrhythmias, moderate to marked decrease in cardiac output (5).

Renal Risk Factors

Preoperative

1. Advanced age—GFR reduced to 50-60% of normal
2. Preexisting renal disease—hypertensive, diabetic nephropathy, diffuse atherosclerosis, renal artery stenosis
3. Angiography—dye insult is nephrotoxic, especially in hypovolemic patients (N.B. elderly, hypertensive diabetic)
4. Ruptured aneurysm with shock—ATN may be established by the time the patient is first seen. One-third develop ATN if they survive surgery.
5. Sepsis, if preexisting, is an important cause of renal insufficiency.

Intraoperative

1. Suprarenal AXC (6)
2. Infrarenal AXC (7,8))
3. Renal artery obstruction (manipulation-induced spasm, atheromatous emboli, direct trauma)
4. Hypotension (inadequate cardiac output, RBF)
5. Complications: DIC, anaphylaxis (transfusion, protamine)

Aortic Cross-clamp: Renal Responses

Gamulin et al. (7) studied 12 patients undergoing infrarenal cross-clamping, with 20% mannitol infused at 100 mL/hr. Application of the cross-clamp increased SVR increased by about 20%, and decreased cardiac output to a similar degree. However, renal vascular resistance increased by 75% and RBF decreased by 40%. Nonetheless, GFR decreased only 20%, reflecting a 15% increase in filtration fraction. These changes persisted at least one hour after cross-clamp release.

Myers et al. (6) studied 30 patients undergoing aortic vascular surgery, 15 with suprarenal and 15 with infrarenal AXC. Mannitol was given to all patients prior to AXC placement. They demonstrated significant reduction in renal blood flow (RBF) during aortic manipulation prior to AXC. There was a marked increase in RBF after AXC release.

The table shows their results with respect to glomerular filtration rate (GFR) in ml/minute in patients with AXC placed suprarenal or infrarenal:

Position of AXC	*Preop*	*1-2 hrs p AXC*	*24 hrs p AXC*
Suprarenal	68	23*	45*
Infrarenal	72	59	84

*Associated with evidence of proximal convoluted tubule (PCT) dysfunction [decreased extraction of para-aminohippurate (PAH)] and distal convoluted tubule (DCT) dysfunction (impaired concentrating ability, water conservation, sodium conservation).

Myers et al. (6) concluded that *suprarenal* AXC causes a form of attenuated acute tubular necrosis (ATN) that is self limiting. Anuria and postoperative azotemia appeared to be related to AXC time of greater than 50 minutes. With *infrarenal* AXC, reduction in GFR is modest and returns to normal in about 24 hours.

PREOPERATIVE ASSESSMENT

Cardiac Assessment

1. History of angina*
2. History, signs of congestive heart failure*
3. Resting ECG changes of ischemia*
4. Preoperative Holter monitoring (9)
5. Stress ECG (treadmill, bicycle, hand ergometer) (10)
6. Thallium scanning (exercise, dipyramidole or dobutamine) (11)
    - assessment of myocardial ischemia

7. Radionuclide scanning (MUGA) (12)
   - left ventricular function (end-diastolic volume, ejection fraction)
8. Cardiac catheterization
   - assess coronary arteries
   - primary coronary artery bypass grafting (CABG). Better prognosis?

Holter Monitoring

Raby et al. (9) studied 176 patients scheduled for vascular surgery. Patients with LBBB, ST-T changes and on digoxin were excluded. 18% had ECG evidence of preoperative ischemia (97% silent); of these 40% had a postop cardiac event. 82% of patients had no preoperative ischemia, with an incidence of 0.7% for a postop cardiac event

Dipyridamole-thallium Scan

Leppo et al. (13) studied 100 patients presenting for major vascular surgery. They excluded those with unstable angina or who had had a recent myocardial infarction. 69 patients underwent exercise testing. Eleven patients were referred for coronary angiography, and 89 underwent vascular surgery. Of these, 15 had a perioperative myocardial infarction. The authors concluded that the finding of thallium redistribution implied a 23-fold increase in perioperative cardiac risk, and a 30-fold increase in risk in diabetic patients.

Their recommendations can be summarized as follows:

Finding	*Action*
normal scan	low risk
redistribution, no other risk factors	proceed with surgery
severe redistribution, ST depression, diabetes	coronary angiography

Dobutamine Stress Test

This is a pharmacologic stress test (tachycardia) using serial doses of dobutamine 5-40 μg/kg/min. New or worsened wall motion abnormalities (WMA) with stress indicates no contractile reserve and/or reversible ischemia The test has highsensitivity/ specificity (≈85%) (14). The test does have the risk of causing acute myocardial ischemia but seems to be remarkably well tolerated.

Cardiac Catheterization

Hertzer et al. (15) at the Cleveland Clinic studied 1000 consecutive patients scheduled for major vascular surgery. 61% had mild to advanced coronary artery disease (CAD); 25% had severe, correctable CAD and 33% of these were asymptomatic. 22% of patients received CABG first (5.3% mortality); 78% of patients proceeded to vascular surgery (2.0% mortality).

Renal Assessment

1. Serum creatinine—may be misleading in cachectic patients; early acute changes missed (e.g., increase from 0.6-1.2 represents 50% reduction in GFR)
2. Creatinine clearance—1-2 hr collection sufficient in catheterized patients. Important if surgery to follow soon after dye study.

Other Organ Systems: Pulmonary and Cerebrovascular Assessment

1. Impaired response to anesthesia—suppression of responses to hypoxemia, hypercarbia
2. Respiratory muscle discoordination and dysfunction
3. CO_2 retention (check total CO_2)—postoperative problems
4. General mental status—may be debilitated, presenile, confused
5. Carotid disease—often asymptomatic. Previous thromboendarterectomy (TEA)
6. Previous stroke

PREOPERATIVE PREPARATION

Cardiovascular

1. Control angina.
2. Consider primary CABG for unstable angina with diffuse, tight coronary lesions.

Renal

1. Defer elective surgery at least 5 days after dye study; assess renal function carefully.
2. Consider use of calcium channel blockers during dye studies (16).
3. Admit patients with severe renovascular hypertension and insufficiency to ICU for preoperative hemodynamic monitoring and stabilization (optimum blood pressure and cardiac output)

Pulmonary

1. Stop smoking
2. Respiratory therapy: incentive spirometry, bronchodilators, antibiotics

Cerebrovascular

1. Question elective surgery in presence of severe cerebrovascular disease.
2. Consider primary carotid TEA with symptomatic disease or >70% narrowing.

MONITORING

1. ECG: Lead II, V5 (early detection of acute ischemia)
2. Arterial line
3. Central venous pressure (CVP)
4. Urinary catheter
5. Pulmonary artery catheter (ischemic heart disease, renovascular hypertension or insufficiency, suprarenal AXC, ruptured aneurysm, sepsis, severe lung disease).
6. Transesophageal echocardiography (TEE) (ischemic heart disease)

ANESTHETIC MANAGEMENT AND POSTOPERATIVE CARE

"Stress-free Anesthesia"

Anesthetic Plan

Premedication

Ensure adequate beta-blockade. Stone et al. (17) studied 128 patients with untreated hypertension. 89 were given a single dose of oral beta-blocker preoperatively, either labetalol 100 mg or atenolol 50 mg. ECG ischemia was documented at intubation and emergence. The incidence of ischemia was 11/39 without beta-blockade (28%), and 2/89 with beta-blockade (2%).

1. *Monitored induction*

- Early detection of BP changes, ischemia, failure

2. *Opioid-based anesthesia (high risk patient)*

- Fentanyl, sufentanil—bolus or infusion: "stress-free" anesthesia—maximal suppression of catecholamines with minimal myocardial depression.
- Avoid nitrous oxide in myocardial ischemia, heart failure. Pancuronium or vecuronium.
- Plan for some period of postoperative ventilation.

3. *Combined general-epidural anesthesia (low-moderate risk patient)*

- Epidural catheter and local anesthetic ± opioid analgesic
- Volume replacement in presence of sympathetic blockade (18)
- Nitrous oxide/oxygen/volatile agent, minimize intraoperative opioids.
- Plan for early postoperative extubation.
- Careful catheter management in presence of perioperative anticoagulation

4. *Aggressive volume replacement*

- Insensible loss + sequestration ≥500 ml/hour
- Anticipate potential for rapid blood loss: RIC, warmer, rapid infuser

5. *Management of aortic cross-clamp (AXC)*

- Management is affected by height of AXC and whether single or bifid graft.
- Use sodium nitroprusside (SNP), nitroglycerin (NTG) ± esmolol during AXC to control BP, HR, decrease SVR and facilitate volume loading. NTG preferred in patients with myocardial ischemia—decreases excessive preload and enhances coronary perfusion.
- Aggressive volume replacement—maintain filling pressures slightly above level before AXC (19).

6. *Management of release of aortic cross-clamp (20)*

- Discontinue vasodilators shortly before AXC release.
- Surgeon should release one limb at a time in bifid grafts.
- Aggressive volume challenge during and after AXC release—anticipate hypotension! Use phenylephrine 50-100 μg IV prn.

IF YOU LOSE CONTROL: ASK THE SURGEON TO PARTIALLY OR COMPLETELY RECLAMP THE AORTA!

7. *Renal protection*

- Adequate volume replacement: best way to maintain RBF is to maintain cardiac output!
- Mannitol 12.5 g IV 15-30 minutes <u>before</u> AXC.
- Dopamine 1-2 μg/kg/min in high-risk patients (questionable benefit)
- Alternate pharmacologic protection:
  IV nicardipine or diltiazem (21); fenoldopam; ANP
- Surgical approaches to renal protection during AXC:
  a. Warm ischemia (<50 minutes)
  b. Renoplegia (chilled crystalloid ± mannitol ± calcium blocker)
  c. Silastic shunts

8. *Prevent hypothermia*

- Many adverse effects: vasoconstriction (impaired peripheral perfusion, increased myocardial afterload, false sense of intravascular volume status); coagulopathy (not detected by lab, which measures at 37°C); shivering and rebound hyperthermia in ICU.

Prevention: Warm OR during induction and line placement, warming blanket, warm prep fluids, warm *all* IV fluids, blood warmer/rapid infuser, heater/humidifier, insulate exposed parts, warm irrigation fluid, forced-air blanket.

But . . . DON'T warm ischemic lower body!

9. *Anticipate coagulopathy*

- Preexisting coagulopathy (Coumadin, liver disease or congestion, malnutrition, uremia); Dilutional coagulopathy (platelets, factors V and VIII).

- DIC (diffuse bleeding surface, hematomas, ischemia).
- Heparin
- Surgical bleeding (not easily assessed once wound closed).

Approach: Correct ACT with protamine (unless peripheral circulation compromised). Consider TEG or Sonoclot. Appropriate indications for antifibrinolytic agents (epsilon aminocaproic acid, tranexamic acid, aprotinin); blood products (platelets, fresh frozen plasma, cryoprecipitate).

10. *Postoperative analgesia*

- Controlled emergence from anesthesia and good postoperative pain relief is essential, especially in the presence of ischemic heart disease.
- Intrathecal morphine 0.3-0.5 mg q 12-24 hr
- Epidural bolus analgesia: morphine 3-5 mg q 12-24 hr (or—Dilaudid, meperidine)
- Epidural infusion analgesia: fentanyl 0.125-2.5 mg/ml + bupivacaine 0.125-0.25% @ 3-8 ml/hr.

IV sedation, mechanical ventilation in ICU: prevent pain-induced hypertension; reduce variables during unstable phase of potential bleeding, rewarming, shivering, hypovolemia, myocardial ischemia, renal insufficiency. Use continuous infusion of fentanyl ± midazolam or propofol.

Other issues: Epidural catheter removal, PCA, ketorolac.
Role of alpha-2 agonists: clonidine, dexmedetomidine.

POSTOPERATIVE PROBLEMS

Early Problems

1. Hypothermia, pain, hypertension
2. Rewarming, hypovolemia, hypotension
3. Hypokalemia, arrhythmias
4. Oliguria
5. Bleeding, thrombosis
6. Pulmonary edema

Later Problems

1. Fluid mobilization
2. Difficult ventilatory weaning

3. CNS status
4. Blood pressure control
5. Pulmonary toilet
6. Gastrointestinal function
7. Ambulation

REFERENCES

1. Crawford ES, Bomberger RA, Glaeser DH, et al: Aortoiliac occlusive disease: factors influencing survival and function following reconstructive operation over a twenty-five year period. Surgery 90:1055-1067, 1981
2. Crawford ES, Saleh SA, Babb JW, et al: Infrarenal abdominal aortic aneurysm: factors influencing survival after operation performed over a 25 year period. Ann Surg 193:699-709, 1981
3. Balastrieri FJ, Johnston WE, Plonk GE, et al: Hemodynamic effects from acute aortic occlusion during surgery. Anesthesiology 63:A97, 1985
4. Meloche R, Pottecher T, Audet J, et al: Hemodynamic changes due to clamping of the aorta. Can Anaesth Soc J 24:20-34, 1977
5. Attia RR, Murphy JD, Snider M, et al: Myocardial ischemia due to infrarenal aortic cross-clamping during aortic surgery in patients with severe coronary artery disease. Circulation 53:961-965, 1976
6. Myers BD, Miller lDC, Mehigan JT, et al: Nature of the renal injury following total renal ischemia in man. J Clin Invest 73:1984
7. Gamulin Z, Forster A, Morel D, et al: Effects of infrarenal aortic cross-clamping on renal hemodynamics in humans. Anesthesiology 61:394-399, 1984
8. Grant RP, Jenkins LC: Modification by preoperative beta-blockade of the renin response to infrarenal aortic cross-clamping. Can Anaesth Soc J 30:480-486, 1983
9. Raby KE, L G, Creager MA, et al: Correlation between preoperative ischemia and major cardiac events after peripheral vascular surgery. N Engl J Med 321:1296-300, 1989
10. Cutler BS, Wheeler HB, Paraskos JA, Cardullo PA: Applicability and interpretation of electrocardiographic stress testing in patients with peripheral vascular disease. Am J Surg 141:501-506, 1981
11. Brewster DC, Okada RD, Strauss HW, et al: Selection of patients for preoperative coronary angiography: use of dipyridamole-stress-thallium myocardial imaging. J Vasc Surg 2:504-510, 1985
12. Pasternack PF, Imparato AM, Riles TS, et al: The value of the radionuclide angiogram in the prediction of perioperative myocardial infarction in patients undergoing lower extremity revascularization procedures. Circulation 72(suppl II):II13-17, 1985
13. Leppo J, Plaja J, Gionet M, et al: Noninvasive evaluation of cardiac risk before elective vascular surgery. JACC 9:269-76, 1987. JACC 9:269-76, 1987
14. Poldermans D, Fioretti PM, Forster T, et al: Dobutamine-atropine stress echocardiography for assessment of perioperative and late cardiac risk in patients undergoing major vascular surgery. Eur J Vasc Surg 8:286-93, 1994

15. Hertzer N: Clinical experience with preoperative coronary angiography. J Vasc Surg 2:510-514, 1985
16. Neumayer HH, Junge W, Kufner A, Wenning A: Prevention of radiocontrast-media-induced nephrotoxicity by the calcium channel blocker nitrendipine: a prospective randomised clinical trial. Nephrology, Dialysis, Transplantation 4:1030-6, 1989
17. Stone JG, Foëx P, Sear JW, et al: Myocardial ischemia in untreated hypertensive patients: effect of a single small oral dose of a beta-adrenergic blocking agent. Anesthesiology 68:495-500, 1988
18. Lunn JK, Dannemiller FJ, Stanley TH: Cardiovascular responses to clamping of the aorta during epidural and general anesthesia. Anesth Analg 58:372-376, 1979
19. Bush HL, LoGerfo FW, Weisel RD, et al: Assessment of myocardial performance and optimal volume loading during elective abdominal aortic aneurysm resection. Arch Surg 112:1301-1306, 1977
20. Silverstein PR, Caldera DL, Cullen DJ, et al: Avoiding the hemodynamic consequences of aortic cross-clamping and unclamping. Anesthesiology 50:462-466, 1979
21. Neumayer HH, Kunzendorf U, Schreiber M: Protective effects of calcium antagonists in human renal transplantation. Kidney International Suppl 36:87-93, 1992

ANESTHESIA FOR CAROTID ENDARTERECTOMY

John C. Drummond, MD, FRCPC

For a time there was uncertainty as to whether carotid endarterectomy (CEA) was beneficial. However, the North American Symptomatic Carotid Endarterectomy Trial (Nascet) published in mid-1991 revealed that "for patients with high-grade stenosis (70-99% narrowing in the luminal diameter) surgery was highly beneficial" (1). A European trial has yielded similar results for patients with 70-99% stenosis (2). The portions of those studies evaluating the benefits in patients with moderate stenosis (30-69%) are ongoing. There has also been confirmation by the NIH sponsored ACAS (Asymptomatic Carotid Artery Stenosis) trial that CEA is beneficial for the asymptomatic patient with diameter stenosis of greater than 60%. These results mean that we will perform more CEA's than in the 1980's.

A Joint Committee of the Society of Vascular Surgery and of the International Society of Cardiovascular Surgery has presented "Practice Guidelines" for CEA (3). Institutions performing CEA should be able to do so with combined stroke-mortality rates of: <3% for neurologically asymptomatic patients; <5% for symptomatic patients; and <7% for those with prior stroke. The "benchmarks" provided by the Nascet and ACAS studies were 2.1% and 2.3%, respectively.

Reduced to its simplest terms, the mission in managing patients undergoing carotid endarterectomy is to A) prevent myocardial infarction and B) prevent stroke. The prevalence of coronary artery disease in this population is substantial (4,5). The question of what cardiovascular evaluation CEA candidates should undergo has been much discussed. It seems excessive to require cardiology consultation for all patients. The investigation of Mackey et al. (6) suggested that "patients at high risk for (perioperative) cardiac death can be identified by clinical criteria." It was their conclusion that risk factors alone (in the absence of overt history or signs of coronary artery disease including previous MI, angina, or EKG abnormalities) should not warrant intensive

T. H. Stanley and P. L. Bailey (eds.), Anesthesiology and the Cardiovascular Patient, 277–288.

evaluation. Urbinati et al. performed two similar surveys and concluded that "silent CAD did not affect the perioperative outcome, but strongly influenced the long-term prognosis" (7,8). This author's rough indications for cardiology evaluation are: 1) congestive failure; 2) unstable angina; 3) angina with activities of daily living or at rest in a patient who has not yet had either a stress-thallium scan or cardiac catheterization; 4) moderate angina in a patient who is not receiving calcium channel blockers (which probably deserves to be considered as first-line management for angina); and 5) the diabetic patient with ischemic EKG changes who has no symptoms and is not yet on anti-anginal medication.

Another preoperative variable that appears to be a correlate of peri-operative morbidity/mortality is hypertension (9-11). There is evidence that the incidence of neurologic deficit in the postoperative period is greater in patients who develop postoperative hypertension (9-10) and that the incidence of both postoperative hypotension and hypertension is greater in patients who have uncontrolled hypertension preoperatively (12). In further support of the significance of preoperative hypertension is the survey by McCrory et al. (13) of the correlates of morbidity and mortality in 1160 patients who underwent CEA in 12 academic medical centers. Events rates were: "death, 1.4%; nonfatal stroke, 3.4%; nonfatal MI, 2.1% . . . . Significant predictors of adverse events were age >75 years, symptom status (ipsilateral symptoms vs asymptomatic or nonipsilateral symptoms), severe hypertension (preop diastolic BP >110 mmHg), CEA performed in preparation for coronary artery bypass surgery, history of angina, evidence of internal carotid artery thrombus, and internal carotid artery stenosis near the carotid siphon." Note that of the items on that list, the only one amenable to preoperative modification is hypertension. Until recently there was little latitude to defer the procedure to control hypertension because we have been presented with predominantly symptomatic patients. The urgency is somewhat less with the asymptomatic patient but at present there are no data to confirm that delaying the procedure to achieve preoperative blood pressure control reduces morbidity and certainly no data to say how long a period of control is required to accrue any benefit.

A small part of hypertension-related post-operative neurologic morbidity is the result of delayed intracerebral hemorrhage. This is a phenomenon that is attributed to a hyperperfusion state that is most likely to develop in patients who had a long-standing, high-grade stenosis prior to CEA. It is the opinion of neurosurgeons that "to minimize the risk of hemorrhage . . . strict maintenance of blood pressure at normotensive . . . levels . . . is advised" in patients who are at risk for this hyper-perfusion state (14,15).

At the University of California at San Diego standard intraoperative monitoring includes the EKG (leads V and II) and an arterial line. The trans-esophageal echo is occasionally used by an appropriately skilled subset of anesthesiologists. CVP or PA catheters are placed very infrequently because of the negligible fluid shifts involved in this procedure.

LOCAL/REGIONAL VS. GENERAL ANESTHESIA

The decision as to whether a local/regional or general anesthetic technique is more appropriate must also be made. It is probable that a substantial majority of the CEA's done in North America are performed under general anesthesia. Nonetheless, a very reasonable case can be made for wider use of local/regional techniques. Among the advantages claimed are 1) shorter operating room time (16, 17); 2) fewer unnecessary shunts (16-18); 3) faster recognition of shunt occlusion or other technical failures; 4) less postoperative cardiovascular instability (19,20); 5) shorter ICU/PACU stays (16); 6) fewer strokes (11,21); 7) fewer myocardial infarctions (19,22,23); 8) shorter overall hospitalization (17,22,24); and 9) lower cost (25). With respect to the rate of shunt utilization, in one large series, the incidence of neurologic changes requiring shunting was 9% (26), while shunts were placed in 15-28% of patients when the decision was based on EEG changes during general anesthesia (27,28). The claims concerning stroke and cardiovascular morbidity rates should not be viewed as well substantiated. For the most part, the study groups have been small and the reports have not been derived from prospective trials in which patients have been randomly assigned to either awake or anesthetized techniques. In fact, there is only one such investigation (29). In that study, which was small (55 patients/group), there was no difference in perioperative complication rates between the two approaches. While not all investigations have identified any advantage of local/regional anesthesia (29,30), only one study has ever claimed a disadvantage. That investigation by Becquemin et al. (23) deserves mention because it appears well-balanced in its view point (in contrast to some reports in which the ardor of the believers in awake CEA is obvious). Their retrospective review of 242 CEAs using general anesthesia (GA) and 145 with local anesthesia revealed a higher incidence of myocardial infarction in the GA group. However, they reported a higher rate of stroke due to "technical imperfection" in the local group. Such strokes were suggested to be the result of unsatisfactory operating conditions arising because inadequate exposure in patients with "short fat necks . . . previous cervical scars . . . high carotid bifurcations . . . high carotid plaques . . . tortuous arteries . . . or in patients who were restless and anxious." They concluded that local/regional anesthesia was best for patients with CAD but that GA was better in the face of unfavorable operating conditions. Corson et al. (248 GA vs 176 regional) also identified advantages of local/regional anesthesia (shorter duration of post-operative hypertension) but cited the need to identify the subset best managed with GA because of anatomic or personality factors.

Local/regional anesthesia is decidedly an acceptable technique. In fact, this reviewer, if faced with the need for a CEA, would go in search of a surgeon-anesthetist team that was comfortable with a local/regional approach. However, it appears inappropriate to impose this approach on all parties. It requires the correct combination of patient, surgeon and anesthesiologist to be accomplished properly. Long operating times and a less than gentle technique will not be well tolerated. Furthermore, the patient with a high carotid bifurcation who requires vigorous retraction under the angle of the mandible be better off with a general anesthesia. The occasional loss of consciousness or episode of restlessness/confusion in association with carotid occlusion may necessitate airway intervention under physically awkward circumstances and the team must be willing and prepared to deal with these occurrences.

Superficial cervical plexus block, deep cervical plexus block, straight local and combinations of the three have all been used successfully. Note that even when a regional block is employed infiltration of the carotid sheath is necessary. The author's further experience has been that careful infiltration with local anesthetic along the ramus and lower border of the mandible will improve the patient's tolerance of retraction under the angle of the mandible (which will be most vigorous when the bifurcation is high).

PREVENTION OF NEUROLOGIC INJURIES

A medical intelligence article by Wong (31) provides an excellent review of the incidence of perioperative stroke and the relevant contributing variables. There are several potential causes of stroke in CEA patients: embolization (during carotid dissection or upon release of occlusion); ischemia during cross-clamping (so-called hemodynamic ischemia); occlusion by intimal dissection (either by the shunt tip during occlusion or by dissection under an intimal flap after reestablishing flow); thrombosis at the arteriotomy site (plus or minus embolization); and hemorrhagic infarction (see above). Postoperative thrombosis and embolism is the most frequent cause (11). Only one-third to one-half of perioperative strokes occur intraoperatively (32,33). As a result, investigations that attempt to manipulate intraoperative variables and examine overall stroke rate as the outcome suffer to some extent from the problem that the intervention can influence only a small fraction of the strokes that occur. This may be why investigations that have attempted to determine whether or not intraoperative monitoring of cerebral function has any relevance to the prevention of stroke have failed to conclusively demonstrate that they do so.

ASSESSING THE ADEQUACY OF CEREBRAL PERFUSION

The discussion of whether or not to monitor some element of cerebral function intraoperatively has covered many printed pages over the last decade. This author is most impressed by the data of Redekop and Ferguson (34). Dr. Ferguson was not initially a "believer" in EEG monitoring (35). However, he recorded (but did not watch or respond to) the EEG during 293 carotid endarterectomies performed without an intravascular shunt. Post hoc he examined the incidence of EEG changes and stroke. Twenty-two of his 293 patients sustained severe EEG changes characterized by substantial increases in low frequency activity and major loss of high frequency (alpha) activity. There were five immediate strokes, and four of the five occurred in patients who fell within the severe EEG change category. These data argue that EEG recording with selective shunting on the basis of severe EEG change is, in fact, appropriate. With that said, it should be made clear that it is not possible to define what severity of EEG change is proof that a stroke will occur. The neurologic threat is clearly the product of both the severity and the duration of the ischemic event (36). Furthermore, the data of Redekop and Ferguson should not be used to support an argument that EEG monitoring is invariably appropriate. They do support the notion that selective shunting (versus a "shunt no one" approach) is appropriate and that there is a small but finite subset of CEA patients who will sustain sufficiently profound ischemia during cross-clamping to cause neuronal damage. There are probably other entirely rational means, in addition to the EEG, of deciding which patients need shunts. In particular, a preoperative assessment aimed at determining whether the Circle of Willis can deliver blood to the side of the endarterectomy should reveal which patients are highly likely to need a shunt. This can be accomplished with either angiography or a transcranial Doppler, though the latter is technically very demanding. Verifying that either the basilar-ipsilateral posterior communicating or anterior communicating-ipsilateral A1 segment are patent should provide proof that there will be blood flow to the occluded side (37,38).

If one is to monitor the EEG, the question, "How many EEG channels is sufficient?" inevitably arises. Does one need the gold standard 16 channels? Will the two channels provided by many processors suffice? There is no definitive answer to the question. However, this author is impressed by the argument that, on the basis of the previously cited results of Redekop and Ferguson (34), it is major EEG change that is the harbinger of impending neurologic damage. Major changes should be detectable with contemporary EEG processors. Note that the efficacy of the EEG in monitoring during CEA will be limited by the skills of the user. The casual user of processed EEG may have a difficult time assuring the technical fidelity necessary for reliable interpretation. One should either use the EEG frequently, or probably not use it at all. Even the skilled user of the EEG should recognize one further limitation. While the EEG should be reliable in identifying major episodes of hemodynamic ischemia (caused by inadequate local perfusion pressure), it is possible that subcortical events will occur and result in neurologic deficit that would not be reflected in the cortical EEG (39,40). These uncommon events are more likely to be embolic in nature and limited in size. However, an anatomically "small" infarction in the internal capsule can have major neurologic consequences.

Somatosensory evoked responses and stump pressure have been advocated as alternative means of giving an indication of inadequate perfusion during carotid endarterectomy. While there are data to suggest that evoked responses may have a yield that is either inferior to (41) or perhaps equal to that of the EEG in detecting ischemia (42,43), few would argue that it is appreciably better than the EEG. The fact that it is monitoring only a limited segment of the nervous system must be a cause for concern. In any event, the relatively cumbersome and labor intensive nature of the methodology makes it less practical than EEG monitoring in most circumstances.

Stump pressure has been subject to much criticism. In short, the problem is that it is very difficult to identify a critical pressure threshold that does not result in either a significant number of false positives or false negatives (44-46). Nonetheless, when stump pressure is employed the commonly used shunting threshold is a mean arterial pressure of 50 mmHg, although lower numbers have been advocated (47). The continued use of stump pressures may reflect the non-availability of technically reliable EEG monitoring in some settings. Some surgeons monitor stump pressure simply to reinforce judgments about the likely quality of collateral flow made on the basis of angiography. They are more likely to shunt when there is a large gradient between the systemic and the stump pressure rather than in response to a specific stump pressure.

The transcranial Doppler is capable of detecting changes in cerebral blood flow velocity and has been applied in the setting of carotid endarterectomy (48). It suffers from the limitation that, for the time being, the values for mean CBFV and/or pulsatility index that correspond to critical degrees of CBF reduction have not been identified. However, the abstract of an investigation by Jørgensen and Schroeder (49) suggests that a ratio of mean CBFV in the MCA during carotid occlusion to mean CBFV prior to occlusion of less than 0.4 may correlate well with the occurrence of ischemic EEG changes. A large scale evaluation of the use of TCD during CEA is ongoing (50).

CHOICE OF ANESTHETIC AGENTS

The appropriate choice of anesthetic agents will be somewhat practitioner dependent. The "right" anesthetic is one that is rational considering the known or likely presence of coronary artery disease and which results in the maintenance of normal to high-normal arterial pressure, especially during periods of carotid occlusion. It is reasonable to maintain high normal mean arterial pressures during the period of carotid occlusion in order to facilitate collateral flow. There are data to suggest that a deep anesthetic supplemented with phenylephrine is more likely to result in myocardial ischemia than will a somewhat lighter anesthetic technique designed to maintain blood pressure near control levels without the use of pressors (51,52). The routine administration of barbiturates or other cerebral protectant anesthetics before and during carotid occlusion does not appear to be appropriate.

Intraoperative infiltration of the carotid sinus nerve (to prevent bradycardia and hypotension with manipulation) was once popular. The contemporary perspective is that this practice may be associated with a greater incidence of hypertension and the practice has been largely abandoned (53). In addition, to reduce postoperative hypertension, surgeons now frequently attempt "nerve-sparing" dissections in order to leave the carotid sinus nerve intact (54).

THE POSTOPERATIVE PERIOD

A somewhat more aggressive approach to the control of hypertension in the immediate postoperative period is probably more important in patients undergoing CEA than many others. This is because of the potential for hypertension to increase the likelihood of neck hematoma formation, myocardial ischemia and, in the small percentage of patients who had a very high grade stenosis with poor collateralization, the occurrence of reperfusion injury.

Attention should also be paid to the possibility of various nerve injuries. Cranial nerve injuries are reported to occur in 10% of CEA patients (55). The most commonly injured nerves are the hypoglossal, the vagus, the recurrent laryngeal nerve, and the accessory nerve. The superior laryngeal and glossopharyngeal nerves may also be injured but in general these latter two are sufficiently remote from the operative site that the incidence is very low. The anesthesiologist is frequently unaware of the potential for injury to any of these nerves, in part, because unilateral injury to any of them is unlikely to cause symptomatology requiring intervention. However, bilateral injuries to either the hypoglossal or the vagus/recurrent laryngeal nerve can result in upper airway obstruction. In the preoperative evaluation of patients who have already undergone a neck procedure (either a previous carotid endarterectomy or an anterior approach to the cervical spine), dysfunction of any one of these nerves should be sought.

Nerves to the carotid sinus may also be damaged. The carotid sinus nerves carry the afferent traffic from both the carotid body and the carotid sinus. Unfortunately, there are no specific signs that will confirm injury to these nerves. However, bilateral deafferentation of the carotid body chemoreceptors has been reported to result in a profound loss of the ventilatory response to hypoxemia in patients who have undergone bilateral carotid endarterectomy and, in addition, to result in as much as a six-torr increase in resting carbon dioxide tension (56). Accordingly, patients undergoing second-side carotid endarterectomy merit close observation, and in all probability, intensive nursing care throughout the entire period where residual effects from general anesthetic agents or narcotic analgesics may exist.

REFERENCES

1. NASCET. North American Symptomatic Carotid Endarterectomy Trial Collaborators. Beneficial effect of carotid endarterectomy in symptomatic patients with high-grade carotid stenosis. N Engl J Med 325:445-453, 1991
2. CEAEuro. European Carotid Surgery Trialists' Collaborative Group. MRC European carotid surgery trial: Interim results for symptomatic patients with severe (70-99%) or with mild (0-29%) carotid stenosis. Lancet 337:1235-1243, 1991
3. Moore WS, Mohr JP, Najafi H, Robertson JT, Stoney RJ, Toole JF. Carotid endarterectomy: Practice guidelines. Report of the Ad Hoc Committee to the Joint Council of the Society for Vascular Surgery and the North American Chapter of the International Society for Cardiovascular Surgery. J Vasc Surg 15:469-479, 1992
4. Rokey R, Rolak LA, Harati Y, Kutka N, Verani MS. Coronary artery disease in patients with cerebrovascular disease: A prospective study. Ann Neurol 16:50-53, 1984
5. Adams HP, Kassell NF, Mazuz H. The patient with transient ischemic attacks—is this the time for a new therapeutic approach? Stroke 15:371-375, 1984
6. Mackey WC, O'Donnell TF Jr, Callow AD. Cardiac risk in patients undergoing carotid endarterectomy: Impact on perioperative and long-term mortality. J Vasc Surg 11:226-234, 1990
7. Urbinati S, Pasquale GD, Andreoli A, et al. Frequency and prognostic significance of silent coronary artery disease in patients with cerebral ischemia undergoing carotid endarterectomy. Am J Cardiol 69:1166-1170, 1992
8. Urbinati S, Pasquale GD, Andreoli A, Lusa AM, Carini G. Preoperative noninvasive coronary risk stratification in candidates for carotid endarterectomy. Stroke 25:2022-7, 1994
9. Asiddao CB, Donegan JH, Whitesell RC, Kalbfleisch JH. Factors associated with perioperative complications during carotid endarterectomy. Anesth Analg 61:631-637, 1982
10. Towne JB, Bernhard VM. The relationship of postoperative hypertension to complications following carotid endarterectomy. Surgery 88:575-580, 1980
11. Riles TS, Imparato AM, Jacobowitz GR, Lamparello PJ, Giangola G. The cause of perioperative stroke after carotid endarterectomy. J Vasc Surg 19:206-16, 1994
12. Bove EL, Fry WJ, Gross WS, Stanley JC. Hypotension and hypertension as consequences of baroreceptor dysfunction following carotid endarterectomy. Surg 85:633-7, 1979
13. McCrory DC, Goldstein LB, Samsa GP, et al. Predicting complications of carotid endarterectomy. Stroke 24:1285-91, 1993
14. Piepgras DG, Morgan MK, Sundt TM Jr, et al. Intracerebral hemorrhage after carotid endarterectomy. J Neurosurg 68:532-536, 1988
15. Reigel MM, Hollier LH, Sundt TM Jr, et al. Cerebral hyperperfusion syndrome: A cause of neurologic dysfunction after carotid endarterectomy. J Vasc Surg 5:628-634, 1987

16. Gabelman CG, Gann DS, Ashworth CJ Jr, W I Carney J. One hundred consecutive carotid reconstructions: Local versus general anesthesia. Am J Surg 145:477-482, 1983
17. Allen BT, Anderson CB, Rubin BG, Thompson RW, Flye MW. The influence of anesthetic technique on perioperative complications after carotid endarterectomy. J Vasc Surg 19:834-43, 1994
18. Evans WE, Hayes JP, Waltke EA, Vermilion BD. Optimal cerebral monitoring during carotid endarterectomy: neurologic response under local anesthesia. J Vasc Surg 2:775-777, 1985
19. Lee KS, Davis CH, McWhorter JM. Low morbidity and mortality of carotid endarterectomy performed with regional anesthesia. J Neurosurg 69:483-487, 1988
20. Corson JD, Chang BB, Leopold PW, et al. Perioperative hypertension in patients undergoing carotid endarterectomy: shorter duration under regional block anesthesia. Circulation 74:I-1/I-4, 1986
21. Corson JD, Chang BB, Shah DM, Leather RP, DeLeo BM, Karmody AM. The influence of anesthetic choice on carotid endarterectomy outcome. Arch Surg 122:807-812, 1987
22. Muskett A, McGreevy J, Miller M. Detailed comparison of regional and general anesthesia for carotid endarterectomy. Am J Surg 152:691-694, 1986
23. Becquemin JP, Paris E, Valverde A, Pluskwa F, Melliére D. Carotid surgery. Is regional anesthesia always appropriate? J Cardiovasc Surg 32:592-598, 1991
24. Luosto R, Kentonen P, Mattila S, et al. Local anaesthesia in carotid surgery. Scand J Thor Cardiovasc Surg 18:133-137, 1984
25. Godin MS, Bell WH, Schwedler M, Kerstein MD. Cost effectiveness of regional anesthesia in carotid endarterectomy. Am Surg 55:656-659, 1990
26. Hafner CD, Evans WE. Carotid endarterectomy with local anesthesia: Results and advantages. J Vasc Surg 7:232-9, 1988
27. Kresowik TF, Worsey MJ, Khoury MD, et al. Limitations of electroencephalographic monitoring in the detection of cerebral ischemia accompanying carotid endarterectomy. J Vasc Surg 13:439-43, 1991
28. Sundt TM, Sharbrough FW, Piepgras DG, Kearns TP, Jr. JMM, O'Fallon W. Correlation of cerebral blood flow and electroencephalographic changes during carotid endarterectomy. Mayo Clin Proc 56:533-543, 1981
29. Forssell C, Takolander R, Bergqvist D, Johansson A, Persson NH. Local versus general anesthesia in carotid surgery. A prospective randomized study. Eur J Vasc Surg 3:503-9, 1989
30. Palmer MA. Comparison of regional and general anesthesia for carotid endarterectomy. Am J Surg 157:329-330, 1989
31. Wong DH. Perioperative stroke. Part I: General surgery, carotid artery disease, and carotid endarterectomy. Can J Anaesth 38:347-73, 1991
32. Steed DL, Peitzman AB, Grundy BL, Webster MW. Causes of stroke in carotid endarterectomy. Surgery 92:634-641, 1982
33. Krul JM, van Gijn J, Ackerstaff RG, Vermeulen FE. Site and pathogenesis of infarcts associated with carotid endarterectomy. Stroke 20:324-328, 1989

34. Redekop G, Ferguson G. Correlation of contralateral stenosis and intra-operative electroencephalogram change with risk of stroke during carotid endarterectomy. Neurosurgery 30:191-194, 1992
35. Ferguson GG. Intra-operative monitoring and internal shunts: Are they necessary in carotid endarterectomy? Stroke 13:287-289, 1982
36. Collice M, Arena O, Fontana RA, Mola M, Galbiati N. Role of EEG monitoring and cross-clamping duration in carotid endarterectomy. J Neurosurg 65:815-819, 1986
37. Schwartz RB, Jones KM, LeClercq GT, et al. The value of cerebral angiography in predicting cerebral ischemia during carotid endarterectomy. Am J Roentgenol 159:1057-1061, 1992
38. Schneider PA, Ringelstein B, Rossman ME, et al. Importance of cerebral collateral pathways during carotid endarterectomy. Stroke 19:1328-1334. 1988
39. Chiappa KH, Burke SR, Young RR. Results of electroencephalographic monitoring during 367 carotid endarterectomies: Use of a dedicated mini-computer. Stroke 10:381-388, 1979
40. Silbert BS, Kluger R, Cronin KD, Koumoundouros E. The processed electroencephalogram may not detect neurologic ischemia during carotid endarterectomy. Anesthesiology 70:356-358, 1989
41. Kearse LA, Brown EN, McPeck K. Somatosensory evoked potentials sensitivity relative to electroencephalography for cerebral ischemia during carotid endarterectomy. Stroke 23:498-505, 1992
42. Lam AM, Manninen PH, Ferguson GG, Nantau W. Monitoring electrophysiologic function during carotid endarterectomy: A comparison of somatosensory evoked potentials and conventional electroencephalogram. Anesthesiology 75:15-21, 1991
43. Schweiger H, Kamp H-D, Dinkel M. Somatosensory-evoked potentials during carotid artery surgery: Experience in 400 operations. Surgery 109:602-609, 1991
44. Kwaan JHM, Peterson GJ, Connolly JE. Stump pressure: An unreliable guide for shunting during carotid endarterectomy. Arch Surg 115:1083-1085, 1980
45. McKay RD, Sundt TM, Michenfelder JD, et al. Internal carotid artery stump pressure and cerebral blood flow during carotid endarterectomy: Modification by halothane, enflurane, and innovar. Anesthesiology 45:390-399, 1986
46. Steed DL, Webster MW, DeVries EJ, et al. Clinical observations on the effect of carotid artery occlusion on cerebral blood flow mapped by xenon computed tomography and its correlation with carotid artery back pressure. J Vasc Surg 11:38-44, 1990
47. Archie JP. Technique and clinical results of carotid stump back-pressure to determine selective shunting during carotid endarterectomy. J Vasc Surg 13:319-326. 1991
48. Jansen C, Vriens EM, Eikelboom BC, et al. Carotid endarterectomy with transcranial Doppler and electroencephalographic monitoring: A prospective study in 130 operations. Stroke 24:665-669, 1993

49. Jørgensen LG, Schroeder TV. Transcranial Doppler identification of cerebral ischemia during carotid endarterectomy. Stroke 23:470, 1992 (abstract)
50. Halsey JH. Transcranial Doppler monitoring in carotid endarterectomy: The risks and benefits of shunting. Progress report of the International Study Group. Stroke 23:470, 1992 (abstract).
51. Smith JS, Roizen MF, Cahalan MK, et al. Does anesthetic technique make a difference? Augmentation of systolic blood pressure during carotid endarterectomy: Effects of phenylephrine versus light anesthesia and of isoflurane versus halothane on the incidence of myocardial ischemia. Anesthesiology 69:846-853, 1988
52. Riles TS, Kopelman I, Imparato AM. Myocardial infarction following carotid endarterectomy: A review of 683 operations. Surgery 85:249-252, 1979
53. Elliott BM, Collins GJ Jr, Youkey JR, et al. Intraoperative local anesthetic injection of the carotid sinus nerve. Am J Surg 152:695-699, 1986
54. Cafferata HT, Merchant RF, DePalma RG. Avoidance of postcarotid endarterectomy hypertension. Ann Surg 196:465-472, 1982
55. Schmidt D, Zuschneid W, Kaiser M. Cranial nerve injury during carotid arterial reconstruction. J Neurol 230:131-135, 1983
56. Wade JG, Larson CP, Hickey RF, Ehrenfeld WK, Severinghaus JW. Effect of carotid endarterectomy on carotid chemoreceptor and baroreceptor function in man. N Engl J Med 282:823-829, 1970

EFFECTS OF DRUGS ON THE VASCULAR SYSTEM

Jerrold H. Levy, M.D.

EFFECTS OF DRUGS ON THE VASCULAR SYSTEM

Introduction

The pharmacologic armamentarium that we administer to maintain hemodynamic stability involves the use of different agents that have direct and indirect effects on the heart and vasculature (1). Because blood pressure is the product of cardiac output x vascular resistance, most of the vasoactive and cardiac drugs we administer to treat hypotension or hypertension act either to increase or decrease heart rate, myocardial contractility (one of the determinants of stroke volume), or vascular resistance (1). This review will focus on pharmacologic therapies affecting the vascular system.

Catecholamines, Alpha$_1$ Adrenergic Responses and Vasoconstriction

Catecholamines are the standard therapeutic agents for the treatment of vasodilation irrespective of the underlying etiology. Although widely used in clinical practice, most physicians are not aware of the mechanism of action of α-adrenergic agents on vascular smooth muscle. Catecholamines and similar agents most often administered as an infusion include dopamine, dobutamine, epinephrine, norepinephrine, phenylephrine and isoproterenol (2). Although catecholamines affect both α and β adrenergic receptors, α_1 adrenergic receptor stimulation produces vasoconstriction by activating membrane phospholipase-C which in turn hydrolyzes phosphatidylinositol 4,5 diphosphate (3). This leads to the secondary activation of two second messengers, diacyl glycerol and inositol triphosphate (3), which increase cytosolic Ca^{2+} by several different mechanisms. These include facilitating release of Ca^{2+} from the sarcoplasmic reticulum and possibly increasing the Ca^{2+} sensitivity of the contractile proteins

T. H. Stanley and P. L. Bailey (eds.), Anesthesiology and the Cardiovascular Patient, 289–293.

in vascular smooth muscle (3). During anaphylactic or septic shock, other vasoactive mediators activate vascular smooth muscle and may produce vascular effects that are unresponsive to catecholamines (4).

Vasodilators and Perioperative Hypertension or Heart Failure

Because a spectrum of different drugs can produce vasodilation, several pharmacologic approaches to producing vasodilation will be considered. Potential therapeutic approaches to treating perioperative hypertension or heart failure with parenteral therapy include: 1) α_1-adrenergic receptor blockade, β_1-adrenergic receptor blockade, ganglionic blockade and calcium channel blockade; 2) stimulation of central α_2 adrenergic receptors or vascular guanylate cyclase and adenylate cyclase; 3) inhibition of phosphodiesterase enzymes; and 4) inhibition of angiotensin-converting enzymes (1). Adenosine in low concentrations is also a vasodilator but is usually administered to inhibit atrioventricular conduction. Losartan, a novel angiotensin II antagonist (AII), has just been released for the treatment of hypertension, but is not available for intravenous use.

Cyclic Nucleotides and Vasodilation (Cyclic AMP)

Increases in cyclic nucleotide formation in vascular smooth muscle produce calcium mobilization out of vascular smooth muscle. Adenosine -3',5'-monophosphate (cyclic AMP) can be increased by prostacyclin, prostaglandin E_1, or β_2 adrenergic receptor stimulation in vascular smooth muscle, or by inhibiting the breakdown of cyclic AMP by phosphodiesterase (4). Increasing cyclic AMP in vascular smooth muscle facilitates calcium uptake by intracellular storage sites, thus decreasing calcium available for contraction. The net effect of increasing calcium uptake is to produce vascular smooth muscle relaxation and, hence, vasodilation. However, most catecholamines with β_2 adrenergic activity (i.e., isoproterenol) and phosphodiesterase inhibitors have positive inotropic and other side-effects that include tachycardia, glycogenolysis, and kaliuresis (1). Prostaglandins (prostacyclin and prostaglandin E_1) are potent inhibitors of platelet aggregation and activation. Catecholamines with β_2 adrenergic activity, phosphodiesterase inhibitors, and prostaglandin E_1 have been used to treat pulmonary hypertension and right ventricular failure (4).

Nitrovasodilators and Endothelium Derived Relaxing Factor (Cyclic GMP)

The vascular endothelium provides endogenous vasodilation by the release of both nitric oxide and prostacyclin (5,6). A spectrum of endogenous mediators can stimulate the vascular endothelium to release an endothelium-derived relaxing factor (EDRF or nitric oxide), which activates guanylyl cyclase to generate cyclic GMP (7,8). The pathophysiology of septic and anaphylactic shock is mediated in part by the excess formation of nitric oxide (4).

Nitrates and sodium nitroprusside, however, generate nitric oxide directly, independent of vascular endothelium (7,8). The active form of any nitrovasodilator is nitric oxide (NO) where the nitrogen exists in a +2 oxidation state. For any nitrovasodilator to be active, it must be first converted to nitric oxide. For nitroprusside, this is easily accomplished because nitrogen is in a +3 oxidation state, with the nitric oxide molecule bound to the charged iron molecule in an unstable manner, thus nitroprusside readily donates its nitric oxide moiety. In the case of nitroglycerin, nitrogen molecules exist in a +5 oxidation state, thus they must undergo several metabolic transformations before they are converted to an active molecule. The reason that nitroglycerin does not produce coronary steal as compared to nitroprusside is that the small intracoronary resistance vessels, those less than 100 microns, lack whatever metabolic transformation pathway required to convert nitroglycerin into nitric oxide (7,8).

The mainstay of therapy for postoperative hypertension is sodium nitroprusside and nitroglycerin, drugs that generate nitric oxide to stimulate guanylate cyclase and generate cyclic GMP in vascular smooth muscle. Although these drugs are effective vasodilators, both are nitric oxide-based agents that produce venodilation which contributes significantly to the labile hemodynamic state. (1) We have all observed the tremendous fluctuations in a patient's blood pressure when sodium nitroprusside is started for the treatment of hypertension in the immediate postoperative period. In the hypertensive patient, intravenous volume administration is often employed to allow nitroprusside to be infused due to the relative intravascular hypovolemia.

Dihydropyridine Calcium Channel Blockers

The use of intravenous dihydropyridine calcium channel blockers produces direct arterial vasodilation and more specific and effective treatment of perioperative peripheral vasoconstriction (1,9). Nifedipine is the prototype of the intravenous dihydropyridines, and the newer, second generation water soluble agents are available including isradipine and nicardipine. Isradipine and nicardipine produce arterial vasodilation without any effects on ventricular filling pressures (i.e., pulmonary artery occlusion pressures or right atrial pressures), no effects on atrioventricular nodal conduction, and no negative inotropic effects (9-16). Nicardipine is the first drug of this class to be available in the United States and offers a novel and important therapeutic option to treat perioperative hypertension. Because calcium channel blockers have longer half lives than nitrovasodilators, rapid loading infusion rates or bolus loading doses need to be administered to obtain therapeutic levels. Bolus nicardipine administration can also be used to treat acute hypertension that occurs during the perioperative period (i.e., intubation, extubation, aortic cross clamping).

Phosphodiesterase Inhibitors

Phosphodiesterase inhibitors are pharmacologic agents that can produce both positive inotropic effects and vasodilation (16). When administered to patients with ventricular dysfunction, they increase cardiac output, while decreasing pulmonary artery occlusion pressure, systemic vascular resistance, and pulmonary vascular resistance. Because of their unique mechanisms of vasodilation, they are especially useful for patients with acute pulmonary vasoconstriction and right ventricular dysfunction. Multiple forms of the drug are currently under investigation The bipyridines (amrinone and milrinone), the imidazolones (enoximone), and the methylxanthines (aminophylline) are the ones most widely available. Papaverine, a derivative isolated from opium, is a nonspecific phosphodiesterase inhibitor and vasodilator used by cardiac surgeons for its ability to dilate the internal mammary artery. These agents will be covered in more detail in another chapter.

REFERENCES

1. Levy JH. The ideal agent for perioperative hypertension. Acta Anaesth Scand 37:20-25, 1993
2. Levy JH, Salmenperra MT. Postoperative circulatory control. In: Kaplan JA, ed. 3rd ed. Philadelphia: W.B. Saunders Co. pp 1168-1193, 1993
3. Lucchesi BR. Role of calcium on excitation contraction in cardiac and vascular smooth muscle. Circulation 80:IV1-13, 1989
4. Levy JH. Anaphylactic Reactions in Anesthesia and Intensive Care (Second ed.) Boston: Butterworth-Heinemann, 1992
5. Ware JA, Heistad DD. Platelet - endothelium interactions. N Engl J Med 328:628-635, 1993

6. Dzau VJ, Gibbons GH, Cooke JP, Omoigui N. Vascular biology and medicine in the 1990s: Scope, concepts, potentials, and perspectives. Circulation 87:705-719, 1993
7. Harrison DG, Bates JN. The nitrovasodilators: new ideas about old drugs. Circulation 87:1461-7, 1993
8. Anderson TJ, Meredith IT, Ganz P, et al. Nitric oxide and nitrovasodilators: similarities, differences and potential interactions. JACC 24:555-66, 1994
9. Begon C, Dartayet B, Edouard A, et al. Intravenous nicardipine for treatment of intraoperative hypertension during abdominal surgery. J Cardiothorac Anesth 3:707-11, 1989
10. Cheung DG, Gasster JL, Neutel JM, et al. Acute pharmacokinetic and hemodynamic effects of intravenous bolus dosing of nicardipine. Am Heart J 119:438-42, 1990
11. David D, Dubois C, Loria Y. Comparison of nicardipine and sodium nitroprusside in the treatment of paroxysmal hypertension following aortocoronary bypass surgery. J Cardiothorac Vasc Anesth 5:357-61, 1991
12. Lambert CR, Grady T, Hashimi W, et al. Hemodynamic and angiographic comparison of intravenous nitroglycerin and nicardipine mainly in subjects without coronary artery disease. Amer J Cardiol 71:420-23, 1993
13. Singh BN, Josephson MA. Clinical pharmacology, pharmacokinetics, and hemodynamic effects of nicardipine. Am Heart J 119:427-33, 1990
14. Leslie J, Brister N, Levy JH, et al. Treatment of postoperative hypertension after coronary artery bypass surgery: double-blind comparison of intravenous isradipine and sodium nitroprusside. Circulation 90:II256-261, 1994
15. Levy JH. Support of the perioperative failing heart with preexisting ventricular dysfunction: currently available options. J Cardiothorac Anaesth 7 (S):46-51, 1993
16. Fleckenstein A. Specific pharmacology of calcium in the myocardium, cardiac pacemakers and vascular smooth muscle. Ann Rev Pharmacol 17:149-66, 1977

DEVELOPMENTS IN CRITICAL CARE MEDICINE AND ANESTHESIOLOGY

1. O. Prakash (ed.): *Applied Physiology in Clinical Respiratory Care.* 1982 ISBN 90-247-2662-X
2. M.G. McGeown: *Clinical Management of Electrolyte Disorders.* 1983 ISBN 0-89838-559-8
3. T.H. Stanley and W.C. Petty (eds.): *New Anesthetic Agents, Devices and Monitoring Techniques.* Annual Utah Postgraduate Course in Anesthesiology. 1983 ISBN 0-89838-566-0
4. P.A. Scheck, U.H. Sjöstrand and R.B. Smith (eds.): *Perspectives in High Frequency Ventilation.* 1983 ISBN 0-89838-571-7
5. O. Prakash (ed.): *Computing in Anesthesia and Intensive Care.* 1983 ISBN 0-89838-602-0
6. T.H. Stanley and W.C. Petty (eds.): *Anesthesia and the Cardiovascular System.* Annual Utah Postgraduate Course in Anesthesiology. 1984 ISBN 0-89838-626-8
7. J.W. van Kleef, A.G.L. Burm and J. Spierdijk (eds.): *Current Concepts in Regional Anaesthesia.* 1984 ISBN 0-89838-644-6
8. O. Prakash (ed.): *Critical Care of the Child.* 1984 ISBN 0-89838-661-6
9. T.H. Stanley and W.C. Petty (eds.): *Anesthesiology: Today and Tomorrow.* Annual Utah Postgraduate Course in Anesthesiology. 1985 ISBN 0-89838-705-1
10. H. Rahn and O. Prakash (eds.): *Acid-base Regulation and Body Temperature.* 1985 ISBN 0-89838-708-6
11. T.H. Stanley and W.C. Petty (eds.): *Anesthesiology 1986.* Annual Utah Postgraduate Course in Anesthesiology. 1986 ISBN 0-89838-779-5
12. S. de Lange, P.J. Hennis and D. Kettler (eds.): *Cardiac Anaesthesia.* Problems and Innovations. 1986 ISBN 0-89838-794-9
13. N.P. de Bruijn and F.M. Clements: *Transesophageal Echocardiography.* With a contribution by R. Hill. 1987 ISBN 0-89838-821-X
14. G.B. Graybar and L.L. Bready (eds.): *Anesthesia for Renal Transplantation.* 1987 ISBN 0-89838-837-6
15. T.H. Stanley and W.C. Petty (eds.): *Anesthesia, the Heart and the Vascular System.* Annual Utah Postgraduate Course in Anesthesiology. 1987 ISBN 0-89838-851-1
16. D. Reis Miranda, A. Williams and Ph. Loirat (eds.): *Management of Intensive Care.* Guidelines for Better Use of Resources. 1990 ISBN 0-7923-0754-2
17. T.H. Stanley (ed.): *What's New in Anesthesiology.* Annual Utah Postgraduate Course in Anesthesiology. 1988 ISBN 0-89838-367-6
18. G.M. Woerlee: *Common Perioperative Problems and the Anaesthetist.* 1988 ISBN 0-89838-402-8
19. T.H. Stanley and R.J. Sperry (eds.): *Anesthesia and the Lung.* Annual Utah Postgraduate Course in Anesthesiology. 1989 ISBN 0-7923-0075-0
20. J. De Castro, J. Meynadier and M. Zenz: *Regional Opioid Analgesia.* Physiopharmacological Basis, Drugs, Equipment and Clinical Application. 1990 ISBN 0-7923-0162-5
21. J.F. Crul (ed.): *Legal Aspects of Anaesthesia.* 1989 ISBN 0-7923-0393-8

DEVELOPMENTS IN CRITICAL CARE MEDICINE AND ANESTHESIOLOGY

22. E. Freye: *Cerebral Monitoring in the Operating Room and the Intensive Care Unit.* 1990 ISBN 0-7923-0349-X
23. T.H. Stanley and R.J. Sperry (eds.): *Anesthesiology and the Heart.* Annual Utah Postgraduate Course in Anesthesiology. 1990 ISBN 0-7923-0634-1
24. T.H. Stanley, M.A. Ashburn, P. G. Fine (eds.): *Anesthesiology and Pain Management.* 1990 ISBN 0-7923-1073-X
25. T.H. Stanley and R.J. Sperry (eds.): *Anesthesia and the Lung 1992.* Annual Utah Postgraduate Course in Anesthesiology. 1992 ISBN 0-7923-1563-4
26. G.M. Woerlee: *Kinetics and Dynamics of Intravenous Anesthetics.* 1992 ISBN 0-7923-1506-5
27. A. Willner (ed.): *Cerebral Damage before and after Cardiac Surgery.* 1993 ISBN 0-7923-1928-1
28. R.J. Sperry, J.O. Johnson and T.H. Stanley (eds.): *Anesthesia and the Central Nervous System.* Annual Utah Postgraduate Course in Anesthesiology. 1993 ISBN 0-7923-2083-2
29. T.H. Stanley and M.A. Ashburn (eds.): *Anesthesiology and Pain Management.* 1994 ISBN 0-7923-2662-8
30. T.H. Stanley and P.G. Schafer (eds.): *Pediatric and Obstetrical Anesthesia.* Annual Utah Postgraduate Course in Anesthesiology. 1995 ISBN 0-7923-3346-2
31. T.H. Stanley and P.L. Bailey (eds.): *Anesthesiology and the Cardiovascular Patient.* 1996 ISBN 0-7923-3895-2

KLUWER ACADEMIC PUBLISHERS – DORDRECHT / BOSTON / LONDON